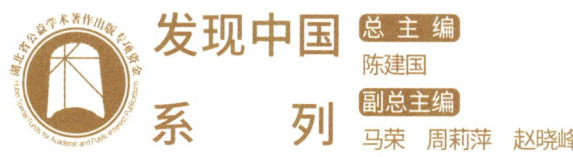

发现中国系列

总主编 陈建国

副总主编 马荣 周莉萍 赵晓峰

中国卫生
（双语版）

主　　编：冯占春　熊巨洋

副 主 编：赵晓峰

英文翻译：洪　涛

华中科技大学出版社
http://press.hust.edu.cn
中国·武汉

图书在版编目（CIP）数据

中国卫生：双语版：汉英对照 / 冯占春，熊巨洋主编. -- 武汉：华中科技大学出版社，2025. 6.
（发现中国系列）. -- ISBN 978-7-5772-1258-6

Ⅰ. R199.2

中国国家版本馆 CIP 数据核字第 20255BG436 号

中国卫生（双语版）
Zhongguo Weisheng（Shuangyu Ban）

冯占春　　熊巨洋　主编

总　策　划：阮海洪
策划编辑：杨玉斌
责任编辑：张瑞芳
封面设计：清格印象
责任校对：刘小雨
责任监印：朱　玢
出版发行：华中科技大学出版社（中国·武汉）　　电话：（027）81321913
　　　　　武汉市东湖新技术开发区华工科技园　　邮编：430223
录　　排：华中科技大学惠友文印中心
印　　刷：湖北金港彩印有限公司
开　　本：787mm×1092mm　1/16
印　　张：20.25
字　　数：593千字
版　　次：2025 年 6 月第 1 版第 1 次印刷
定　　价：168.00 元

编委会

主　　编　冯占春　熊巨洋
副 主 编　赵晓峰
参编人员　（按音序排）
　　　　　　付　谦　刘晨曦　卢　珊　唐尚锋　唐玉清
　　　　　　吴泰来　徐　娟　叶　婷　张　研

总　　序

纵观人类历史，教育兴则国家兴，教育强则国家强。如今，随着经济全球化的深入推进，教育对外开放已成为推动国家发展的重要战略。党的十八大以来，有关高等教育国际化发展的重要文件密集出台，国际交流与合作已被列入高校五大职能之一，华中科技大学积极响应号召，发布一系列纲领性文件，深入推进国际化办学，高度重视来华留学生教育工作。"发现中国系列"正是在这一背景下为来华留学生打造的经典著作，可以说既是时代之需，也是责任之举。

我们身处的时代，是一个交通高度发达、人员往来密切、文化交流日益频繁的时代。在这个时代，如何讲好中国故事，让世界更好地了解中国，成为摆在我们面前的重要课题。我们深知，来华留学生具有"贯通中外"的优势，是中外友好往来的特殊使者，是沟通中国与世界的重要桥梁。向来华留学生全面系统讲述中国经济社会发展情况，有助于赋能来华留学生讲好中国故事，增强中华文明的国际传播力和影响力。

近年来，习近平总书记多次饱含深情给海外学子、留学归国人员、来华留学生回信，认真学习这些回信让我深受启发，倍感鼓舞。一方面，我曾是海外学子，于1995年出国留学，先后在德国、美国学习工作6年多，这些经历让我更了解来华留学生的学习和生活需求；另一方面，留学归国20多年来，我一直在高校从事科研教学和管理工作，在担任华中科技大学副校长期间更是分管国际交流与合作工作多年，来华留学生教育工作是我的重要工作职责之一。我见证和亲历了我国高等教育事业和科技事业的飞速发展，面对日益庞大的来华留学生队伍，深感骄傲和自豪，同时也感到责任重大。

当前，我国社会正处于高质量发展的新阶段，以高水平对外开放促进高质量发展已成为时代要求，在经济领域如是，在教育领域亦然。我相信，高水平的教育对外开放既是推动高校"双一流"建设的动力，也是开辟高校国际合作新领域的契机。因而，在国际化工作中，我们始终坚持从国际维度布局，在国际坐标定位，以国际名校为标杆，大力拓展与国际顶尖大学的实质性合作，在扩大我校来华留学生规模的基础上，进一步提升来华留学生教育质量。

"发现中国系列"选取了中国的经济发展、医疗卫生、数字化建设等民生热点，通过阐述各大领域的发展历程、技术创新、政策演变、深层逻辑、国际合作等内容，全面介绍现代化建设的中国质量和中国速度，不仅是对中国现代化建设的生动记录，更是对中华文明精神标识和文化精髓的提炼展示。

该系列每一本书都由相关领域的权威专家担任主编，在这里，我要特别感谢各位主编的大力支持与辛勤付出。他们既是深耕科研的顶尖专家学者，对我国乃至国际的经济与科技发展态势有敏锐的感知，具有丰富的图书编写经验，对内容的把握高屋建瓴，又是拥有丰富教学经验的一线教师,了解来华留学生的需求,深谙授业之道,在人才培养上有独特的见解。我相信,这样一套契合时代背景、精选热点主题、洞悉读者需求的双语系列图书,能很好地向广大来华留学生展示全面、立体、真实的中国,赋能他们讲好中国故事,当好友谊使者,搭起合作桥梁。

据我所知,"发现中国系列"已与世界知名出版机构施普林格达成英文版出版协议,将面向全世界出版发行。这也意味着,我们将站在一个更为广阔的舞台上讲述中国故事,宣介中国智慧、中国方案,有助于推进对外文化交流、加强国际传播能力建设,构建中国叙事体系。

未来,"发现中国系列"还会陆续编写、出版,为来华留学生的教育工作逐步夯实基础,一步一个脚印、稳扎稳打做好我校国际化建设工作。我很期待来华留学生和海外读者能从"发现中国系列"中认识中国、了解中国、爱上中国,也很希望该系列能够成为中外文化交流的一道亮丽风景线,为推动构建人类命运共同体贡献我们的智慧和力量。

陈建国

华中科技大学原副校长

Series Editor's Preface

Throughout the history of mankind, when education in a country thrives, the country will thrive, and strong education makes a strong nation. Today, as economic globalization continues to deepen, the opening-up of education has become an essential strategy for national development. Since the 18th National Congress of the Communist Party of China, numerous important documents concerning the internationalization of higher education have been issued, with international exchange and cooperation now being one of the five major functions of universities. Huazhong University of Science and Technology (HUST) has actively responded to this call by releasing a series of guiding documents to promote the internationalization of education, and placing significant emphasis on the education of international students in China. The "Introduction to China's S&T Innovation" is a classic collection of works created for international students in China in this context, which can be said to be both a need of the times and a responsibility.

We live in an era characterized by advanced transportation, frequent interpersonal exchanges, and increasingly dynamic cultural interactions. In this era, how to tell China's stories well and let the world understand China better has become an important issue for us. We are fully aware that international students in China possess the unique advantage of being "bridges between China and the world," serving as special envoys of friendship between China and the world and important connectors between China and the world. By providing international students with a comprehensive understanding of China's economic and social development, we can empower them to tell China's stories well, thereby enhancing the international dissemination of Chinese civilization.

In recent years, Xi Jinping, General Secretary of the Central Committee of the Communist Party of China, has written numerous heartfelt letters to overseas students, returning scholars, and international students in China. Studying these letters has deeply inspired and encouraged me. On the one hand, as a former overseas student who studied abroad in Germany and the United States for over six years starting in 1995, I have gained a deep understanding of the academic and living needs of international students in China. On the other hand, since returning from studying abroad over 20 years ago, I have been engaged in research, teaching, and administrative work at universities. During my tenure as Vice President of Huazhong University of Science and Technology, I was responsible for international exchange and cooperation for many years, with international student education being one of my primary responsibilities. I have witnessed and experienced the rapid development of China's higher education and scientific research. As the number of international students in China continues to grow, I feel proud and honored, and at the same time, I also feel a great sense of responsibility.

At present, China is in a new phase of high-quality development, where promoting high-quality development through high-level opening-up has become a requirement of the times, both in the economic and educational fields. I believe that high-level opening-up of education is not only a driving force for the "Double First-Class" initiative in Chinese universities, but also an opportunity to explore new areas of international cooperation for universities. Therefore, in our internationalization efforts, we have consistently adopted an international perspective, positioning ourselves within a global framework, benchmarking against world-class universities, and actively expanding substantial cooperation with top international institutions. While expanding the scale of international students in China, we have also worked to further improve the quality of their education.

The "Introduction to China's S&T Innovation" selects key topics related to China's economic development, medical and health care, digitalization construction and other hot spots of China's livelihood. By explaining the development process, technological innovations, policy evolution, underlying logic, and international cooperation in these fields, the series provides a comprehensive introduction to the quality and speed of China's modernization efforts. It not only serves as a vivid record of China's modernization, but also highlights the spiritual symbols and cultural essence of Chinese civilization.

Each book in this series is edited by authoritative experts in the relevant field. Here, I would like to extend my heartfelt gratitude to the chief editors for their strong support and hard work. They are leading scholars deeply engaged in scientific research, with keen insights into the trends of economic and technological development in China and internationally. They possess rich experience in book compilation and a profound understanding of the content. Furthermore, they are front-line educators with extensive teaching experience, who understand the needs of international students in China, know the ways of teaching, and have unique insights into talent cultivation. I am confident that this series, which fits the background of the times, carefully selects hot topics, and understands readers' needs, will be able to present a comprehensive, multidimensional, and authentic China to international students. It will empower them to tell a good story about China, act as good envoys of friendship, and build bridges of cooperation.

As far as I know, the "Introduction to China's S&T Innovation" has reached an agreement with Springer, a world-renowned publishing house, to publish the English version, which will be distributed worldwide. This also means that we will stand on a broader stage to tell China's stories, promote Chinese wisdom and solutions, and contribute to advancing cultural exchanges, strengthening international communication capabilities, and shaping a Chinese narrative.

Looking ahead, the "Introduction to China's S&T Innovation" will continue to be developed and published, laying a solid foundation for the education of international students in China. We will continue to advance the internationalization of our university step by step. I look forward to seeing international students and overseas readers get to know, understand, and fall in love with China through the "Introduction to China's S&T Innovation." I also hope that this series will become a beautiful landscape of cultural exchange between China and the world, contributing our wisdom and strength to the building of a community with a shared future for mankind.

Chen Jianguo
Former Vice President of Huazhong University of Science and Technology

序　言

当你们翻开"发现中国系列"之《中国卫生（双语版）》时，或许正在思考一个深刻的问题：如何让一个拥有14亿多人口的发展中国家，在有限的资源条件下，实现人人享有基本卫生保健服务？这正是中国医疗卫生体制改革（以下简称"中国医改"）向世界贡献的中国智慧。作为这场改革的亲历者和参与者，我们很荣幸能通过本书，向全球特别是发展中国家的同仁分享我们的实践与思考。

中国医改不是实验室里的理想模型，而是一场在广袤土地上展开的民生实践。2009年新医改启动时，中国面临着城乡差距大、资源分布不均、传染病与慢性病双重负担等典型的发展中国家困境。但通过10余年的探索，中国构建了全球最大的基本医疗保障网，居民个人卫生支出占比从2012年的34.34%下降到2021年的27.60%，人均预期寿命从2011年的74.8岁增长到2021年的78.2岁。这些数字背后凝结着五项关键的经验。

以公平性统领制度设计　中国医改强势破解城乡二元结构，将新型农村合作医疗制度与城镇居民基本医疗保险制度整合为统一的城乡居民基本医疗保险制度；截至2023年底，基本医疗保险参保人数约为13.34亿人，参保覆盖面稳定在95%以上。中央财政对中西部地区的专项补助，使最偏远的山村也能享有基本医疗服务。这种"托底式公平"，让健康权成为最普惠的民生福祉。

用基层网络筑牢健康防线　截至2021年底，中国90%的城乡居民15分钟内可到达最近医疗点。这不是依靠兴建超级医院，而是通过"县乡村一体化"机制，让3.5万个乡镇卫生院和59.9万个村卫生室成为"健康守门人"。基层首诊、双向转诊的分级诊疗模式，使大医院门诊量降低，县域内就诊率超过90%。

让预防优于治疗成为国家行动　中国建立了全球最大的传染病网络直报系统及疾病和健康危险因素监测网络，将高血压、糖尿病、慢性阻塞性肺疾病等慢性病管理纳入国家基本公共卫生服务。爱国卫生运动从"除四害"升级为健康城市创建，例如这一举措有效降低了江苏启东这一肝癌高发区的肝癌发病率。

以技术创新破解资源瓶颈　通过"互联网＋医疗健康"，三甲医院专家可实时指导5 000千米外的新疆乡村医生的诊疗工作。中国积极推广人工智能辅助诊断系统，并在部分贫困县试点应用，有效降低了基层误诊率。中药配方颗粒技术让传统验方走进现代药房，惠及广大的慢性病患者。

用制度创新激发系统活力　福建三明的"三医联动"改革证明，医疗、医保、医药协同改革，可以在不增加财政负担的前提下实现服务质量提升。这种改革智慧正在转化为国家层面的支付方式改革和药品集中带量采购制度，为患者节约费用超过千亿元。

当然，中国医改仍在路上。老龄化社会的"银发浪潮"、疾病谱系的深刻变化、群众对优质医疗的更高期待，都在催生着新的变革。但我们坚信，只要坚守"以人民健康为中心"的初心，任何挑战都将转化为进步的阶梯。

对于发展中国家同仁，中国经验的核心启示在于：健康治理没有放之四海而皆准的模板，但存在普遍的价值坐标——将健康视为社会投资而非消耗性支出，将制度优势转化为资源整合能力，用适宜技术架起理想与现实的桥梁。例如，中非"光明行"活动在津巴布韦、马拉维、莫桑比克等多国相继开展，为 2 000 多名非洲白内障患者带来光明；同时，中国与东盟国家签订的首个人工智能合作创新平台落地老挝。这些实践生动展现了全球健康治理中的东方智慧。

期待本书能成为一把钥匙，为读者开启理解中国医改的大门，更期盼各国读者从中获得启迪，共同谱写人类健康事业的新篇章。

2025 年 2 月 27 日于武汉

Preface

When you open *China's Health System* (*Bilingual Edition*) of "Introduction to China's S&T Innovation," you might be pondering a profound question: How can a developing country with a population of over 1.4 billion achieve universal access to basic health care services under limited resources? This is precisely the Chinese wisdom that China's medical and health system reform has contributed to the world. As witnesses and participants in this reform, we are honored to share our practices and reflections with global peers, especially those from developing countries, through this book.

China's medical and health system reform is not an ideal model conceived in a laboratory but a practical endeavor unfolding across a vast land. When the new medical reform was launched in 2009, China faced typical challenges of developing countries, such as significant urban-rural disparities, uneven resource distribution, and the dual burden of infectious and chronic diseases. However, through over a decade of exploration, China has built the world's largest basic medical insurance network. The proportion of personal health expenditure dropped from 34.34% in 2012 to 27.60% in 2021, and the average life expectancy increased from 74.8 years in 2011 to 78.2 years in 2021. Behind these figures lie five key experiences.

Prioritizing equity in system design China's medical and health system reform has vigorously addressed the urban-rural dual structure by integrating the new rural cooperative medical care system with the basic medical insurance system for non-working urban residents into a unified basic medical insurance system for rural and non-working urban residents. By the end of 2023, the number of people covered by basic medical insurance reached approximately 1.33 billion, with a coverage rate stable at over 95%. Central government subsidies to central and western regions ensure that even the most remote villages have access to basic medical services. This "bottom-line equity" approach has made the right to health a universal benefit.

Strengthening health defenses with grassroots networks By the end of 2021, 90% of urban and rural residents in China could reach the nearest medical facility within 15 minutes. This was achieved not by building super hospitals but through a "county-township-village integration" mechanism, turning 35 000 township health centers and 599 000 village clinics into "health gatekeepers." The hierarchical diagnosis and treatment model, featuring primary care first diagnosis and two-way referrals, has reduced outpatient visits to large hospitals, with over 90% of patients treated within their counties.

Making prevention a national priority   China has established the world's largest direct reporting system for infectious disease epidemics and a monitoring network for diseases and health risk factors. Chronic diseases such as hypertension, diabetes, and chronic obstructive pulmonary disease have been incorporated into the national basic public health services. The Patriotic Health Campaign has evolved from the Elimination of the Four Pests to the creation of healthy cities. For example, this initiative has effectively reduced the incidence of liver cancer in Qidong, Jiangsu Province—a region previously known as a high-risk area for liver cancer.

Breaking resource bottlenecks with technological innovation   Through "Internet + Healthcare," experts from Grade-A tertiary hospitals can guide rural doctors in Xinjiang, 5 000 kilometers away, in real time. China has actively promoted AI-assisted diagnostic systems, and piloted their use in some impoverished counties, effectively reducing misdiagnosis rates at the grassroots level. Traditional Chinese medicine formula granule technology has brought ancient prescriptions into modern pharmacies, benefiting a vast number of chronic disease patients.

Inspiring systemic vitality through institutional innovation   The "Triple Linkage" reform in Sanming, Fujian Province, demonstrates that coordinated reforms in health care, medical insurance, and medicine can improve service quality without increasing financial burdens. This reform wisdom is now being translated into national-level payment reforms and centralized drug bulk-buying systems, saving patients over 100 billion yuan.

Of course, China's medical and health system reform is still ongoing. The "silver wave" of an aging society, profound changes in disease patterns, and higher public expectations for quality health care are all driving new transformations. However, we firmly believe that as long as we adhere to the principle of "putting people's health at the center," any challenge can become a stepping stone to progress.

For our peers in developing countries, the core lesson from China's experience is that there is no one-size-fits-all template for health governance, but there are universal values: treating health as a social investment rather than a consumptive expense, transforming institutional advantages into resource integration capabilities, and bridging ideals and reality with appropriate technologies. For example, the Chinese Brightness Action in Africa has been carried out in Zimbabwe, Malawi, Mozambique, and other countries, restoring sight to over 2 000 African cataract patients. Meanwhile, the first AI cooperation and innovation platform between China and ASEAN countries has been established in Laos. These practices vividly demonstrate the Eastern wisdom in global health governance.

We hope this book will serve as a key to unlocking the door to understanding China's medical and health system reform for its readers. Furthermore, we hope that readers from around the world will gain inspiration from it and work together to write a new chapter in the advancement of global health and well-being.

Written in Wuhan on February 27, 2025

目录

Contents

1　中国卫生体系概况

中国的基本政治制度包括中国共产党领导的多党合作和政治协商制度、民族区域自治制度、基层群众自治制度。中国行政机关由中华人民共和国国务院（简称"国务院"）及其领导的地方各级人民政府组成。地方卫生行政部门受本级人民政府领导，并接受上级卫生行政部门指导。20 世纪 80 年代初期以来，随着中国经济的快速增长、城镇化进程的迅速推进、工业化的高速发展、人口的大规模流动，以及人口老龄化程度的加深，与生活方式和老龄化相关的疾病已成为中国最重要的健康问题之一。

1.1　中国卫生体系背景

1.1.1　地理与人口背景

中华人民共和国于 1949 年 10 月 1 日成立，陆地总面积约 960 万平方千米，居世界第三位，海域总面积约 473 万平方千米。截至 2022 年，中国共有 34 个省级行政区划单位，包括 4 个直辖市（北京、上海、天津、重庆）、23 个省（包括台湾）、5 个自治区和 2 个特别行政区（香港特别行政区和澳门特别行政区）；在省级以下，中国设 333 个地级行政区划单位、2 843 个县级行政区划单位，以及 38 602 个乡级行政区划单位。

中国是世界人口大国。2020 年，中国人口（不含港、澳、台）达到 14.12 亿人，约占世界总人口的 18%；女性人口占比为 48.8%；2010—2020 年人口年平均增长率为 0.5% 左右。按照世界卫生组织的标准，中国在 1999 年已经进入老龄化社会，2021 年 65 岁及以上人口占总人口的 14.2%。近几十年来，中国人口受教育水平明显提高。中国高中（含中专）及以上受教育人口占比从 1990 年的 9.4% 提高到了 2020 年的 30.6%，而文盲率从 1990 年的 15.9% 下降到了 2020 年的 2.7%。

自 20 世纪 80 年代中期开始，中国城镇化建设快速推进，人口流动趋于活跃。2011 年，中国城镇人口达到 6.91 亿人，首次超过农村人口。2020 年，中国城镇人口达到 9.02 亿人，占全国人口的 63.9%。同年，中国流动人口达到 3.76 亿人，占全国人口的 26.6%，人口流动方向主要是从农村流向城市。中国人口分布很不均衡，东部和中部地区人口密集，西部高原地区人口稀少。2020 年，中国人口密度为 147 人/平方千米。

1.1.2　人群健康状况

与世界上其他大多数国家一样，中国人口和疾病模式已经从高出生率、高死亡率、传染病和营养不良为主向低出生率、低死亡率、慢性病为主转变。这突出表现在以下几个方面。

人均预期寿命。中国居民的人均预期寿命有了很大增长，从 1949 年的 35 岁提高到 1996 年的 70.8 岁和 2021 年的 78.2 岁。

儿童死亡率。中国婴儿死亡率从 1980 年的 46.9‰下降到 2021 年的 5.0‰，5 岁以下儿童死亡率从 1980 年的 62.7‰下降到 2021 年的 7.1‰。城乡儿童死亡率差距正在缩小，但是差距仍然存在。1995 年农村婴儿死亡率比城市婴儿死亡率高 2.9 倍，而 2021 年高 0.8 倍；1995 年农村 5 岁以下儿童死亡率比城市高 3.1 倍，而 2021 年高 1.1 倍。

孕产妇死亡率。中国孕产妇死亡率从 1990 年的 88.8/10 万下降到 2021 年的 16.1/10 万。城乡孕产妇死亡率差距逐渐缩小。1990 年，中国农村地区孕产妇死亡率是城市地区的 2.5 倍，而 2021 年两者基本持平，其中农村地区孕产妇死亡率(16.5/10 万)比城市地区(15.4/10 万)略高。

死因构成。自 20 世纪 90 年代开始，中国人口死因构成的最大变化是恶性肿瘤、脑血管疾病和心脏病等疾病的占比不断上升，而传染病、慢性呼吸道疾病和消化系统疾病的占比不断下降。伴随此转变，非传染性慢性疾病已经成为中国主要的疾病负担。在每年各种疾病导致的死亡中，恶性肿瘤、心脏病、脑血管疾病为排名前三的死因，这三类疾病的致死人数占总死亡人数的近 70%。

传染病。包括霍乱、麻风、肺结核、血吸虫病和疟疾等在内的传染病，曾经是影响中国居民健康水平的最主要疾病。而通过建立疾病预防控制体系、开展预防接种和爱国卫生运动等防控措施，中国成功降低了传染病发病率，并使得重点传染病得到了有效控制，例如严重急性呼吸综合征(SARS)、人感染高致病性禽流感、手足口病、输入性脊髓灰质炎，以及人感染 H7N9 禽流感等。2019 年，中国甲类传染病共报告发病 21 例，死亡 1 例，其中鼠疫报告发病 5 例、死亡 1 例，霍乱报告发病 16 例、死亡 0 例。目前中国主要传染病包括病毒性肝炎、肺结核、艾滋病等。2021 年，中国病毒性肝炎发病率为 87/10 万，肺结核发病率为 45.4/10 万，而艾滋病为 4.27/10 万。2021 年，中国艾滋病、肺结核和病毒性肝炎死亡人数分别为 19 623 人、1 763 人、520 人。

1.2 中国卫生体系基本构成

2009 年，《中共中央 国务院关于深化医药卫生体制改革的意见》出台，这是中国新一轮医药卫生体制改革(简称"新医改")的纲领性文件。在该文件指导下，中国近年来以"一个目标、四梁八柱"(图 1-1)为原则构建起中国卫生体系框架。其中，"一个目标"是建立基本医疗卫生服务制度。"四梁"指的是覆盖城乡居民的公共卫生服务体系、医疗服务体系、医疗保障体系、药品供应保障体系。"八柱"指的是医药卫生管理体制、医药卫生机构运行机制、多元卫生投入机制、医药价格形成机制、医药卫生监管体制、医药卫生科技创新机制和人才保障机制、医药卫生信息系统、医药卫生法律制度。

1.2.1 主要组成体系

1.2.1.1 公共卫生服务体系

在中国，公共卫生服务主要由基层医疗卫生机构和专业公共卫生机构提供。中国建立

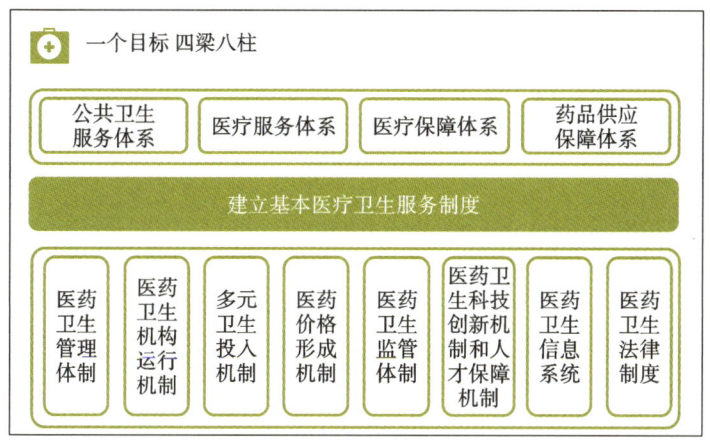

图 1-1 中国卫生体系建设的"一个目标、四梁八柱"

了以社区卫生服务中心(站)、乡镇卫生院、村卫生室等城乡基层医疗卫生服务网络为基础,由疾病预防控制、健康教育、妇幼保健、精神卫生、应急救治、采供血、卫生监督等专业公共卫生机构负责具体业务指导的公共卫生服务体系。中华人民共和国国家卫生健康委员会(简称"国家卫生健康委")设医政司、基层卫生健康司、医疗应急司等 19 个内设机构及机关党委(党组巡视工作领导小组办公室)、离退休干部局,主要负责开展公共卫生、医疗服务、卫生应急等方面的监督管理工作。地方卫生行政部门内设相关机构,负责地方的公共卫生管理工作。

1.2.1.2 医疗服务体系

在中国,医疗服务体系由二、三级综合医院,专科医院和基层医疗卫生机构等医疗卫生机构共同组成。其中,二、三级综合医院主要提供门诊和住院医疗服务,专科医院可以提供与精神疾病和口腔疾病等相关的医疗服务,社区卫生服务中心(站)、乡镇卫生院和村卫生室等基层医疗卫生机构负责为辖区居民提供基本医疗服务。城市和农村居民都可以自主选择到各类医疗卫生机构就诊。

1.2.1.3 医疗保障体系

中国实施以基本医疗保险为主体,医疗救助为托底,补充医疗保险、商业健康保险、慈善捐赠、医疗互助等共同发展的多层次医疗保障体系。其中,基本医疗保险包括城镇职工基本医疗保险和城乡居民基本医疗保险,前者覆盖城市就业人口,后者覆盖城市非就业人口及农村人口。近年来,基本医疗保险基本实现了人口的覆盖(参保覆盖率稳定在95%以上),但是其对费用的报销比例仍有待提高。

医疗救助是中国多层次医疗保障体系的托底层次。医疗救助体系通过政府拨款和社会捐助等多渠道筹集资金,主要是为城乡低保家庭成员、五保户(农村地区无劳动能力、无生活来源又无法定赡养、抚养、扶养义务人,或者其法定赡养、抚养、扶养义务人无赡养、抚养、扶养能力的老年人、残疾人和未满 16 周岁的未成年人,由政府保吃、保穿、保医、保住、保葬)和其他经济困难家庭人员提供资助,以确保贫困人口享有基本医疗服务。医疗救助以住院救助为主,同时兼顾门诊救助。

城乡居民大病保险是在基本医疗保障的基础上,对大病患者发生的高额医疗费用给予进一步保障的一项制度性安排,是基本医疗保障制度的拓展和延伸。为避免城乡居民发生家庭灾难性医疗支出,根据规定,大病保险补偿政策的实际支付比例不低于50%,同时按医疗费用高低分段制定支付比例,原则上医疗费用越高支付比例越高。

随着中国社会主义市场经济体制的进一步完善和居民收入的提高,居民的医疗卫生服务需求在不断增加,商业医疗保险在医疗保障体系中发挥的作用也越来越重要。当前商业医疗保险市场中,学生医保、补充医疗保险以及包含医疗险、意外险、财产险及人寿险在内的综合保险较为常见。

1.2.1.4 药品供应保障体系

从20世纪80年代至今,经过40余年的法制建设,中国已经建立了一个由法律法规、部门规章和其他规范性文件构成的较为完整的药品管理法律法规体系,包括《中华人民共和国药品管理法》《中华人民共和国中医药法》《药品注册管理办法》《药品生产质量管理规范》《药品经营质量管理规范》等。中国从1995年开始陆续实施《药品生产质量管理规范》《药品经营质量管理规范》《中药材生产质量管理规范》等认证制度,并于2006年实行"飞行检查"制度,以加强对药品生产和经营质量的监督管理。此外,国家药品监督管理局是中国药品监督管理行政机构,省、自治区、直辖市人民政府药品监督管理部门负责本行政区域内的药品监督管理工作,对药品及其生产、流通、消费环节实施统一监督管理。国家中医药管理局负责中药材监管等工作。

在解决药品可及性问题的过程中,中国在建立和完善医药管理制度和医疗保障制度等方面采取了一系列措施,在一定程度上降低了药价、激励了新药研发、改善了药品可及性。近年来,中国为保障药品可及性而采取的重大举措包括建立国家基本药物制度、完善国家基本药物目录遴选和调整机制、进行药品采购机制改革,以及推进政府举办的基层医疗卫生机构按购进价格实行零差率销售基本药物等。截至2013年,中国所有省份已经实现了基本药物制度在政府办基层医疗卫生机构的全覆盖。为了解决市场供应不足或供应不稳定的问题,对于用量小且临床必需的基本药物品种实行定点生产,也从一定程度上保证了药品供应。

传统上,中国的药品流通主要是从生产企业流向批发企业,再流向医院药房或者零售企业,最终到达消费者。但是从2009年建立国家基本药物制度工作正式实施以后,中国开始实行基本药物的省级集中招标采购,这改变了基层医疗卫生机构原有的药品流通方式。此外,自2018年底进行国家组织药品集中采购和使用试点(也称"4+7"试点)以来,中国已累计开展了十批国家组织药品集中带量采购工作;同时各地方也以省级或省际联盟的形式积极开展药品集中带量采购工作。在中国,几乎所有的医疗机构都拥有药房,这些药房负责机构药品的销售;医院是药品销售的主要渠道。

1.2.2 体系支持制度

1.2.2.1 医药卫生管理体制

中华人民共和国全国人民代表大会(简称"全国人大")是中国最高国家权力机关,其常设机关为全国人民代表大会常务委员会(简称"全国人大常委会")。全国人大行使的主要职权包括修改宪法,监督宪法的实施,制定和修改刑事、民事、国家机构的和其他的基本法律等。全国人民代表大会教育科学文化卫生委员会于1983年设立,主要负责审议全国人大主席团或全国人大交付的有关教科文卫等方面的议案和法律草案、质询案;向全国人大主席团或全国人大常委会提出属于人大职权范围内同教科文卫委员会有关的议案；参与教科文卫体人口等方面立法工作；在全国人大常委会领导下，依法对教科文卫等方面的法律进行视察与监督等。

国家卫生健康委隶属于国务院，是中国最高卫生行政机关。国家卫生健康委及由其管理的国家中医药管理局和国家疾病预防控制局是中国最主要的卫生行政管理机构。根据职责划分，在国务院的其他组成部门中，中华人民共和国国家发展和改革委员会（简称"国家发展改革委"）、民政部、财政部、人力资源和社会保障部（简称"人力资源社会保障部"）等部门也在中国卫生治理中承担规划、筹资、保险管理等相应职责。国务院部委管理的国家局中，国家药品监督管理局等机构也参与中国卫生治理工作。

在卫生治理中，中国各级行政机构的具体职责存在差异，形成自上而下的分级管理体系。地方政府各工作部门受同级人民政府统一领导，并且依照法律或行政法规的规定受上级主管部门的业务指导或者领导。省、市、县各级卫生行政机关是同级人民政府的卫生行政职能部门，在同级人民政府的直接领导下，负责本行政区域内的卫生行政管理工作，并接受上级卫生行政机关的业务指导。中国卫生管理组织体系分为国家、省、市、县四级，乡（镇）一般不设独立的卫生行政部门。

在中国，非政府组织也会参与卫生体系各领域的工作，包括慈善组织、基金会以及各类专业协会等。专业协会，如中华医学会、中华中医药学会、中华预防医学会、中国医师协会、中华护理学会等，在卫生治理中发挥一定作用；主要职责包括组织在职培训或继续教育，向政府及有关部门反映医药工作者的意见、建议和要求，组织专家协助政府对相关法规政策进行论证等。

1.2.2.2　医药卫生机构运行机制

这里主要介绍医院及基层医疗卫生机构两个方面。其中，公立医院占有绝大部分的卫生资源，提供主要的门诊和住院服务。早在十几年前，中国便开始实施医院改革试点，并逐步建立起相应的机构运行机制。2010年，中国启动公立医院综合改革试点，主要内容包括探索医药分开模式、破除"以药补医"的医院补偿机制，以及医务人员工资分配制度和药品采购制度等方面的改革。2012年，中国开始推进县级公立医院综合改革试点。试点的主要内容包括改革补偿机制，如将公立医院补偿由服务收费、药品加成收入和政府补助三个渠道改为服务收费和政府补助两个渠道，破除"以药补医"等。2012年后，为加快形成多元办医格局，中国进一步提出大力促进非公立医疗机构发展；具体政策包括要求地方政府出台鼓励社会资本办医的实施细则，鼓励公立医院资源丰富的地区利用社会资本参与部分公立医院转制等。中国还在进一步探索和建立医院运行机制。这些运行机制对医院行为的影响目前还缺乏全国范围内的客观评价。

另一方面，2009年中国开始进行基层医疗卫生机构运行体制改革，实施了包括双向转诊制度、基层首诊制度等在内的相关制度，以及基层医疗卫生机构和人员绩效考核机制、基层医疗卫生机构收入分配机制等。2012年，中国明确提出基层医疗卫生机构人员收入分配以服务数量和质量为基础、向核心和骨干卫生技术人员倾斜等机制。

近年来，中国基层医疗卫生机构的设施条件已得到改善，但基层卫生技术人员短缺及能力不足问题仍然存在。为此，中国已实施建设基层医疗卫生队伍、免费为农村基层医疗卫生机构定向培养卫生人员等策略，并出台建立全科医生制度等措施。

1.2.2.3 多元卫生投入机制

在中国，政府卫生支出、社会卫生支出和个人卫生支出是卫生筹资及投入的主要来源。从卫生总费用的筹资来源看，政府卫生支出占GDP（国内生产总值）比例在1980—1995年呈下降趋势，而2005—2012年该比例上升了近一倍；然而，政府卫生支出占政府总支出的比例从1995年的5.7%下降到了2000年的4.5%，尽管该比例2005年开始缓慢上升到4.6%，2012年进一步上升至6.7%，但仍处于较低水平。中国个人卫生支出占卫生总费用的比例较高，2001年达到峰值60%后开始逐渐下降，2012年下降到34.3%，为1990年以来的最低水平。个人卫生支出也是私人卫生费用的主要构成之一，所占比例逐年下降，从2000年的95.6%下降到了2012年的78.0%。

1.2.2.4 医药价格形成机制

在中国，药品价格管理有政府定价、政府指导价和市场调节价三种形式。列入国家基本医疗保险药品目录的药品以及国家基本医疗保险药品目录以外具有垄断性生产经营特征的药品，实行政府定价或者政府指导价；其他药品实行市场调节价。《中华人民共和国药品管理法》针对上述三种定价形式制定了较为详细的定价方法。国务院药品价格主管部门和省级政府药品价格主管部门根据中央和地方定价目录，分别制定并公布本级药品定价目录。政府药品价格主管部门负责对实行政府指导价和市场调节价的药品的实际购销价格、流通差价率变化情况实施监测。2009年，新医改开始研究取消药品加成，提高医疗机构公益性，减轻药品费用负担。2012年7月开始执行的《药品流通环节价格管理暂行办法》管控批发环节差价率（额）、非营利性医疗机构销售环节差价率（额），规定药品批发环节的实际差价按照"低价高差率，高价低差率"的方法，实行差率（额）控制，以及逐步取消医疗机构销售药品加成。

另一方面，医疗机构可向卫生行政管理部门申请营利性或非营利性医疗机构执业登记，非营利性医疗机构在税费等方面享有一定的优惠政策。中国对非营利性医疗机构提供的基本医疗服务价格实行政府指导价，而对营利性医疗机构实行市场调节价。针对非营利性医疗机构，2012年，国家发展改革委、卫生部、国家中医药管理局发布《关于规范医疗服务价格管理及有关问题的通知》，正式出台《全国医疗服务价格项目规范（2012年版）》，全面规范医疗服务价格管理。

1.2.2.5 医药卫生监管体制

中国医药卫生监管体制通常包括三种形式：一是设立标准，强制执行；二是提供意见，政策引导；三是设定禁止类事项。卫生监督主要通过由政府设置（出台）规定进行限制（规制）来执行，即具体规制活动由有关政府部门执行，其所属事业单位等也可承担部分规制活动，但需政府授权。中央人民政府主要负责国家层面的卫生事业发展的总体设计和安排，各级地方政府在辖区范围内行使法律法规赋予的卫生监督职能。国家卫生健康委、财政部、人力资源社会保障部、民政部、国家发展改革委和国家药品监督管理局等机构是参与卫生监督的主要国家机构。地方政府也设立了相应部门。这些机构和部门根据各自职能开展相应的卫生监督活动，为明确医疗保障范围和水平、规范医疗卫生服务行为、确保医疗服务质量与安全等提供了保障。

对于专业技术要求较高的监督职能，政府也会委托相关的专业技术协会、行业协会制定标准，参与组织实施标准，并对标准实施情况进行监督。例如，中国医师协会除了开展医师相关技术培训外,还会组织医师定期考核,推进行业自律维权,并为政府提供制定政策和法律法规的相关信息。这些行业协会也在各地设立分会,以保证工作的上下协调、联合互动。各行业协会制定协会内部的相关章程、会员管理规定等,凡参与协会工作的组织或个人都必须遵守相关规定,这也起到了行业监督的作用。

1.2.2.6　医药卫生科技创新机制和人才保障机制

中国政府高度重视医药卫生科技进步,把医药卫生科技创新作为国家科技发展的重点,努力攻克医药卫生科技难关,为人民群众健康提供技术保障。近年来,中国不断增加医学科研投入、整合优势医学科研资源、实施医药卫生科技重大专项计划、鼓励自主创新,并加强对重大疾病防治技术和新药研制关键技术等的研究,在医学基础和应用研究、高技术研究、中医和中西医结合研究等方面有了一定的突破。

人才保障方面,自 1949 年以来,中国逐步建立了包括院校医学教育、毕业后医学教育和继续医学教育等在内的连续统一的医学教育体系。

在中国,院校医学教育包括本科、专科等层次。高中毕业生参加普通高等学校招生全国统一考试(简称“高考”)后,根据考试成绩的高低进入不同层次的学校接受不同的医学教育。医学教育除了培养临床医生以外,也培养其他类别的卫生技术人员,包括护理人员、卫生管理人员、药剂人员以及医学检验人员等。中国院校医学教育也包括研究生教育。本科毕业生通过推荐或参加统一考试获得研究生学习资格。硕士研究生和博士研究生学制为 2～4 年不等,毕业后分别被授予硕士和博士学位。

住院医师规范化培训属于毕业后医学教育,是指医学专业毕业生在完成医学院校教育之后,以住院医师的身份在认定的培训基地接受以提高临床能力为主的系统化、规范化培训。住院医师规范化培训是临床医师培养所特有和必经的教育阶段,对于提高医疗质量、确保医疗安全具有不可替代的重要意义。

继续医学教育,是指在完成院校医学教育和毕业后医学教育之后进行的在职进修教育。其旨在使在职卫生人员不断学习同本专业有关的新知识和新技术,跟上医学科学的发展。中国的继续医学教育实行学分制。在职卫生人员必须每年参加继续教育活动,完成一定的学分。

中国于 1998 年颁布《中华人民共和国执业医师法》,宣布实行医师执业注册制度。卫生技术人员需要通过全国统一的医师资格考试,并获得由国家卫生健康委统一颁发的医师资格证书。只有获得医师资格证书,并经注册取得医师执业证书的人员才具有独立从事医疗活动的资格。受县级以上人民政府卫生行政部门委托的机构应当按照医师执业标准,对医师的业务水平、工作成绩和职业道德状况进行定期考核。目前,医师只能在其注册的医疗机构行医,但中国正在制定和推行医师多点执业制度。中国的卫生技术人员职称设三个级别:初级、中级和高级。

1.2.2.7　医药卫生信息系统

医药卫生信息系统是卫生体系的重要组成部分,中国新医改将卫生信息化作为重要任务和重要支撑与保障。从业务领域看,中国医药卫生信息系统主要包括医院信息系统、公共卫生信息系统、医疗保障信息系统、综合卫生管理信息平台以及区域卫生信息平台等内容。上述医药卫生信息系统中,除医疗保障信息系统中的城镇职工和城镇居民基本医疗保险信息系统主要由人力资源和社会保障部门管理外,其余信息系统均主要由卫生行政部门负责管理。

中国医药卫生信息系统管理主要包括制定医药卫生信息管理政策法规和医药卫生信息事业发展规划,建立全面系统的信息资源开发和共享机制,推进医药卫生信息标准工作的规范统一,加强医药卫生信息基础设施和网络建设,以及强化医药卫生信息安全等。目前,中国以业务应用为主线的信息系统对于提高业务效率和决策水平起到了重要作用。随着信息技术的普及、扩展型网络和先进数据挖掘技术的发展,越来越多的数据和信息迅速积累。

1.2.2.8 医药卫生法律制度

中国特色社会主义法律体系是以宪法为统帅,以法律为主干,以行政法规、地方性法规为重要组成部分,由宪法相关法、民法商法、行政法、经济法、社会法、刑法、诉讼与非诉讼程序法等多个法律部门组成的有机统一整体。

《中华人民共和国宪法》对居民健康权益有明确规定:"中华人民共和国公民在年老、疾病或者丧失劳动能力的情况下,有从国家和社会获得物质帮助的权利。国家发展为公民享受这些权利所需要的社会保险、社会救济和医疗卫生事业。"根据卫生法律的调整对象,中国医药卫生法律制度分为医药卫生机构法律制度、医药卫生职业法律制度、医药卫生服务法律制度等。这些法律制度主要就某一具体领域进行规范指导。中国目前尚缺乏可以统帅卫生法律体系、连接宪法与具体卫生法律法规的综合性法律。

中国目前没有专门的卫生法,只有以公共卫生与医政管理为主的单个法律法规构成的相对完整的卫生法体系。医疗方面主要包括《中华人民共和国基本医疗卫生与健康促进法》《中华人民共和国传染病防治法实施办法》《中华人民共和国精神卫生法》《中华人民共和国药品管理法》等法律法规。除此之外,还有大量地方性法规、部委和地方政府规章与规范性文件等。

1.3 中国卫生体系发展历程

1949年新中国成立以来,中国卫生体系经历了不同的发展阶段,最终形成了目前的卫生体系。中国卫生体系的建立与发展,特别是组织与治理模式的变革与中国政治、经济、行政管理等体制变革息息相关。中国的社会经济发展与改革可分为不同阶段,在不同阶段卫生体系发展呈现不同特征。从新中国成立到改革开放前,中国卫生体系以计划经济为基础,主要依靠公共筹资来发展,这一时期存在卫生资源短缺和卫生服务提供能力不足等突出问题;从改革开放开始到2002年,中国卫生体系逐步过渡到以市场经济为主,各级政府动员社会各方面力量筹集发展卫生事业的资金,卫生资源不断增加,卫生服务提供能力快速提升,但同期政府投入责任弱化,2000年左右个人卫生支出占卫生总费用的比重接近60%;2003年以后,中国不断强化各级政府投入责任,加大了政府卫生投入力度,到2021年,个人卫生支出占卫生总费用的比重下降到了27.6%。

1.3.1 第一阶段:新中国成立至改革开放前(1949—1978年)

新中国成立之初,中国经济发展水平低下,政府将实现社会公平作为核心价值理念之一,并将其贯穿到社会主义政治制度、经济制度、分配制度的设计过程中,逐渐形成了以高度集中为特征、以行政管理为主要手段的计划经济体制。国家通过行政手段管理社会经济事务,在收入分配上,实行"按劳分配"的分配制度。在政府强有力的统一规划和组织下,自上而下的卫生行政管理组织体系得以形成,卫生体系也得以建立并快速发展:形成了包括医疗、预防、保健、康复、教学、科研等在内的比较完整的卫生体系,尤其是以农村合作医疗和农村三级医疗卫生服务网络为代表的农村卫生服务体系得到了世界卫生组织的高度评价。中国医疗卫生服务体系的基本框架大体上也形成于这个时期。由于当时社会经济发展水平的限制,中国卫生体系的特征是"低水平、广覆盖",筹资和报销水平较低,统筹单位通常是市或县。总体而言,卫生人员受教育水平较低,医疗服务提供能力和服务质量不高。公共筹资的医疗保险覆盖了大部分城市居民,但补偿水平非常低,农村合作医疗的情况尤其如此。当时,"缺医少药"情况比较严重,这一方面是因为当时卫生人员数量总体不足,另一方面是因为尽管可通过短期培训等方式培养较多的初级卫生人员(如赤脚医生),但其服务能力相对较低,而高质量卫生人员较为缺乏;同时,计划经济条件下卫生技术人员收入与服务质量没有直接联系,卫生技术人员提供医疗卫生服务的积极性较低,服务效率不高。在改革开放之前的一段时期,中国卫生体系内的各种矛盾日益凸显。

1.3.2 第二阶段:改革开放初步阶段(1979—2002 年)

1978 年召开的中共十一届三中全会开启了中国从计划经济向社会主义市场经济的转轨,作出了把党和国家的工作中心转移到经济建设上来、实行改革开放的历史性决策。这一时期中国的政治体制、行政管理体制、经济体制和财政体制发生了巨大变革,对卫生体系产生了深刻影响。

第一,政治体制改革。1982 年公布施行的《中华人民共和国宪法》确立了新时期中国政治体制和经济发展的纲领。1987 年召开的中共十三大提出,建立高度民主、法制完备、富有效率、充满活力的社会主义政治体制,是政治体制改革的长远目标。1979—2002 年,中国政治体制改革的内容主要是党政分开、权力下放、精简机构。

第二,行政管理体制改革。中国行政管理体制改革是随着计划经济体制向社会主义市场经济体制的转型与经济体制改革同步进行的。随着中国经济、社会事业的发展,中国政府开始简政放权。地方政府开始承担更多的卫生职责,在医疗机构方面体现为大部分医疗机构开始成为"自主经营、自负盈亏"的独立经营实体。

第三,经济体制改革。1979—2002 年,中国经济体制改革的核心是资源配置由行政分配逐步过渡到市场发挥基础性作用。在医疗卫生服务领域,很多卫生要素越来越市场化,主要由市场调节,但医疗服务价格主要采取政府定价形式。

第四,财政体制改革。1994 年,中国启动了"分税制"的财政体制改革,中央政府的财力集中程度提高,而地方政府收入下降,财政支出压力明显加大。政府财权的不断上移与卫生领域政府事权的层层下放之间出现了矛盾,政府对卫生的投入力度受到较大影响。

为解决计划经济时期人民卫生需求与医疗卫生服务效率之间的矛盾,改革开放后,参照经济体制改革的做法,卫生领域也开始更多地引入市场机制,包括改变医疗机构的收入分配办法、调整医药价格政策和收费标准等,医疗卫生服务主要围绕居民需求展开;此外,开始允许私人资本开设诊所等医疗机构并提供医疗卫生服务,同时部分公立医疗机构转为私有化。1979—2002 年,中国卫生事业快速发展,卫生机构、卫生人员、医疗床位和设备数快速增加,卫生服务提供能力显著增强。但是由于体制机制改革不到位，医疗机构趋利倾向日趋严重，进而导致医药费用过快上涨、医患矛盾升级等问题。2001 年，中国居民个人卫生支出占卫生总费用的比重高达 60%，达到历史最高水平，而政府卫生支出占比只有不到 16%。同时，政府对公共卫生的投入力度不足、农村卫生服务体系及医疗保障制度建设滞后等问题日益凸显。这些问题的出现使得医药卫生体制改革和卫生事业发展问题被列入了中央人民政府的重要议事日程。

1.3.3　第三阶段：改革开放深化阶段（2003 年至今）

这一时期中国的政治、经济、财政等各项改革进入攻坚阶段，经济继续保持较高的增长速度，但面临一些不协调问题，如贫富差距、城乡二元制、社会保障覆盖率低等突出问题。2003 年，中共十六届三中全会提出了科学发展观，强调以人为本、统筹经济社会发展。2007 年，中共十七大提出，要"继续解放思想，坚持改革开放，推动科学发展，促进社会和谐，为夺取全面建设小康社会新胜利而奋斗"，其中推动卫生发展是重要内容之一。

2003 年 SARS 疫情在中国全国蔓延，中国卫生体系经历了严峻的挑战。SARS 疫情暴发之后，中国政府开始反思中国卫生体系中存在的问题，努力解决卫生工作中存在的"重医轻防""重城轻乡"等弊端，加强公共卫生服务体系建设，大力推进农村卫生和城市社区卫生建设。2003 年之后，新型农村合作医疗（简称"新农合"）制度进入加速发展时期，但是医疗卫生体系内市场和政府职能定位还未完全明确，仍存在医疗机构过分依靠市场竞争维持自身发展，以及"看病难、看病贵"情况突出等问题，同时群众多层次的需求也未得到很好的满足。

为解决卫生领域存在的矛盾和问题，实现人人享有基本医疗卫生服务的目标，2009 年新医改正式启动，并明确长远目标：到 2020 年，覆盖城乡居民的基本医疗卫生制度基本建立。新医改进一步明确了政府在卫生领域的责任，并明确提出政府卫生投入增长幅度要高于经常性财政支出增长幅度等要求，例如 2009 年人均基本公共卫生服务经费标准不低于 15 元，到 2011 年不低于 20 元。此外，公立医院改革试点在部分城市开始实施。基本医疗保障筹资和补偿水平不断提高，2021 年城乡居民基本医疗保险人均财政补助标准达到每人每年不低于 580 元，是 2009 年的 7.25 倍。2021 年，政府卫生支出占卫生总费用的比重达到了26.91%。此外，中国还加大了鼓励社会资本办医的力度，放宽社会资本举办医疗机构的准入范围，并改善社会资本举办医疗机构的执业环境，使得民营医院从 2009 年的 6 240 个增加到 2021 年的 24 766 个。与第二阶段的改革（1979—2002 年）鼓励社会资本相比，第三阶段主要强调在保证政府举办的医疗机构公益性和非营利性的前提下，鼓励社会资本和私人资本进入医疗卫生领域，以满足群众多层次需求，同时更加注重政策环境的改善。

2018 年，国务院开始了改革开放以来的第八次机构改革，将国家卫生和计划生育委员会等多个机构的职责整合，组建国家卫生健康委。保留全国老龄工作委员会，日常工作由国家卫生健康委承担。民政部代管的中国老龄协会改由国家卫生健康委代管。国家中医药管理局由国家卫生健康委管理。

案例 农村三级医疗卫生服务网络

20世纪50年代至70年代,中国通过建设以县级医疗卫生机构为龙头、乡镇卫生院为主体、村卫生室为基础的三级医疗卫生机构,建立了比较系统的农村三级医疗卫生服务网络,有效地保障了农民的健康水平,这一举措被世界卫生组织誉为发展中国家解决医疗卫生问题的典范。农村三级医疗卫生服务网络主要承担着预防保健、基本医疗、卫生监督、健康教育等任务,为农民获得基本医疗卫生服务提供保障,可缓解"看病难、看病贵"问题,并推进实现农村医疗卫生发展目标,使农民"小病不出村、常见疾病不出乡、大病不出县"。

目前,中国农村三级医疗卫生服务网络基本健全。截至2021年底,全国县(区、市)、乡镇、行政村共设县级医院1.7万个、乡镇卫生院3.5万个、村卫生室59.9万个。健全完善乡村医疗卫生体系,是筑牢亿万农民群众健康的"第一道防线",是全面推进乡村振兴的应有之义。目前,中国要求进一步深化改革,促进乡村医疗卫生体系健康发展,包括坚持和加强中国共产党对乡村医疗卫生工作的全面领导、强化县域内医疗卫生资源统筹和布局优化、发展壮大乡村医疗卫生人才队伍和提高农村地区医疗保障水平等;要求到2025年实现目标任务,即乡村医疗卫生机构功能布局更加均衡合理、基础设施条件明显改善,乡村医疗卫生人才队伍发展壮大、人员素质和结构明显优化,乡村医疗卫生体系运行机制进一步完善,乡村医疗卫生体系改革发展取得明显进展等。

2 中国的卫生工作方针与健康中国行动

在中国,卫生工作方针是卫生健康事业发展的指导思想,具有全局性和统领性特点,是中国共产党和中央人民政府领导卫生工作的基本方针。健康中国行动是中国卫生工作方针在特定时期的重点任务,旨在促进人民健康和全面发展。了解和掌握卫生工作方针和健康中国行动的基本内容,以及制定卫生工作方针和卫生发展战略的基本原则,对于指导卫生系统的改革和发展具有至关重要的意义。

2.1 中国的卫生工作方针

工作方针是指导工作或事业发展的纲领。卫生工作方针是中国指导卫生健康事业发展的基本原则,是制定各项卫生制度和卫生政策的主要依据。

2.1.1 中国卫生工作方针的发展与内容

新中国成立以来,中国政府结合基本国情、卫生健康事业发展基本规律和人民群众的健康需要,制定了不同时期的卫生工作方针。实践证明,这些卫生工作方针能够适应中国特定时期的卫生健康事业发展形势,指引不同历史时期卫生健康事业发展的方向和道路,促进国家卫生健康事业的良性发展。

2.1.1.1 新中国成立初期卫生工作四大方针(1949—1977 年)

(1)卫生工作四大方针的形成

1949 年 9—10 月,全国卫生行政会议召开。此次会议根据当时严重缺医少药、医疗卫生条件极差和传染病流行的状况,初步确立了全国卫生建设的工作方针,即"预防为主,卫生工作的重点放在保证生产建设和国防建设方面,面向农村、工矿,依靠群众,开展卫生保健工作"。1950 年 8 月,中央人民政府卫生部和中央人民政府人民革命军事委员会卫生部联合召开第一届全国卫生会议,讨论确定了中国卫生工作的总方针和总任务,并确定了卫生工作的三大原则,即面向工农兵、预防为主、团结中西医。1950 年 9 月,中央人民政府政务院第 49 次政务会议正式批准了卫生工作的三大原则。1952 年 12 月,第二届全国卫生会议又将"卫生工作与群众运动相结合"列入其中,形成了卫生工作的四大原则。这四大原则也被称为卫生工作的四大方针。

(2)卫生工作四大方针的基本内容

面向工农兵。面向工农兵明确了卫生工作的方向和服务对象。卫生工作必须为人民群众服务,这是一个重大原则问题。工人和农民作为中国人口的主体,构成了人民民主政权的根基,同时也是新中国生产建设的中坚力量。他们所面临的健康挑战尤为严峻,但在卫生保障方面获得的支持却相对有限。此外,军人作为中国共产党领导的国家武装力量基本成员,是中国国防建设的基石。没有军人的参与,中国的建设发展和人民的和平生活将无法得到充分保障。

预防为主。预防为主代表了一种最为经济、人道、主动且有效的疾病防治策略,这与广大人民群众的根本利益相一致。所有医疗、预防和保健机构及全体从业人员,均应将预防工作作为其主要职责之一,以确保实现疾病预防和健康促进的目标。

团结中西医。团结中西医旨在将中西医从业人员团结起来,共同为人民群众提供健康服务;通过充分发挥中西医各自的专业优势,促进中西医之间的相互学习与共同发展,实现医疗资源的最优配置和医疗服务质量的全面提升。

卫生工作与群众运动相结合。卫生工作的实施必须紧紧依靠群众,应发动和动员广大人民群众积极参与到与疾病的斗争中来。这种群众性的参与不仅能够促进卫生意识的普及和健康习惯的养成,而且能加快卫生健康事业的发展步伐,尤其是在基层医疗卫生机构的建立和卫生人员的培训方面。

这些方针充分反映了中国特色社会主义卫生健康事业的性质和特征,符合中国的基本国情、人民健康的需要和卫生健康事业发展的规律。在这些方针的指导下,中国卫生工作取得了巨大成就。

2.1.1.2　新时期卫生工作方针(1978—2015 年)

(1)新时期卫生工作方针的形成

1978 年召开的中共十一届三中全会开启了中国改革开放历史新时期。随着社会主义市场经济体制的稳步建立以及社会、经济、文化、科学技术的深入改革与发展,新中国成立初期确立的卫生工作方针面临着与新时期卫生工作发展形势不相适应的挑战。为了应对这一挑战,1997 年出台的《中共中央 国务院关于卫生改革与发展的决定》中明确提出了适应新时期要求的卫生工作方针。

(2)新时期卫生工作方针的基本内容

新时期卫生工作方针为“以农村为重点,预防为主,中西医并重,依靠科技与教育,动员全社会参与,为人民健康服务,为社会主义现代化建设服务”。这一方针的提出,体现了中国对农村卫生工作的特别关注,强调了预防在卫生工作中的核心地位,同时强调了中西医并重的发展理念。它还突出了科技与教育在提升卫生服务专业水平中的关键作用,并号召全社会广泛参与,以实现更广泛的人民健康服务目标,进而为社会主义现代化建设提供坚实的健康保障。此方针体现的卫生工作战略重点是以农村为重点、预防为主、中西医并重,基本策略是依靠科技与教育、动员全社会参与,根本宗旨是为人民健康服务、为社会主义现代化建设服务。

以农村为重点。农村卫生工作一直是中国高度重视的重点领域。尽管自改革开放以来,中国的农村卫生工作取得了很大的进展——县、乡、村三级医疗预防保健网络建设得到了进一步加强,农村卫生队伍也在逐步调整和充实,但仍面临许多困难和问题。因此,必须大力加强农村卫生工作,以遏制因病致贫和因病返贫对农村经济和社会发展的制约。

预防为主。新时期卫生工作方针继续将预防作为主要内容。各级医疗、预防和保健机构都应贯彻预防为主的方针,切实做好三级预防工作。

中西医并重。新时期提出的中西医并重方针，是对团结中西医方针的继承和发展，也是振兴中医药并将其推向世界的政策保证。它要求中西医加强团结，相互学习，取长补短，共同提高，并积极探索中西医结合发展的途径和方法。

依靠科技与教育。依靠科技与教育是落实科学技术是第一生产力思想和科教兴国战略的具体表现，也是新中国成立以来卫生工作长足发展的基本经验总结。

动员全社会参与。动员全社会参与是卫生工作与群众运动相结合方针的进一步发展和完善。动员全社会参与包括各级党政领导的重视、社会各部门的协作配合以及广大人民群众的积极参与等内容。

为人民健康服务，为社会主义现代化建设服务。卫生健康事业是一项惠及全体社会成员的公共事业，其发展必须始终坚持两个核心方向：一是致力于保障和提升广大人民群众的健康水平，二是积极支持和促进社会主义现代化建设进程。坚持为人民健康服务，意味着卫生工作要不断满足人民群众日益增长的健康需求，通过提供全面、优质的医疗服务，保障人民享有健康的权利。同时，为社会主义现代化建设服务则要求卫生健康事业的发展与国家的整体发展战略相协调，通过提高人民的健康水平，为国家的经济发展、社会进步和文化繁荣贡献力量。

新时期卫生工作方针有效克服了中国卫生健康事业存在的许多困难和问题，指引了社会主义市场经济体制下卫生健康事业发展的正确道路。通过明确战略重点、基本策略和根本宗旨，卫生工作可以更好地服务人民，促进社会主义现代化建设，改善人民健康状况，促进社会和谐稳定。

2.1.1.3　新时代卫生与健康工作方针（2016年至今）

（1）新时代卫生与健康工作方针的形成

中共十八大以来，中共中央把全民健康作为全面小康的重要基础，并强调将健康放到优先发展的战略位置。中国卫生工作的重心逐渐转向管健康、促健康，以及制定和实施健康中国行动。2016年8月19日至20日，全国卫生与健康大会在北京召开。在本次会议上，习近平总书记深刻阐述了健康中国建设的重大意义，并明确了新时代卫生与健康工作方针，即"以基层为重点，以改革创新为动力，预防为主，中西医并重，将健康融入所有政策，人民共建共享"。随后，中共中央、国务院于2016年10月25日印发《"健康中国2030"规划纲要》，发出建设健康中国的号召，并明确了建设健康中国的大政方针和行动纲领。

（2）新时代卫生与健康工作方针的基本内容

以基层为重点。以基层为重点是新时代卫生与健康工作方针适应中国经济社会发展新形势的重要体现。随着中国城镇化进程的不断推进，传统的农村地区正逐步实现城镇化转型，农民的身份也随之转变为居民。在此背景下，将卫生工作的重点从"农村"转向"基层"，不仅更加准确地反映了当前的社会结构和人口分布，也更好地适应了人民群众对医疗卫生服务的新需求。以基层为重点意味着，卫生资源的配置、医疗卫生服务的提供以及健康促进活动，都应更多地关注基层。这要求加强基层医疗卫生机构的服务能力，提高基层卫生人员的专业水平，完善基层医疗服务网络，确保基层群众能够享受到便捷、高效、优质的医疗服务。同时，以基层为重点也强调了卫生工作要与基层社会治理相结合，应动员和依靠基层群众参与到卫生工作中来，形成政府主导、社会参与、群众受益的良好局面。

以改革创新为动力。以改革创新为动力标志着新时代卫生与健康工作方针的重要演进。它超越了传统的"依靠科技与教育"的范畴,将文化和制度创新亦纳入卫生工作的核心动力之中。这体现了对创新、协调、绿色、开放、共享五大发展理念的全面贯彻,是推动中国卫生健康事业持续发展的必由之路。

预防为主,中西医并重。预防为主,中西医并重是中国卫生工作的重要原则。当前,中国传染病防治形势仍然严峻,非传染性慢性疾病的死亡率也在上升。心脑血管疾病、恶性肿瘤和其他慢性病已成为城乡居民的主要死因。在卫生工作中,应全面实施预防策略,以有效降低慢性病的发生率和死亡率。这一策略的实施,旨在构建一个更加完善的医疗卫生体系,提高人民群众的健康水平,为实现健康中国目标奠定坚实的基础。中国将发挥中医药在预防和治疗方面的优势,加快推进中医药的现代化和产业化,促进中西医药相互补充和协调发展,高质量推进中医药事业和产业发展,推动中医药走向世界。

将健康融入所有政策。将健康融入所有政策是实现中国大健康理念的具体行动,体现了对健康影响因素的全面认识和应对。当前,全球范围内已经形成共识,即健康状态与贫困、教育、环境、就业等多重社会因素存在密切的联系。为了保障健康成果的可持续性,中国必须将大健康理念贯穿于政府的各项政策之中,树立维护健康是政府各部门共同责任的理念,并实施综合性的健康管理。

人民共建共享。人民共建共享将卫生工作与群众运动相结合、动员全社会参与方针进一步完善,增加了"共享"理念。卫生健康事业涉及社会的各个方面,关系到千家万户,是一项系统工程。因此,只有社会各部门积极配合、人民群众广泛参与,才能实现人人参与、人人有责、人人享有的目标。各级党委和政府则肩负着重大责任。只有坚持人民共建共享,才能确保健康成果的可持续性。

2.1.2　制定卫生工作方针的基本原则

在中国,卫生工作方针的制定主要坚持以下原则:

坚持中国共产党对卫生健康工作的全面领导。这反映了中国发展卫生健康事业的坚定意志,以及中国共产党全心全意为人民服务的根本宗旨。只有坚持党对卫生健康工作的全面领导,才能确保卫生健康工作得到有效推进和落实。

坚持卫生健康事业的公益属性。中国卫生健康事业具有福利性和公益性特征。福利性强调政府对卫生健康事业发展和人民健康的责任,特别是保护弱势群体的责任;公益性则强调政府、社会和个人共同承担发展卫生健康事业和保护人民健康的责任。在不同的经济体制下,中国卫生健康事业的性质不同。计划经济时期的卫生健康事业属于福利事业,而建立社会主义市场经济体制后,卫生健康事业发展成为一种不以营利为目的的具有一定福利性质的社会公益事业。

保障卫生健康事业在经济社会发展中的基础性地位。卫生部门通过提供医疗、预防、保健和康复等服务来保护人们的生命安全和身心健康、参与生产力的完善和劳动力的修复,并促进经济社会发展。这种功能是其他任何部门都代替不了的。卫生与教育、文化、科技和体育具有同等重要的地位,它们是上层建筑中分工不同的部分。应保障卫生健康事业在经济社会发展中的基础性地位,并给予其足够的支持和关注。

坚持以计划和规划为主导的卫生改革导向。坚持以计划和规划为主导的卫生改革导向,体现了中国政府对卫生健康事业的责任和担当,强调国家对卫生领域的宏观调控和管理。而以市场为导向的卫生改革,可能会忽视基层医疗卫生服务的均衡发展,使得一些贫困地区和弱势群体难以获得基本医疗卫生服务。在卫生领域,市场力量难以完全替代政府的职责和作用。政府应当保障和提高公共卫生服务的质量并扩大服务的覆盖面,通过计划和规划来引导医疗卫生资源的合理配置和流动,确保人民群众的基本医疗卫生服务需求得到满足。

坚持把保障人民健康放在优先发展的战略位置。坚持把保障人民健康放在优先发展的战略位置,是制定卫生工作方针的重要原则之一。它强调了保障人民健康的重要性,并将保障人民健康放在经济、社会、国防等各个方面的发展之前,以确保人民的健康状况得到充分关注、人民的健康权益得到充分保障。这一原则促进了卫生健康事业的稳步发展,有利于提高全民健康水平和国家整体素质,同时也有助于促进社会和经济的持续发展。因此必须从卫生工作的属性、宗旨、规律等方面入手,深刻认识"没有全民健康,就没有全面小康""努力全方位全周期保障人民健康"的重大意义。

2.2　健康中国行动

2.2.1　卫生发展战略

卫生发展战略是为满足人民健康需求而制定的长远谋划。它是经济社会发展战略的重要领域,必须与经济社会发展战略保持协调。中国卫生发展战略以提高人民健康水平为核心,要求强化基本医疗卫生服务建设,并实现内涵与外延发展相结合。该战略的主导原则是坚持公平与效率相统一,并保证全体人民享有基本医疗卫生服务。

2.2.1.1　卫生发展战略的意义

推动经济发展和社会进步。推动经济发展和社会进步是卫生发展战略的重要目标之一。通过提高人民健康水平和强化基本医疗卫生服务建设,卫生工作可以促进劳动力的修复和提高生产效率,从而为经济发展提供有力支撑。同时,卫生工作还可以减少疾病和健康问题对社会的负面影响,提高人民群众的生活质量,增强社会稳定和社会发展的可持续性。

指导卫生健康事业科学发展。制定和实施科学的卫生发展战略可以确保卫生健康事业朝着正确的方向发展,提高卫生工作的科学性、针对性和有效性,从而更好地服务人民群众、提高整体健康水平。同时,科学的卫生发展战略还能够刺激卫生领域进行更多的创新性研究,提升卫生健康事业的发展水平和国际竞争力,为卫生健康事业的长期发展奠定坚实基础。

促进卫生健康事业目标的实现。卫生发展战略的制定可以帮助管理者顺应客观规律和客观形势,抓住环境带来的机遇,变被动应付为主动作为,促进卫生健康事业目标的实现。

体现卫生健康事业发展重点。卫生发展战略的制定能够让卫生健康事业的发展更有针对性并且更加高效。它聚焦于当前和未来最紧迫的健康问题,要求优先发展和提高卫生服务质量和水平,有助于满足人民群众的健康需求。通过明确卫生健康事业的发展重点,卫生发展战略能够引导资源的合理配置和使用,并促进卫生健康事业的长足发展。

提高国民健康素质。中国既面临发展中国家面临的传统健康问题,又面临发达国家面临的健康问题,同时城乡、地区和人群之间的健康差异较大。卫生发展战略以解决危害城乡居民健康的主要问题为重点,通过出台切实可行的国家健康行动计划,加强对影响国民长远健康问题的有效干预,进而维护和增进国民健康。

2.2.1.2　卫生发展战略的特征

卫生发展战略具有全局性、长远性、领导性、纲领性、适应性和前瞻性等特征,这些特征共同构成了中国卫生健康事业科学发展的理论基础和实践指南。

全局性。卫生发展战略需从宏观角度出发,全面考虑卫生政策的制定、资源的投入、人才的培养等关键要素。它应涵盖医疗服务、健康教育、疾病预防控制等卫生领域的各个方面,并着眼于未来,为卫生健康事业的可持续发展奠定坚实基础。

长远性。卫生发展战略应是中长期规划,并关注卫生健康事业的整体生存和发展。它要求制定长期目标,持续加强基础设施建设和人才培养,并以科学发展的理念推动卫生健康事业的持续进步。

领导性。卫生行政主管部门在卫生健康事业发展中扮演领导角色,负责明确发展方向、制定战略目标、出台相关政策和计划,并组织和监督各项工作的实施,进而确保卫生健康事业协调稳定发展。

纲领性。作为指导卫生健康事业发展的纲领性文件,卫生发展战略为制定卫生发展目标、政策,以及资源配置、管理和服务规划提供了全面指导。

适应性。卫生发展战略应具备灵活性和适应性,以满足社会变化和多元化的卫生需求。卫生部门需及时调整卫生服务模式,提升卫生服务水平,不断创新和推广适应性强的卫生技术和方针,扩大卫生服务的覆盖面,并提高卫生服务质量。

前瞻性。卫生发展战略的制定者应具备前瞻性思维,预见未来可能出现的新问题、新情况和新挑战,并制定相应的应对策略。这有助于卫生健康事业朝着更有针对性和更可持续的方向发展,避免盲目跟风,确保卫生健康事业发展更加顺畅和健康。

2.2.1.3　制定卫生发展战略的基本原则

坚持为人民健康服务的宗旨、全面提高人民健康水平是中国卫生发展战略的核心。围绕这个核心,卫生发展战略的制定应遵循以下基本原则:

坚持以人为本。将提高人民健康水平作为国家发展的核心目标,全面纳入经济社会发展规划。健康不仅是个人和家庭幸福的基础,也是国家和民族发展的重要基石。通过优先发展卫生健康事业,全方位守护人民群众的健康,可以提升社会对健康的重视程度,确保经济社会发展战略目标的实现。

坚持公平优先,兼顾效率。确保不同人群都能公平地享有基本卫生服务,同时注重卫生资源的有效利用,以最少的卫生资源投入实现最大的健康效果。此外,还应注重政府责任与市场机制的结合,动员全社会力量参与,形成有序竞争机制,并满足人民多样化的健康需求。

坚持统筹兼顾,突出重点。在制定卫生发展战略时,要全面考虑,平衡各方面利益,突出关键领域,加强协同合作,增强卫生健康事业发展的整体性和协调性。通过制定全面系统的规划,实现卫生资源的合理配置,提升卫生资源的利用效率,解决卫生领域的根本矛盾。

坚持预防为主,防治结合。强调从源头上预防和控制疾病的发生,减少医疗资源的浪费。同时,强调预防与治疗相结合,注重疾病的早期诊断和治疗,推动医学模式从"以病为本"向"以人为本"、从"治疗为主"向"预防为主"、从"以病人为中心"向"以健康为中心"转变。

坚持保基本、强基层、建机制。确保提供基本的公共卫生和医疗服务,满足人民群众的基本医疗需求。加强基层卫生服务能力,推进分级诊疗制度建设,将服务和资源重点放在基层。建立健全卫生健康事业发展体制机制,加强卫生政策法规的制定与实施,促进卫生健康事业的科学化、规范化和制度化发展。

2.2.2 健康中国行动的内容与沿革

新中国成立以来,不同时期制定的卫生工作方针,共同促进了中国卫生发展战略的形成。健康中国行动是中国卫生发展战略的核心内容,也是当前中国的主要卫生发展战略。健康中国行动是全面建成小康社会的重要内容之一。健康既是发展的目的,也是发展的源泉;是促进人的全面发展的必然要求,是经济社会发展的基础条件,是民族昌盛和国家富强的重要标志,也是广大人民群众的共同追求。

2.2.2.1 健康中国行动的发展过程

20世纪70年代,世界卫生组织提出"2000年人人享有卫生保健"的战略目标,之后中国政府承诺实现该目标。1988年,该目标被纳入2000年中国社会经济发展总目标。1997年,《中共中央 国务院关于卫生改革与发展的决定》确定了农村卫生、预防保健、中西医并重为中国卫生工作的战略重点。中共十八届五中全会和中共十九大报告进一步确立了人民健康的重要地位。

2.2.2.2 健康中国行动的主要特点

健康中国行动坚持目标导向和问题导向,突出了战略性、系统性、指导性和操作性,具有以下鲜明特点:

突出大健康的发展理念。当前中国居民主要健康指标总体上优于中高收入国家的平均水平,但随着工业化、城镇化、人口老龄化发展以及生态环境、生活方式变化,维护人民健康面临一系列新挑战。据世界卫生组织研究,人的行为方式和环境因素对健康的影响越来越突出,"以疾病治疗为中心"难以解决人的健康问题,也不可持续。因此,健康中国行动确立了"以促进健康为中心"的"大健康观""大卫生观",提出将这一理念融入公共政策制定实施的全过程,统筹应对广泛的健康影响因素,全方位、全生命周期维护人民群众健康。

着眼长远与立足当前相结合。健康中国行动围绕全面建成小康社会、实现"两个一百年"奋斗目标的国家战略,充分考虑与经济社会发展各阶段目标相衔接、与联合国2030年可持续发展议程要求相衔接,同时针对当前突出问题,创新体制机制,从全局高度统筹卫生计生、体育健身、环境保护、食品药品、公共安全、健康教育等领域政策措施,形成促进健康的合力。

目标明确、可操作。健康中国行动围绕总体健康水平、健康影响因素、健康服务与健康保障、健康产业、促进健康的制度体系等方面设置了若干主要量化指标,使目标任务具体化,工作过程可操作、可衡量、可考核,并据此提出健康中国"三步走"的目标,包括"到2020年,主要健康指标居于中高收入国家前列""到2030年,主要健康指标进入高收入国家行列""到2050年,建成与社会主义现代化国家相适应的健康国家"。

2.2.2.3 健康中国行动的目标

第一,到2020年,建立覆盖城乡居民的中国特色基本医疗卫生制度,健康素养水平持续提高,健康服务体系完善高效,人人享有基本医疗卫生服务和基本体育健身服务,基本形成内涵丰富、结构合理的健康产业体系,主要健康指标居于中高收入国家前列。

第二,到 2030 年具体实现以下目标:

人民健康水平持续提升。人民身体素质明显增强,2030 年人均预期寿命达到 79 岁,人均健康预期寿命显著提高。

主要健康危险因素得到有效控制。全民健康素养大幅提高,健康生活方式得到全面普及,有利于健康的生产生活环境基本形成,食品药品安全得到有效保障,消除一批重大疾病危害。

健康服务能力大幅提升。优质高效的整合型医疗卫生服务体系和完善的全民健身公共服务体系全面建立,健康保障体系进一步完善,健康科技创新整体实力位居世界前列,健康服务质量和水平明显提高。

健康产业规模显著扩大。建立起体系完整、结构优化的健康产业体系,形成一批具有较强创新能力和国际竞争力的大型企业,成为国民经济支柱性产业。

促进健康的制度体系更加完善。有利于健康的政策法律法规体系进一步健全,健康领域治理体系和治理能力基本实现现代化。

第三,到 2050 年,建成与社会主义现代化国家相适应的健康国家。

2.2.2.4　健康中国行动的内容

健康中国行动的总体战略是以人的健康为中心,按照从内部到外部、从主体到环境的顺序,依次针对个人生活与行为方式、医疗卫生服务与保障、生产与生活环境等健康影响因素,提出普及健康生活、优化健康服务、完善健康保障、建设健康环境、发展健康产业等五个方面的战略任务。

第一,普及健康生活。从健康促进的源头入手,强调个人健康责任,通过加强健康教育,提高全民健康素养,广泛开展全民健身运动,塑造自主自律的健康行为,引导群众形成合理膳食、适量运动、戒烟限酒、心理平衡的健康生活方式。

第二,优化健康服务。以妇女儿童、老年人、贫困人口、残疾人等人群为重点,从疾病的预防和治疗两个层面采取措施,强化覆盖全民的公共卫生服务,加大慢性病和重大传染病防控力度,实施健康扶贫工程,创新医疗卫生服务供给模式,发挥中医治未病的独特优势,为群众提供更优质的健康服务。

第三,完善健康保障。通过健全全民医疗保障体系,深化公立医院、药品、医疗器械流通体制改革,降低虚高价格,切实减轻群众看病负担,改善就医感受。加强各类医保制度整合衔接,改进医保管理服务体系,实现保障能力长期可持续。

第四,建设健康环境。针对影响健康的环境问题,开展大气、水、土壤等污染防治,加强食品药品安全监管,强化安全生产和职业病防治,促进道路交通安全,深入开展爱国卫生运动,建设健康城市和健康村镇,提高突发事件应急能力,最大程度减少外界因素对健康的影响。

第五,发展健康产业。区分基本和非基本,优化多元办医格局,推动非公立医疗机构向高水平、规模化方向发展。加强供给侧结构性改革,支持发展健康医疗旅游等健康服务新业态,积极发展健身休闲运动产业,提升医药产业发展水平,不断满足群众日益增长的多层次多样化健康需求。

案例　《健康中国行动(2019—2030 年)》

　　为了有效推动《"健康中国 2030"规划纲要》的实施和目标实现,2019 年 6 月,国家卫生健康委制定了《健康中国行动(2019—2030 年)》。2019 年 7 月,国务院成立健康中国行动推进委员会,负责统筹推进《健康中国行动(2019—2030 年)》的组织实施、监测和考核相关工作。《健康中国行动(2019—2030 年)》围绕疾病预防和健康促进两大核心,提出将开展 15 项重大专项行动,促进以治病为中心向以健康为中心转变,努力使群众不生病、少生病。这 15 项专项行动为:健康知识普及行动、合理膳食行动、全民健身行动、控烟行动、心理健康促进行动、健康环境促进行动、妇幼健康促进行动、中小学健康促进行动、职业健康保护行动、老年健康促进行动、心脑血管疾病防治行动、癌症防治行动、慢性呼吸系统疾病防治行动、糖尿病防治行动、传染病及地方病防控行动。

3 中国医疗服务体系

中国的医疗卫生机构主要包括医院和基层医疗卫生机构等。自改革开放以来,中国的医院数量保持持续增长的趋势。截至 2021 年末,中国有 36 570 个医院,是 1978 年的 3.9 倍,其中民营医院数量占 67.7％。与此相应,中国医院床位数也经历了持续的增长。2021 年,每千人口医疗卫生机构床位数达到 6.7 张。虽然大型医疗设备主要集中在二级及以上医院,但是基层医疗卫生机构的设备配置也在逐年改善。信息化建设方面,医院管理信息系统、临床信息系统以及区域卫生信息系统均取得了快速发展。卫生领域的政府投入集中在基层医疗卫生机构、基本医疗保障等方面。

中国的卫生人力资源发展迅速。2021 年,每千人口卫生技术人员数达到 7.97 人,但护理人员相对短缺。中国公立医疗卫生机构的卫生技术人员有清晰的职业生涯发展规划,其职业发展前景相对广阔。但在卫生技术人员的配备上,城乡之间存在一定差距。2021 年,城市地区每千人口卫生技术人员数为 9.87 人,而农村地区为 6.27 人。中国卫生人力资源发展面临的其他挑战还包括基层缺少足够的卫生人员,卫生技术人员的受教育水平较低等。虽然中国已初步建立包括院校医学教育、毕业后医学教育和继续医学教育等在内的连续统一的医学教育体系,但该体系仍有待完善,医学教育质量仍有待加强。

3.1 中国医疗服务体系概况

3.1.1 医疗卫生机构及其类型

中国的医疗卫生机构可以分为四类:医院、基层医疗卫生机构、专业公共卫生机构和其他医疗卫生机构。这里主要介绍医院概况。

中国的医院既提供住院服务,也提供门诊服务。根据医院服务的对象或疾病类型,医院可分为综合医院、专科医院等。综合医院提供针对各类人群和各类疾病的综合医疗服务,专科医院如儿童医院、耳鼻喉医院、妇产科医院、口腔医院等则提供专科医疗服务。中国的医院包括西医医院和中医医院等。大多数医院可提供西医服务。在中国,几乎每个县城都有中医医院,并提供中医服务。在一些少数民族地区,也存在民族医医院,比如藏医院、蒙医院。根据所有制的不同,中国的医院可分为公立医院和民营医院。目前,公立医院是中国医疗服务体系的主体。民营医院在近些年也取得了一定的发展。大多数民营医院为营利性医院,也有一部分为非营利性医院。

1989 年,中国开始实施医院分级管理制度。根据医院的规模和功能等综合水平,中国将医院划分为三级。

一级医院是直接向拥有一定人口的社区提供预防、医疗、保健、康复服务的基层医院。一级医院承担的职责主要包括提供预防保健（社区卫生防疫、妇幼保健、计划生育手术和技术指导、健康教育等）、医疗服务（社区内常见病、多发病的门诊及住院诊治，社区康复医疗等）等。

二级医院是向多个社区提供综合医疗服务并承担一定教学、科研任务的地区性医院。二级医院承担的职责主要包括提供医疗服务（对社区提供全面、连续的医疗、护理、预防保健和康复服务），与医疗相结合开展教学、科研工作，以及指导地区内基层医疗卫生机构做好社区治疗、预防保健、康复和精神卫生等工作。

三级医院是向多个地区提供高水平专科医疗服务并承担高等教学、科研任务的区域性以上的医院。三级医院承担的职责主要包括提供专科医疗服务、解决危重疑难病症、接受二级转诊、对下级医院进行业务技术指导和人才培训，完成培养各种高级医疗专业人才的教学任务和承担省级以上科研项目，以及参与和指导一、二级预防工作。

自改革开放以来，中国的医院数量保持持续增长的趋势。1978 年，中国只有 9 293 个医院；到 2021 年，医院总数量达到 36 570 个，是 1978 年的 3.9 倍。其中，综合医院、中医医院和专科医院的数量都有明显增长。2021 年中国所有医院中，公立医院数量占 32.3%，民营医院数量占 67.7%。

3.1.2 医疗卫生机构资金投入

中国的医疗卫生机构多为公立医疗卫生机构，而公立医疗卫生机构的建设及设备购买等事项理应由政府负责。但 20 世纪 80 年代至 90 年代，中国的医疗卫生机构逐渐开始尝试引入市场化运作机制，政府对公立医疗卫生机构的财政投入逐渐减少，公立医疗卫生机构的财政自主权逐渐扩大。许多医院和基层医疗卫生机构可以利用自己的业务收入进行基础建设，或购买医疗设备。有些医疗卫生机构甚至举债进行房屋建设和设备购买。

2009 年新医改启动以来，中国政府加大了对基本医疗保障和基层医疗卫生机构的投入。2016—2021 年，中国财政卫生健康支出从 13 159 亿元增长到 19 142.68 亿元，包括中央财政投入 223.51 亿元。2016—2020 年，中央财政共下达城乡居民医保补助资金 14 484 亿元，城乡居民医保财政补助标准从 2016 年的每人每年 420 元提高到 2020 年的每人每年550 元。2016—2020 年，中央财政共安排公立医院综合改革补助资金 508 亿元，支持各地巩固破除以药补医成果。2018 年和 2019 年，中国将城乡居民医保年人均新增财政补助的一半用于提高大病保险保障能力。2017 年，中国全面推开公立医院综合改革，全国所有公立医院全部取消药品加成。2019 年，中国取消公立医院医用耗材加成。各级政府投入对于医疗卫生机构的硬件设施建设起到不同的作用。在基层医疗卫生机构的房屋和设备等硬件设施建设方面，中央政府和省级政府投入发挥主要作用；县级政府由于财政能力较弱，除了负责发放卫生技术人员的工资之外，对于硬件设施建设的投入较少，在西部欠发达地区情况尤其如此。

此外，虽然中国政府加大了对二级及以上公立医院的投入，但投入力度不如基层医疗卫生机构。因此，二级及以上公立医院仍然需要利用业务收入或其他筹资渠道，加强硬件设施建设。中国鼓励社会资本办医，日益增多的民营医疗卫生机构主要依靠社会资本投资房屋和设备等硬件设施的建设。

3.1.3　医疗卫生机构规模现状

床位数可反映一个医院的经营规模。根据中国卫生统计官方资料,医院床位数通常按以下类别统计:0~49张、50~99张、100~199张、200~299张、300~399张、400~499张、500~799张,以及800张及以上。2021年末,中国全国医疗卫生机构共有床位944.8万张,其中医院741.3万张(占78.5%)、基层医疗卫生机构171.2万张(占18.1%)、专业公共卫生机构30.2万张(占3.2%);城市和农村医疗卫生机构床位数基本持平,各占52.6%和47.4%。在医院中,公立医院床位占70.2%,民营医院床位占29.8%。

与医院数量的变化趋势一致,中国医院的床位数也经历了持续的增长,且增长速度超过了医院数量的增长速度。1978年,中国医院床位数只有110万张,而2021年增长到了741.3万张,是1978年的6.7倍。基层医疗卫生机构的床位数也有了明显增长,但增长速度低于医院。考虑到人口的增长,我们以每千人口拥有床位数来看医疗卫生机构床位数的变化趋势,2007年每千人口拥有床位数是2.83张,2021年达到6.70张,14年内涨幅达到136.7%。

中国城乡医疗卫生机构床位数差异不大。近年来,城乡医疗卫生机构床位配置差异逐渐缩小。2010年,城市地区每千人口医疗卫生机构床位数约为5.94张,是农村地区的2.28倍,而2020年这一数值是1.78倍。2021年,城市和农村地区的每千人口医疗卫生机构床位数分别是7.47张和6.01张。此外,因地区、级别的不同,不同医疗卫生机构之间在床位配置以及所提供的服务方面也存在一定差异。

病床使用率和出院者平均住院日可反映医院床位的使用情况。病床使用率是实际占用的总床日数与实际开放的总床日数之比。出院者平均住院日是出院者占用总床日数与出院人数之比。2021年,中国全国医院病床使用率为74.6%,医院出院者平均住院日为9.2日。

中国不同级别医院的病床使用率存在明显差异。2021年的数据显示,中国三级医院的病床使用率为85.3%,二级和一级医院则分别为71.1%和52.1%。中国医院出院者平均住院日在1992年左右达到峰值,为16.2日;此后总体呈下降趋势,到2021年降为9.2日。

3.1.4　卫生人力资源现状

截至2021年底,中国的卫生人员总数为1 398.3万人,其中卫生技术人员为1 124.2万人。同年,每千人口执业(助理)医师、注册护士分别为3.04人、3.56人,每万人口全科医生、专业公共卫生机构人员分别为3.08人、6.79人。

从1949年开始,中国卫生人员总数总体保持上升趋势。20世纪50年代,卫生人员数量快速增长,每年递增约11万人。20世纪60年代,卫生人员数量停滞不前,在180万人上下波动。20世纪70至80年代卫生人员数量又快速增长,每年递增约15万人,90年代后递增速度变慢。2001—2003年,卫生人员数量出现负增长。2005年以后,卫生人员数量再次快速增长,每年递增均超过20万人,其中2021年比2020年增加50.8万人(增长了3.8%)。

3.1.4.1　卫生人力资源的结构和分布

新中国成立初期,中国医护比约为10∶1。但是护士数量的增长速度明显比医生数量的增长速度快。到 2021 年,中国医护比达到 1：1.17。中国卫生技术人员通常以女性居多,2018 年中国卫生技术人员中女性占 71.8%,其中注册护士这一职业更是高达 97.7%。近年来,中国卫生技术人员的年龄结构以中青年为主。2018 年,中国卫生技术人员中 25～54 岁的人员占 83.3%;55 岁及以上的人员占 11%,与 2017 年(9.2%)相比有所上升。中国卫生技术人员的学历通常分为研究生、本科、大专、中专等几个层次。近年来,中国卫生技术人员的学历不断提升,2020 年拥有大学本科及以上学历的卫生技术人员占 42%,而 2005 年这一比例只有 17.1%。

3.1.4.2　卫生人员教育

自 1949 年开始,中国逐步建立了包括院校医学教育、毕业后医学教育和继续医学教育等在内的连续统一的医学教育体系。从 20 世纪 90 年代起,中国医学教育快速发展。尤其是在 1999 年出台的高等教育扩招政策的鼓励下,中国医学院校的办学规模迅速扩大。2019 年高等医学教育的招生数量为 2000 年的 6.7 倍。高等医学院校数量由新中国成立初期的 44 个,发展到 2020 年的 192 个。从新中国成立初期到 2019 年,高等医学院校在校生数量由 1.52 万人增长到 331.5 万人。此外,2019 年中等医学教育在校生达到 115.5 万人。

3.1.4.3　卫生人员职业生涯

中国的卫生技术人员职称设为三个级别:初级、中级和高级。以医生为例,中专和大专医学生毕业后,可通过考核获取医士资格,本科毕业生则可获得医师(或住院医师)资格。医士和医师均属于初级职称,工作满一定年限(如 5 年)后,可通过一定程序晋升为主治医师(中级职称)。高级职称包括副主任医师和主任医师。其他卫生人员也有相应的职业发展体系。医学院附属医院的卫生人员由于有教学、科研和指导研究生的任务,还有副教授和教授职称。若所在医疗机构有相应的晋升岗位(或职称晋升名额),符合晋升条件的卫生人员可向该机构提出申请。医疗机构审核通过后,上报上级卫生行政部门和人事部门批准。晋升中级职称(如主治医师)需要通过由省级统一组织的考试,考试内容包括专业知识、外语和计算机等。晋升高级职称(如副主任医师和主任医师),则需要进行答辩。省级卫生行政部门和人事部门邀请相关领域专家组成专业委员会,对申请人的资格和能力进行审核。省级人事部门根据答辩结果,最终决定是否同意申请人晋升。

3.2　中国各级医疗服务现状及发展方向

3.2.1　居民就诊路径

在中国,城市和农村居民都可以自主选择到各类医疗卫生机构就诊,见图 3-1 及图 3-2。但是随着医疗卫生机构级别的提高,医疗费用和居民自付医疗费用的比例也相应增加。此外,基层医疗卫生机构多设在居民区内,一般不需要等待就可以获得治疗,因此居民在自我判断病情较轻时多选择在基层医疗卫生机构就诊。

3.2.2　基层医疗服务

中国基层医疗服务主要由社区卫生服务中心(站)、乡镇卫生院、村卫生室等基层医疗

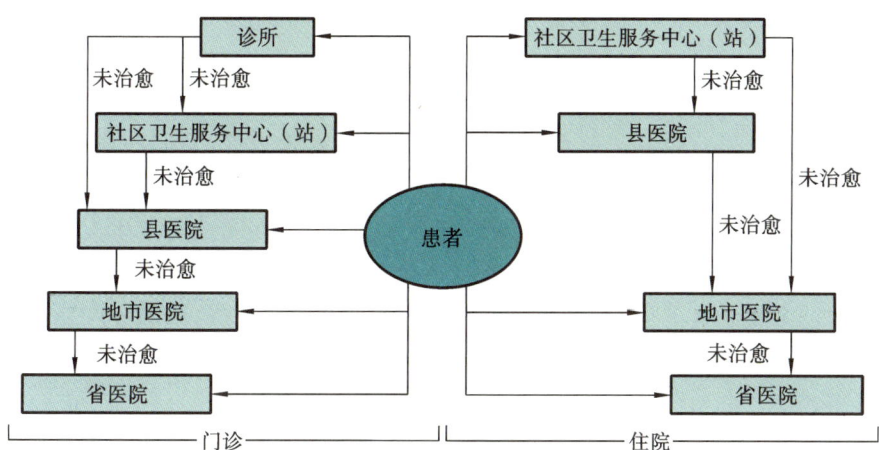

图 3-1 城市居民就诊路径

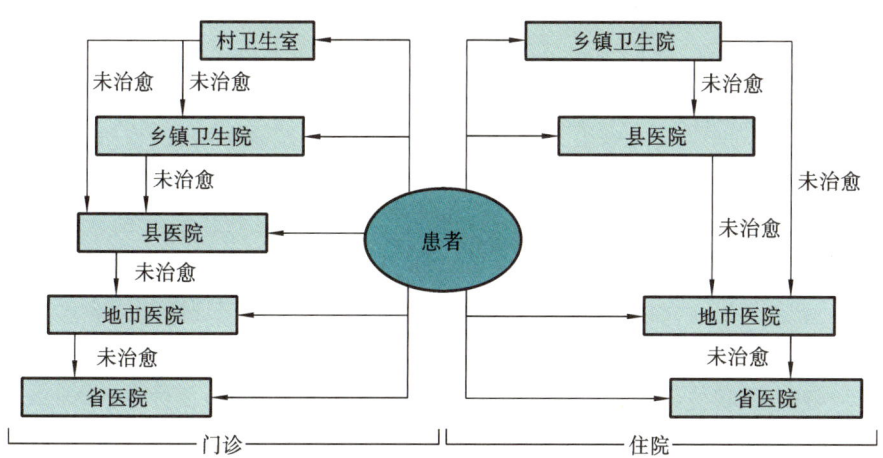

图 3-2 农村居民就诊路径

卫生机构提供。社区卫生服务中心对其下设的社区卫生服务站实行一体化管理,其他社区卫生服务站接受社区卫生服务中心的业务管理。村卫生室接受乡镇卫生院的业务管理和技术指导,在部分已实现乡村卫生服务一体化的地区由乡镇卫生院对村卫生室实行统一管理。

社区卫生服务中心(站)和乡镇卫生院主要负责为当地居民提供健康教育、预防、保健、康复服务和一般常见病、多发病的诊疗服务。村卫生室为农村居民提供基本的医疗服务。卫生行政部门负责对基层医疗卫生机构实施日常监督与管理,疾病预防控制中心、妇幼保健院(所、站)、专科疾病防治院(所)等预防保健机构负责对基层医疗卫生机构所承担的公共卫生服务工作进行业务评价与指导。

截至 2021 年末,中国基层医疗卫生机构中,社区卫生服务中心(站)有 36 160 个(其中社区卫生服务中心 10 122 个,社区卫生服务站 26 038 个),乡镇卫生院 34 943 个,诊所和医务室 271 056 个,村卫生室 599 292 个;卫生人员中,社区卫生服务中心(站)卫生技术人员共59.2 万人,乡镇卫生院卫生技术人员 128.5 万人,村卫生室人员 136.3 万人。

中国基层医疗卫生机构诊疗量总体上呈现增长趋势。2021 年,中国基层医疗卫生机构诊疗量为 42.5 亿人次（占全国总诊量的 50.2%），与 2020 年相比增加了 1.3 亿人次；基层医疗卫生机构住院量为 3 592 万人次（占总住院量的 14.5%），与 2020 年相比减少了 115 万人次。

目前，中国基层医疗服务在人才队伍建设方面仍然任重道远，卫生技术人员数量不足、素质不高、工作不稳定等问题仍是制约基层医疗卫生机构进一步改善服务和提高水平的"瓶颈"问题。为了强化基层医疗服务能力，中国各地区正在积极推进农村卫生人员在职在岗培训，实施农村卫生人员培训规划和订单定向医学生免费培养项目；在城市大力开展社区卫生人员岗位培训，实施社区卫生人员培训项目和以全科医生为重点的基层医疗卫生队伍建设规划；在体系建设上，完善以社区卫生服务为基础的城市医疗卫生服务体系，逐步推进落实社区首诊、分级诊疗和双向转诊制度。

3.2.3　二、三级医院提供的医疗服务

中国的二级医院包括一般市、县医院及直辖市的区级医院，以及具有一定规模的工矿、企事业单位的职工医院。三级医院包括全国、省、市直属的市级大医院，以及医学院校的附属医院。截至 2021 年末，中国有三级医院 3 275 个，二级医院 10 848 个。中国二、三级医院按照提供服务类别的不同分为综合医院、中医医院、中西医结合医院、民族医医院、专科医院和护理院。综合医院一般设有内科、外科、妇产科、儿科、耳鼻喉科、眼科、皮肤科、中医科等专科，还设有检验科、影像科等医技部门。中医医院、中西医结合医院和民族医医院主要提供与中医和民族医有关的医疗服务。专科医院是为诊治各类专科疾病而设置的医院，如妇产科医院、传染病医院、肿瘤医院、口腔医院、职业病医院等。而护理院是为患者提供长期医疗护理、康复促进、临终关怀等服务的医疗机构。

中国于 2009 年启动新医改，根据相关文件，政府鼓励和引导社会资本办医，鼓励医疗卫生技术人员在公立医院与民营医院之间自由流动执业。近年来，中国民营医院数量不断增加。2021 年，中国公立医院占医院总量的 32.3%，而民营医院占 67.7%。

2021 年中国总诊疗量中，医院 38.8 亿人次（占 45.8%），基层医疗卫生机构 42.5 亿人次（占 50.2%），其他医疗卫生机构 3.4 亿人次（占 4%）。2021 年，中国医院病床使用率为 74.6%，其中公立医院为 80.3%。2021 年，中国医院出院者平均住院日为 9.2 日（其中公立医院 9.0 日），与上年比减少 0.3 日（其中公立医院减少 0.3 日）。2005 年以来，中国一些大型综合医院开始开设日间病房，为患者提供无须住院的日间急诊手术和日间病床服务。目前，日间照护服务在中国还处在发展阶段。

在过去一段时间里，医疗费用高和服务质量参差不齐的问题在中国部分二、三级医院中较为突出。为改善这一局面，2010 年，中国开始启动城市公立医院综合改革试点，力求在完善服务体系、创新体制机制、加强内部管理、加快形成多元化办医格局等方面实现突破。2012 年，中国全面启动县级公立医院综合改革试点工作，并探索公立医院补偿机制等方面的改革方法。

3.2.4　二、三级医院提供的医疗服务与基层医疗服务间的关系

为了引导一般性诊疗工作在基层开展及促进医疗资源合理配置，中国在 2006 年出台了

双向转诊制度,鼓励患者首选基层医疗卫生机构就诊,必要的时候由基层医疗卫生机构负责将患者转到二、三级医院就诊,待患者病情稳定后再由这些医院将患者下转到基层医疗卫生机构进行康复治疗等后续治疗。2009年新医改启动以来,中国开始探索建立二、三级医院与城乡基层医疗卫生机构的分工协作机制,二、三级医院负责在技术、人员和管理等方面带动基层医疗卫生机构的发展。为了实现这一目标,中国开始探索医疗联合体(简称"医联体")建设,以推动分级诊疗格局的形成。

3.2.5　中医服务和民族医医疗服务

中国大部分综合性医疗机构和基层医疗卫生机构都设有中医科,提供以草药、针灸、按摩等传统疗法为主的中医服务。这些服务都不同程度地被纳入城镇职工基本医疗保险、城镇居民基本医疗保险和新农合的补偿范围内。截至2021年,中国中医类医疗卫生机构总数77 336个,其中中医类医院5 715个,中医类门诊部、诊所71 583个,中医类研究机构38个。除此之外,还有大量的私人传统医疗诊所和个体行医者提供中医服务。全国中医药卫生人员总数达88.4万人,其中中医类别执业(助理)医师73.2万人、中药师(士)13.6万人。全国中医类医疗卫生机构总诊疗人次12亿人次,中医类医疗卫生机构出院人次3 800.2万人次。

《中华人民共和国中医药条例》规定,开办中医医疗机构,应当符合国务院卫生行政部门制定的中医医疗机构设置标准和当地区域卫生规划,并按照《医疗机构管理条例》的规定办理审批手续,取得医疗机构执业许可证。中医从业人员,应当依照有关卫生管理的法律、行政法规、部门规章的规定通过资格考试,并经注册取得执业证书后,方可从事中医服务活动。

截至2015年底,中国有中医类医院3 966个,其中民族医医院253个、中西医结合医院446个;中医类别执业(助理)医师45.2万人(含民族医医师、中西医结合医师);中医类门诊部、诊所42 528个,其中民族医门诊部、诊所550个,中西医结合门诊部、诊所7 706个。2015年,全国中医类医疗卫生机构总诊疗人次达9.1亿人次,中医类医疗卫生机构出院人次2 691.5万人次。

根据《"十四五"中医药发展规划》,中国将建设优质高效中医药服务体系,提升中医药健康服务能力,建设高素质中医药人才队伍,建设高水平中医药传承保护与科技创新体系,推动中药产业高质量发展,发展中医药健康服务业,推动中医药文化繁荣发展,加快中医药开放发展,深化中医药领域改革,强化中医药发展支撑保障。

除传统的中医疗法外,中国还存在大量的少数民族传统疗法,研究这一领域的学科被称为"民族医学"。部分民族医学疗法与传统中医学相似,如草药、拔罐、针灸等。此外,两者都有其特有的疗法。中国的民族医学有藏医、蒙医、苗医等数十种类别。截至2019年,中国共有中西医结合医院699个、民族医医院312个。民族医疗服务除在民族医医院内开展外,更多地在寺院(如在藏传佛教寺院中设立的教育和行医机构叫曼巴扎仓)、诊所等场所,或以个体行医的形式开展。民族医学往往以口传身授甚至祖传等较为保守的方式来进行教学,保留了更多自成体系的独特传统疗法和技能,但其应用的广泛程度与中医学不可同日而语。通常,对民族医师的管理方式参照对中医医师的方式进行。

3.3   中国医疗服务体系的高质量发展

3.3.1   医联体

建设医联体是中国推进分级诊疗制度的重大举措。2017 年，《国务院办公厅关于推进医疗联合体建设和发展的指导意见》印发，明确在县域主要组建医疗共同体，加强医疗卫生与养老服务相结合，为患者提供一体化、便利化的疾病诊疗—康复—长期护理连续性服务。

一方面，通过调整优化医疗资源布局，医联体可以有效将优质资源和技术服务逐级下沉到基层，并通过专家下沉、对口帮扶、远程医疗等各种形式和手段，提升基层医疗服务能力；另一方面，作为医疗资源上下贯通、双向转诊的重要渠道，医联体可以逐步破除行政区划、财政投入、医保支付、人事管理等方面的壁垒和障碍，促进优质医疗资源上下贯通。

在医联体的组织模式方面，中国提出了四种成熟的模式。一是在城市主要组建医疗集团，主要是以三级公立医院为核心，联合社区卫生服务机构、护理院、康复中心等各类医疗机构，提供各种类型的服务，以满足患者在不同阶段的健康、医疗和康复需求。二是在县域主要组建医疗共同体，重点探索以县医院为龙头、乡镇卫生院为枢纽、村卫生室为基础的县乡一体化管理。对人、财、物以及防、保、康等进行高度的统筹管理和密切分工合作，构建三级联动的县级医疗服务体系。三是针对各种专科疾病，鼓励具有优势专科医疗资源的医疗机构牵头，开展跨区域的医疗联盟。同时，充分发挥国家在专科医疗方面的资源优势，以专科协作为纽带，提升基层对专科疾病的治疗水平并畅通双向转诊的渠道。四是在边远贫困地区发展远程医疗协作网，充分利用远程医疗、远程教学、远程培训等现代化高科技手段，延伸上级医疗机构的医疗技术和服务能力，扩大服务半径，满足一些基层地区，特别是偏远、贫困地区的医疗需求。

当前，中国医联体建设全面推开，所有三级公立医院均参与医联体建设，双向转诊成效初步显现，区域医疗资源实现共享，医疗服务能力明显提升。截至 2019 年，全国 118 个城市规划建设了 607 个城市医联体网格，在 567 个县（市、区）推进了县域医疗共同体建设试点。截至 2020 年底，全国医疗卫生机构双向转诊患者 2 507.5 万例次。"十三五"期间下转患者人次数逐年增长，年均增长率达 38.4%。2020 年，上转患者人次数首次出现下降，"上转容易、下转难"问题逐渐缓解。全国第六次卫生服务统计调查数据显示，双向转诊患者中 46.9% 为医联体内转诊，高于其他转诊方式。

3.3.2   基层医疗卫生机构改革

中国基层医疗卫生机构发展面临着许多挑战。过度依赖药品收入影响了其提供合理的卫生服务。建立合理的补偿机制和增加政府投入是中国基层医疗卫生机构改革的重点。此外，基层医疗卫生机构需要加强人力资源和其他条件的建设。

基层医疗卫生体系建设。2009—2011 年，改革的主要目标是完善县乡村三级医疗卫生服务网络；重点支持城乡基层医疗卫生机构，包括县乡村卫生机构和城镇社区卫生机构建设；支持边远地区村卫生室和困难地区城市社区卫生服务中心建设。2012 年后，中国继续强化对乡镇卫生院的建设,并加强基层医疗卫生机构中医药服务能力建设。

基层医疗卫生队伍建设。2009—2011 年,中国开始实施免费为农村基层医疗卫生机构定向培养卫生人员的计划。2011 年,《国务院关于建立全科医生制度的指导意见》出台,明确了逐步建立统一规范的全科医生培养制度、改革全科医生执业方式等政策措施。2012 年医改提出加强以全科医生为重点的基层人才队伍建设,继续为中西部乡镇卫生院和基层部队定向免费培养医学生。对基层医疗卫生机构人员进行在岗培训是提高卫生人员能力的重要内容。新医改以来,中国各级政府纷纷投入资金组织各种形式的在岗培训。此外,中国还实施了城市医院对口支援农村医院的政策,即要求每个城市三级医院与 3 个左右的县级医院建立长期技术援助关系,以提升县级医院服务能力。

基层医疗卫生机构补偿机制建设。明确政府补助、服务收费(包括医疗保险收费和公共卫生服务补偿)等作为基层医疗卫生机构主要补偿方式。最重要的是,药品加成不再是基层医疗卫生机构主要的补偿渠道。对政府负责举办的乡镇卫生院、城市社区卫生服务中心(站)按国家规定核定的基本建设、设备购置、人员经费及所承担公共卫生服务的业务经费,采取项目补助或者购买服务等方式给予补偿;对非政府举办的基层医疗卫生机构提供的公共卫生服务,采取政府或者基本医疗保险购买服务的方式给予补偿;明确财政对村卫生室实施基本药物制度的补偿。

基层医疗卫生机构运行机制建设。实施的改革措施包括建立双向转诊制度、基层首诊制度、基层医疗卫生机构和人员绩效考核机制,以及基层医疗卫生机构收入分配机制等。2012 年,中国明确提出基层医疗卫生机构人员收入分配以服务数量和质量为基础、向核心和骨干卫生技术人员倾斜等机制。

3.3.3　未来发展

中国自 2009 年新医改实施以来,在基层医疗卫生机构服务能力提升和公立医疗卫生机构改革等方面取得了显著进展。同时,由于其复杂性和系统性,卫生改革也面临着许多挑战,需要长期坚持。针对出现的新问题要不断完善改革内容,并有效推进改革政策和措施的落实。

中国公立医院改革需持续深化,重点在于解决医疗服务体系问题,从体系建设和发展的角度推动改革。同时,发展健康产业、实现多元化办医格局,也是未来的重要发展方向。面对持续的健康和人口转型问题,中国需要一个更加有效的医疗服务体系来应对慢性病的挑战,并满足不断增长的健康需要。中国医疗服务体系改革的重点主要包括以下四个方面:

第一,深化医药卫生体制改革,包括深化基层医疗卫生机构综合改革,健全网络化城乡基层医疗卫生服务运行机制;完善合理分级诊疗模式,建立社区医生和居民契约服务关系;充分利用信息化手段,促进优质医疗资源纵向流动;加强区域公共卫生服务资源整合等。主要任务是建立功能清晰、定位准确、相互协作的医疗卫生服务体系,发挥不同功能和级别医疗卫生机构的作用。这需要整合医疗卫生服务体系,包括医疗和公共卫生服务机构的整合以及区域内医疗卫生机构的制度衔接和纵向整合,以提高整个体系的能力,并应对主要健康挑战。

第二,加快公立医院改革,包括创新体制机制、调动医务人员积极性等,其中理顺医药价格、建立科学补偿机制是重点。县级公立医院改革是未来几年的重点工作,改革内容主要包括坚持公益性,履行政府办医职责;深化分配制度改革,充分调动医务人员积极性;建立现代医院管理制度,加强内部管理;推进支付制度改革;优化资源配置,加强行业监管等。

　　第三,加强医疗卫生人才队伍建设和医疗卫生信息化建设。医疗卫生人才队伍的质量、结构和分布一直是制约中国医疗卫生服务能力提升的最重要因素之一。中国已建立住院医师规范化培训制度、全科医师培养制度,并推进稳定乡村医生队伍政策。在医疗卫生信息化建设方面,中国正在研究建立全国统一的电子健康档案、电子病历、药品器械、医疗服务、医疗保险等信息标准体系,并推进医疗卫生信息技术标准化建设。

　　第四,鼓励社会办医,优先支持社会力量举办非营利性医疗卫生机构,包括在区域卫生规划和医疗卫生机构设置规划中给社会办医留有合理发展空间,建立以非营利性医疗卫生机构为主体、营利性医疗卫生机构为补充的社会办医体系,完善社会办医税收等方面的优惠政策措施,推动完善医师多点执业政策,保证非公立医疗卫生机构办医质量等。

4 中国公共卫生管理体系和公共卫生服务体系

中国已经建立了较完善的公共卫生管理体系和公共卫生服务体系。在公共卫生管理方面,各级卫生健康委、国家疾病预防控制局以及各级疾病预防控制中心负责制定和落实公共卫生事业发展规划和公共卫生政策。在公共卫生服务方面,服务内容不断充实和完善,公共卫生服务网络不断健全,从各级疾病预防控制中心到社区卫生服务中心(站)、乡镇卫生院和村卫生室等机构负责为城乡居民提供传染病防控、慢性病防治、健康教育、食品安全监测和监督、劳动场所卫生监测、突发公共卫生事件处理、妇女儿童保健等公共卫生服务。

2003 年 SARS 疫情暴发以来,中国政府增加了对公共卫生机构和公共卫生服务项目的财政支持。近几年,中国政府又进一步对公共卫生管理体系和机构职能进行了调整,这极大地促进了中国公共卫生服务体系的完善。

4.1 中国公共卫生管理体系

中国公共卫生管理体系主要由国家卫生健康委、国家疾病预防控制局和中国疾病预防控制中心等国家级卫生管理机构,以及省、市、县各级上述机构构成,它们分别承担不同的管理职责。卫生健康委总体负责公共卫生行政管理,疾病预防控制局负责贯彻落实疾病预防控制政策和决策部署,疾病预防控制中心负责技术支持和工作执行。从国家层面到省、市、县层面,各级规划管理和政策制定机构的职能逐步具体化,各项决策部署逐步可操作化。地方公共卫生政策有时是国家政策的有力补充。

4.1.1 国家卫生健康委

国家卫生健康委主要负责组织拟订国民健康政策,拟订卫生健康事业发展法律法规草案、政策、规划,制定部门规章和标准并组织实施,以及协调推进深化医药卫生体制改革,研究提出深化医药卫生体制改革重大方针、政策、措施的建议等工作。2022 年,中共中央办公厅、国务院办公厅将国家卫生健康委的部分职责,如制定并组织落实传染病预防控制规划、国家免疫规划以及严重危害人民健康公共卫生问题的干预措施等划入国家疾病预防控制局。

目前国家卫生健康委下设的医疗应急司、基层卫生健康司、食品安全标准与监测评估司、妇幼健康司、职业健康司等机构,主要负责公共卫生相关服务内容的行政管理。具体来说,医疗应急司负责组织协调传染病疫情应对工作,承担医疗卫生应急体系建设,组织指导各类突发公共事件的医疗救治和紧急医学救援工作,拟订医疗安全、医疗监督、采供血机构管理及行风建设等行业管理政策、标准并组织实施,以及拟订重大疾病、慢性病防控管理政策规范并监督实施。基层卫生健康司下设的基本公共卫生处负责对基层公共卫生进行相应的行政管理。食品安全标准与监测评估司负责组织拟订食品安全国家标准,开展食品安全风险监测、评估和交流等工作。妇幼健康司负责拟订妇幼卫生健康政策、标准和规范,推进妇幼健康服务体系建设等工作。职业健康司负责拟订职业卫生、放射卫生相关政策、标准并组织实施等工作。

4.1.2　国家疾病预防控制局

2022年1月,根据国家卫生健康委职能配置调整方案,中国撤销了国家卫生健康委疾病预防控制局,并成立了国家疾病预防控制局。新成立的国家疾病预防控制局是由国家卫生健康委管理的国家局,为副部级。

国家疾病预防控制局的主要职责包括组织拟订传染病预防控制及公共卫生监督的法律法规草案、政策、规划、标准,领导地方各级疾病预防控制机构业务工作,制定并组织落实国家免疫规划以及严重危害人民健康公共卫生问题的干预措施,统筹规划并监督管理传染病医疗机构及其他医疗机构疾病预防控制工作,规划指导传染病疫情监测预警体系建设,负责传染病疫情应对相关工作,协同指导疾病预防控制科研体系建设,负责传染病防治、环境卫生、学校卫生、公共场所卫生、饮用水卫生监督管理等。目前,中国各省也在积极组建省级疾病预防控制局。

4.1.3　中国疾病预防控制中心

在中国,疾病预防控制中心分为国家级、省级、设区的市级和县级四级,各级之间工作重点有一定差异。中国疾病预防控制中心为国家级,是国家疾病预防控制局直属事业单位。中国疾病预防控制中心的主要职责包括开展疾病预防控制、突发公共卫生事件应急、环境与职业健康、营养健康、老龄健康、妇幼健康、放射卫生和学校卫生等工作;组织制定国家公共卫生技术方案和指南,承担公共卫生相关卫生标准综合管理工作;开展传染病、慢性病、职业病、地方病、突发公共卫生事件和疑似预防接种异常反应监测及国民健康状况监测与评价,开展重大公共卫生问题的调查与危害风险评估;开展疾病预防控制、突发公共卫生事件应急、公众健康关键科学研究和技术开发;指导地方实施国家疾病预防控制规划和项目,开展对地方疾病预防控制机构的业务指导,参与专业技术考核和评价相关工作等。

4.1.4　其他公共卫生管理及业务指导机构

4.1.4.1　中国疾病预防控制中心精神卫生中心

中国疾病预防控制中心精神卫生中心是全国精神卫生业务技术中心。在中国疾病预防控制中心的业务领导下,受中国疾病预防控制中心委托,其主要承担以下职责:为国家制定与精神障碍预防控制相关的法律、法规、规章、政策、标准、技术规范和规划等提供科学依据和决策咨询;指导建立国家精神障碍监测系统,对常见精神障碍的发生、分布和发展规律进行流行病学监测,建立数据库,定期分析监测结果;组织制定常见精神疾病的防治方案,对方案实施进行质量监控和效果评估;承担精神障碍防治信息的报告、管理和预测、预报;负责精神卫生工作人员的业务指导与技术培训,承担卫生工作中与精神障碍预防控制有关的技术指导;开展与精神卫生相关的应用性科学研究,引进、开发和推广新技术、新方法等。

4.1.4.2　中国疾病预防控制中心妇幼保健中心

中国疾病预防控制中心妇幼保健中心是全国性妇幼保健业务技术指导中心。其主要职责包括开展妇幼健康工作,为国家制定妇幼健康法律法规、政策、规划、项目等提供技术支撑和咨询建议;组织制定妇幼健康技术方案、指南和标准;开展妇幼健康相关领域科学研究,对妇女儿童健康状况及影响因素进行监测、评估、评价;承担妇幼健康信息化建设,负责相关数据的收集、管理和应用服务技术支持;开展地方妇幼健康工作业务指导,组织业务培训,推广新技术、新方法,参与妇幼健康服务专业技术考核和评价相关工作;开展妇幼健康教育、健康科普和健康促进相关工作;开展妇幼健康领域的研究生教育和继续教育;开展妇幼健康相关领域的国际交流与合作等。

4.1.4.3　中国健康教育中心

中国健康教育中心是国家卫生健康委直属事业单位,负责全国健康教育与卫生健康新闻宣传工作的技术指导,开展相关理论与实践的研究,承担全国健康教育与卫生健康新闻宣传大型活动的组织实施及信息管理、媒体联系、业务培训等有关技术和服务性工作。具体来说,其职责包括组织开展健康教育与健康促进、卫生健康宣传领域的理论、方法与策略的研究,为政府制定相关的法律、法规、部门规章和技术规范等提供技术咨询及政策建议;协助开展健康教育与健康促进、卫生健康宣传以及人口宣传教育活动的组织实施、业务培训和有关技术指导工作;协助开展国家卫生健康委新闻发布和重大宣传活动的组织协调工作,开展相关政策宣传;组织开展健康教育政策宣传和健康科普工作实用技术研究与推广,开发健康科普信息,开展健康科普活动和控烟履约政策研究及相关宣传工作,协助开展国家健康科普资源库和专家库建设和内容维护相关工作等。

4.1.4.4　采供血机构

中国的采供血机构分为血站和单采血浆站。血站包括一般血站和特殊血站,是不以营利为目的,采集、提供临床用血的公益性卫生机构。一般血站分为血液中心、中心血站和中心血库。特殊血站包括脐带血造血干细胞库等血库。采供血机构设置规划应与当地经济发展状况、人口、医疗资源和区域医疗机构设置规划相适应。根据《中国卫生健康统计年鉴(2022)》,2021年中国共有采供血机构628个,其中城市365个、农村263个。血液中心、中心血站和中心血库由地方人民政府设立,特殊血站根据全国的规划设置在省级行政区域范围内。

血液中心由省、自治区人民政府所在地的城市和直辖市规划设置。中心血站由设区的市级人民政府所在地的城市规划设置。中心血库设置在中心血站服务覆盖不到的县级综合医院内。三者的主要职责均包括按照省级人民政府卫生行政部门的要求,在规定范围内开展无偿献血者的招募、血液的采集与制备、临床用血供应以及医疗用血业务指导等工作。

4.1.4.5　专科疾病防治机构

专科疾病包括各类传染病、职业病、精神病、皮肤病与性病等。从机构的级别设置上划分,中国专科疾病防治机构包括专科疾病防治院、专科疾病防治所、专科疾病防治站。从防治疾病的类型上划分,中国专科疾病防治机构包括传染病防治机构、结核病防治机构、职业病防治机构、口腔病防治机构、精神病防治机构、皮肤病与性病防治机构、地方病防治机构、药物戒毒所等。

4.2　中国公共卫生服务体系

中国公共卫生服务体系由专业公共卫生服务网络和医疗卫生机构提供的公共卫生服务组成（图 4-1）。专业公共卫生服务网络包括疾病预防控制、健康教育、妇幼保健、精神卫生、应急救治、采供血、卫生监督和专业防治等专业公共卫生服务，其中专业防治服务的具体内容包括传染病防治、口腔病防治、皮肤病与性病防治、结核病防治、职业病防治、地方病防治、血吸虫病防治等。在医疗服务体系中，具有"医防一体"功能的基层医疗卫生机构（在城市即社区卫生服务机构，在农村则是乡镇卫生院、村卫生室）既为辖区居民提供基本医疗服务，同时也提供基本公共卫生服务。此外，医院也提供公共卫生服务，比如传染病医院、精神病医院等专科医院，以及综合医院的公共卫生相关科室（如传染病科、发热门诊等）。

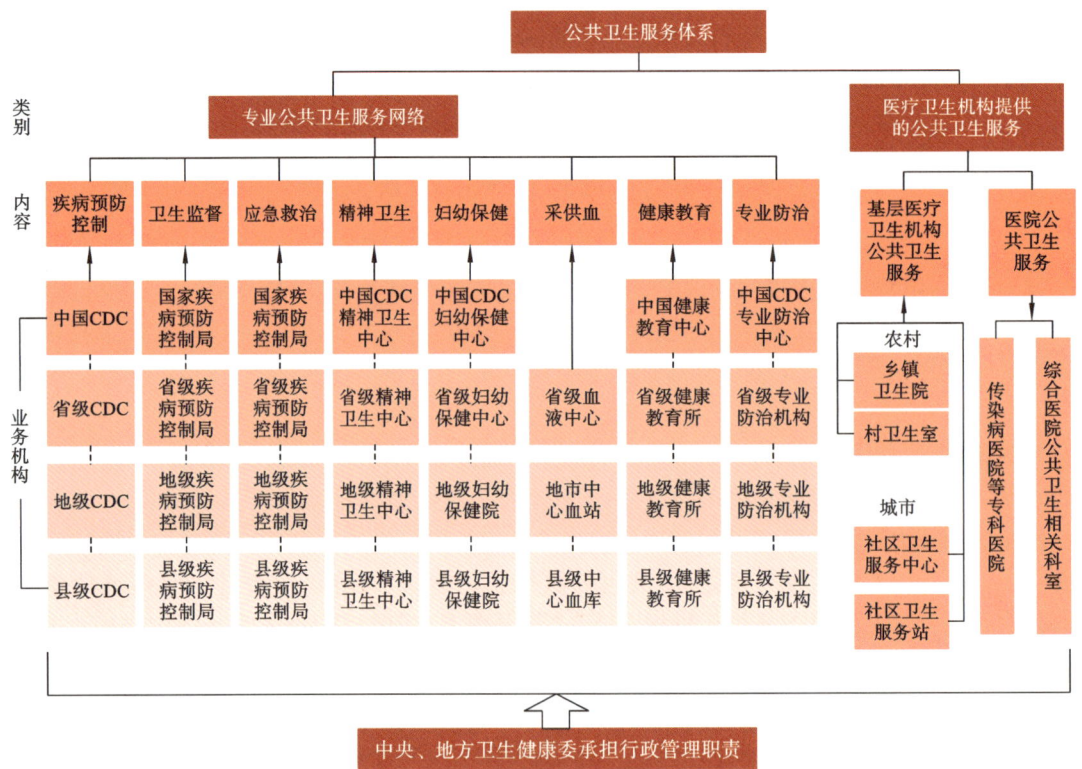

图 4-1　中国公共卫生服务体系

注：CDC 为 Center for Disease Control and Prevention（疾病预防控制中心）的缩写

数据来源：参考《转型中的中国卫生体系》（孟庆跃等，2015），增加了 2015 年后机构变更相关内容

在中国，公共卫生服务的具体内容包括传染病防治、疫情监测和卫生应急网络建设、妇幼卫生监测与干预、慢性病防治、地方病防治、职业病防治、环境与健康监测、健康教育和健康促进等。以下是对公共卫生服务具体内容的介绍。

4.2.1　基本公共卫生服务

中国自 2009 年启动基本公共卫生服务均等化改革,向全体居民免费提供基本公共卫生服务,并持续推动基本公共卫生服务覆盖全体居民。基本公共卫生服务明确为中央与地方共同财政事权,由中央和地方财政共同承担支出责任。2022 年,中国基本公共卫生服务经费人均财政补助标准达到了 84 元。中国的基本公共卫生服务面向社区层面,具体公共卫生服务项目的提供由覆盖城乡的社区服务网络完成。截至 2021 年底,年内在基层医疗卫生机构接受健康管理的 65 岁及以上老年人达 11 941.2 万人,接受健康管理的高血压患者达 10 938.4 万人,接受健康管理的 2 型糖尿病患者达 3 571.3 万人,以乡镇街道为单位的预防接种率一直保持在 95% 以上,基本公共卫生服务项目已经实现人口全覆盖。

目前中国国家基本公共卫生服务项目共包含 28 项,近年来部分项目变化情况见表 4-1。基本公共卫生服务主要通过社区卫生服务中心(站)、乡镇卫生院、村卫生室等城乡基层医疗卫生机构免费为全体居民提供。中国国家基本公共卫生服务项目内容每年都会有相应的变化,由国家卫生健康委会同国家中医药管理局、国家疾病预防控制局、财政部等部门根据经济社会发展情况、公共卫生服务需要和财政承受能力等因素适时调整。

表 4-1　中国国家基本公共卫生服务项目 2009—2022 年的变化情况

年份	项目序号或变动情况	项目名称
2009	1	城乡居民健康档案管理
	2	健康教育
	3	0～36 个月儿童健康管理
	4	孕产妇健康管理
	5	老年人健康管理
	6	预防接种
	7	传染病报告和处理
	8	高血压患者健康管理
	9	2 型糖尿病患者健康管理
	10	重性精神疾病患者管理
2011	项目新增	卫生监督协管
	项目更名	"传染病报告和处理"更名为"传染病及突发公共卫生事件报告和处理"
	项目更名	"0～36 个月儿童健康管理"更名为"0～6 岁儿童健康管理"
2013	项目合并	项目 8、项目 9 合并为"慢性病患者健康管理"
	项目新增	中医药健康管理
	项目更名	"城乡居民健康档案管理"更名为"建立居民健康档案"
	项目更名	"0～6 岁儿童健康管理"更名为"儿童健康管理"
2015	项目新增	结核病患者健康管理

续表

年份	项目序号或变动情况	项目名称
2017	项目新增	免费提供避孕药具
	项目新增	健康素养促进行动
2018	项目取消	免费提供避孕药具
	项目取消	健康素养促进行动
2019	除上述 12 项外新增 19 项不限于基层医疗卫生机构实施的项目(原属重大公共卫生和计划生育项目)	地方病防治,职业病防治,重大疾病与健康危害因素监测,人禽流感、SARS 防控项目,鼠疫防治项目,国家卫生应急队伍运维保障,农村妇女"两癌"检查项目,基本避孕服务项目,贫困地区儿童营养改善项目,贫困地区新生儿疾病筛查项目,增补叶酸预防神经管缺陷项目,国家免费孕前优生健康检查项目,地中海贫血防控项目,食品安全标准跟踪评价项目,健康素养促进项目,国家随机监督抽查项目,老年健康与医养结合服务,人口监测项目,卫生健康项目
2022	取消 2019 年新增的 19 项服务项目中的 3 项	根据中国财政部等 5 部委联合印发的《关于修订基本公共卫生服务等 5 项补助资金管理办法的通知》,重大疾病与健康危害因素监测、国家随机监督抽查项目以及人口监测项目不再列入基本公共卫生服务

数据来源:国家卫生健康委

4.2.2 传染病防治

《中华人民共和国传染病防治法》规定对传染病实行分类管理。法定传染病分为甲、乙、丙三类,共 40 种,其中甲类 2 种(鼠疫、霍乱)、乙类 27 种、丙类 11 种。中国坚持在政府统一领导下,实行预防为主的传染病防治政策。各级疾病预防控制机构承担具体的传染病疫情监测、流行病学调查和疫情报告等工作。公立和民营医疗卫生机构承担责任范围内的传染病疫情报告和临床治疗工作。

目前,威胁中国居民健康的传染病主要有肺结核、艾滋病和病毒性肝炎等。2021 年,全国共报告法定传染病发病 623 万例,死亡 22 198 人;报告发病率为 442.16/10 万,报告死亡率为 1.57/10 万;报告死亡数居前 5 位的分别是艾滋病、肺结核、病毒性肝炎、狂犬病和流行性出血热,占甲、乙类传染病报告死亡总数的 99.7%。自 2007 年中国实施扩大国家免疫规划项目以来,中国免疫规划疫苗种类由 6 种扩大到 14 种,可预防 15 种传染病。中国已经消灭了天花,实现了无脊髓灰质炎目标,并消除了新生儿破伤风。

4.2.3 疫情监测和卫生应急网络建设

2003 年 SARS 疫情暴发后,中国逐步建立了全球规模最大的传染病疫情和突发公共卫生事件网络直报系统,实现了包括乡镇卫生院在内的各级各类医疗卫生机构可直接向国家报告传染病疫情和突发公共卫生事件的目标,平均报告时间由之前的 5 天缩短至 4 小时以内。这套系统覆盖中国16.8万个各类医疗卫生机构,用户数达35万,使得全国法定传染病报告及时率达到99%以上。多年来,该系统的有效运行降低了传染病的漏报率,显著提高了传染病报告的及时性。目前,中国100%的县级以上疾病预防控制机构、98%的县级以上医疗卫生机构和94%的基层医疗卫生机构实现了法定传染病实时网络直报。近来,该系统进一步提高了中国卫生统计工作的效率,为疾病感染者的密接追踪、流调溯源、疫情研判、大数据比对分析等提供了有力的数据支撑。

4.2.4　妇幼卫生监测与干预

中国已经建立了较完善的妇幼卫生保健网络。2021年末,中国共有妇幼保健机构3 032个,其中省级26个、地(市)级377个、县(区、县级市)级2 554个;妇幼保健机构卫生技术人员达到45.4万人。在妇幼卫生信息化建设方面,中国先后建立了妇幼卫生年报信息系统、妇幼卫生监测信息系统和妇幼保健机构监测信息系统。中国积极推动住院分娩,保障母婴安全。2021年,中国孕产妇产前检查率达97.6%,产后访视率达96%,住院分娩率为99.9%(市100%,县99.9%),基本实现全部住院分娩;3岁以下儿童系统管理率达92.8%。中国通过开展筛查工作,防治妇女常见病。截至2020年,中国"两癌"筛查工作已经覆盖了全国近2 600个县(市、区),累计开展免费筛查近2亿人次,其中宫颈癌筛查1.3亿人次、乳腺癌筛查6 400万人次。2023年,中国发布了《加速消除宫颈癌行动计划(2023—2030年)》,以积极响应世界卫生组织提出的"加速消除宫颈癌全球战略",加快中国宫颈癌消除进程,保护和增进广大妇女健康。该行动计划中提出如下目标:到2025年,试点推广适龄女孩HPV(人乳头瘤病毒)疫苗接种服务,适龄妇女宫颈癌筛查率达到50%,宫颈癌及癌前病变患者治疗率达到90%。到2030年,持续推进适龄女孩HPV疫苗接种试点工作,适龄妇女宫颈癌筛查率达到70%,宫颈癌及癌前病变患者治疗率达到90%。

近年来,中国生殖健康和出生缺陷综合防治工作进一步加强。中国积极推进婚前保健服务,2018年共有1 020万名新婚夫妇接受了婚前医学检查,婚检率达到61.1%;实施国家孕前优生健康检查项目,2010—2018年共为8 349万名计划怀孕夫妇提供免费检查;实施增补叶酸预防神经管缺陷项目,2009—2018年免费为近1.02亿生育妇女补服了叶酸;逐步扩大产前筛查和产前诊断覆盖面,2018年唐氏综合征产前血清学筛查率达61.1%;加强地中海贫血防控,截至2018年在南方10个省份为164.5万对夫妇提供免费筛查,有效减少了重型地中海贫血患儿出生;稳步扩大新生儿疾病筛查覆盖面,2017年全国新生儿遗传代谢病筛查率达97.5%,2018年启动新生儿先天性心脏病筛查。

4.2.5　慢性病防治

中国常见慢性病主要有心脑血管疾病、糖尿病、恶性肿瘤、慢性呼吸系统疾病等。为了做好慢性病预防控制工作,遏制慢性病导致的过早死亡率快速上升的势头,中国自2012年起开始制定国家防治慢性病规划。中国在《中国防治慢性病中长期规划(2017—2025年)》中提出如下目标:到2020年,慢性病防控环境显著改善,降低慢性病过早死亡率,力争30~70岁人群心脑血管疾病、癌症、慢性呼吸系统疾病和糖尿病过早死亡率较2015年降低10%。到2025年,慢性病危险因素得到有效控制,实现全人群全生命周期健康管理,力争30~70岁人群心脑血管疾病、癌症、慢性呼吸系统疾病和糖尿病过早死亡率较2015年降低

20%。逐步提高居民健康期望寿命,有效控制慢性病疾病负担。

为了实现上述目标,中国提出,建立疾病预防控制机构、医院、专科疾病防治机构和基层医疗卫生机构在慢性病防治中的分工负责和分级管理机制,明确职责和任务。疾病预防控制机构和专科疾病防治机构协助卫生行政部门做好慢性病及相关疾病防控规划和方案的制定和实施,提供业务指导和技术管理;医院开展慢性病相关信息登记报告,提供慢性病危重急症患者的诊疗、康复服务,为基层医疗卫生机构开展慢性病诊疗、康复服务提供技术指导,建立和基层医疗卫生机构之间的双向转诊机制;基层医疗卫生机构负责相关慢性病防控措施的执行与落实。此外,中国明确,健康教育机构负责研究慢性病健康教育策略方法,传播慢性病防治核心信息,并指导其他机构开展慢性病健康教育活动;妇幼保健机构负责提供与妇女儿童有关的慢性病预防咨询指导。

目前,中国防治慢性病的一项重要工作就是抓好慢性病综合防控示范区建设,推动慢性病综合防控示范区创新发展。中国于 2010 年启动慢性病综合防控示范区工作。在示范区内,通过开展社区调查诊断,明确本地区主要健康问题和危险因素,应用适宜技术,发展适合当地的慢性病防控策略、措施和长效管理模式。关于推动慢性病综合防控示范区创新发展,《中国防治慢性病中长期规划(2017—2025 年)》中提出如下措施:以国家慢性病综合防控示范区建设为抓手,培育适合不同地区特点的慢性病综合防控模式。示范区建设要紧密结合卫生城镇创建和健康城镇建设要求,与分级诊疗、家庭医生签约服务相融合,全面提升示范区建设质量,在强化政府主体责任、落实各部门工作职责、提供全人群全生命周期慢性病防治管理服务等方面发挥示范引领作用,带动区域慢性病防治管理水平整体提升。

4.2.6 地方病防治

地方病是由生物地球化学因素、生产生活方式等原因导致的呈地方性发生的疾病,多发生在老、少、边、穷地区,是病区群众因病致贫、因病返贫的重要原因。地方病防治是一项十分复杂的社会系统工程,也是一项重大民生工程。在中国,各级疾病预防控制机构和地方病防治专业机构负责地方病监测、健康教育、防控措施制定及效果评估等工作,并协调有关部门落实普及碘盐、改水等防控措施。中国曾是地方病流行较为严重的国家。全国都不同程度上存在地方病危害,主要有碘缺乏病、水源性高碘甲状腺肿、地方性氟中毒、地方性砷中毒、大骨节病和克山病等。但经过多年努力,目前大多数地区的地方病危害得到了有效控制或消除。通过 2018 年启动的地方病防治专项三年攻坚行动,中国保持持续消除碘缺乏危害,基本消除燃煤污染型氟砷中毒、大骨节病和克山病危害,有效控制饮水型氟砷中毒、饮茶型地氟病和水源性高碘危害,防治目标与脱贫攻坚任务同步完成,地方病防治取得历史性成就。然而,地方病为生物地球化学性疾病,必须长期巩固、维持防治措施,才能防止其卷土重来。因此未来,中国将在地方病防治专项三年攻坚行动基础上,进一步提高全国地方病综合防治能力,健全长效预防与救治管理机制,解决目前地方病防治中存在的重点和难点问题,持续巩固提升防治成果,保护人民群众身体健康。

4.2.7 职业病防治

职业健康是健康中国建设的重要基础和组成部分,事关广大劳动者健康福祉与经济发展和社会稳定大局。中国目前在保障劳动者健康方面面临新的形势和要求:一是新旧职业病危害日益交织叠加,职业病和工作相关疾病防控难度加大等;二是职业健康管理和服务人群、领域不断扩展,劳动者日益增长的职业健康需求与职业健康工作发展不平衡不充分的矛盾突出;三是职业病防治支撑服务和保障能力亟待加强,职业健康信息化建设滞后等;四是职业健康基础需要进一步夯实,部分地方政府监管责任和用人单位主体责任落实不到位等。

中国实行职业卫生监督制度。国务院安全生产监督管理部门、卫生行政部门、劳动保障行政部门依法负责全国职业病防治的监督管理工作。职业病的诊断和职业健康检查工作由经省级卫生行政部门批准的医疗卫生机构承担。一旦发生急性职业病危害事故,用人单位应立即采取应急救援和控制措施,并及时报告所在地卫生行政部门和有关部门。卫生行政部门负责组织医疗救治工作。职业病患者的诊疗、康复费用以及伤残和丧失劳动能力的职业病患者的社会保障按照用人单位参加的国家工伤保险的规定执行,如果用人单位没有参加工伤保险,患者的医疗和生活保障将由用人单位承担。

2021年,中国出台了《国家职业病防治规划(2021—2025年)》,规划提出如下目标:到2025年,职业健康治理体系更加完善,职业病危害状况明显好转,工作场所劳动条件显著改善,劳动用工和劳动工时管理进一步规范,尘肺病等重点职业病得到有效控制,职业健康服务能力和保障水平不断提升,全社会职业健康意识显著增强,劳动者健康水平进一步提高。

4.2.8　环境与健康监测

2007年,中国出台了《国家环境与健康行动计划(2007—2015)》,这是中国环境与健康领域的第一个纲领性文件。2022年,中国政府制定的《"十四五"环境健康工作规划》提出如下目标:到2025年,基本掌握全国重点地区高环境健康风险源分布特征,环境健康风险监测布局初步形成;进一步完善环境健康标准体系,研制一批环境健康风险评估技术规范和模型计算软件;在10～15个地区开展环境健康管理试点,环境健康管理实现多层次、多样化和特色化发展;打造专业化队伍,累计开展业务培训5万人次;营造全社会支持参与环境健康工作的良好氛围,全国居民环境健康素养水平达到20%以上。

4.2.9　健康教育和健康促进

中国已初步建立以健康教育专业机构为主导,以城乡基层医疗卫生机构为基础,包括其他医疗卫生机构和学校、企业、机关、事业单位等重点场所在内的健康教育体系。健康教育专业机构包括健康教育中心、健康教育所和健康教育站。中国健康教育中心负责全国健康教育与卫生健康新闻宣传工作的技术指导,开展相关理论与实践的研究,承担全国健康教育与卫生健康新闻宣传大型活动的组织实施及信息管理、媒体联系、业务培训等有关技术和服务性工作。地方上设立健康教育所或健康教育站,负责地方的健康教育具体业务工作。为了促进城乡居民健康,中国政府部门、社会团体和企业联合或独立开展了多项健康教育和健康促进活动,涉及烟草控制、妇幼健康、儿童营养、肝炎防治等方面。

中国已经建立了常规监测和健康体检相结合的人群健康监测方式。常规监测主要指基层医疗卫生机构开展的基本公共卫生服务中有关人群健康监测的常规性工作。这些监测工作主要由乡镇卫生院和社区卫生服务中心负责组织实施,村卫生室、社区卫生服务站分别在乡镇卫生院和社区卫生服务中心的业务管理下开展具体的健康监测工作。近年来,健康体检在中国得到了快速发展,健康体检主要由依附于医院的体检机构提供,另外一些独立于医院之外的专业体检机构也可提供健康体检服务。

此外，中国也开展了一些专项健康监测项目，如自1959年开始开展的中国居民营养与健康状况监测项目。近年来，中国居民死因监测、肿瘤随访登记、慢性病与营养监测等项目也相继开展，监测点覆盖面逐年扩大，各项工作不断规范，涵盖发病、患病、死亡和危险因素等信息的慢性病监测和信息管理平台正逐步形成。

案例（一）　血吸虫病防治案例

世界卫生组织资料显示，截至2021年，全球有78个国家报告存在血吸虫病传播，其中51个国家的传播程度为中度或高度，需要针对人群和社区进行大规模血吸虫病预防性化疗。2021年，全球至少有2.51亿人需要获得血吸虫病预防性治疗。血吸虫病是由裂体吸虫属血吸虫引起的一种慢性寄生虫病。血吸虫病防治项目是中国重大传染病防治项目之一。据统计，新中国成立初期，中国有血吸虫病患者1 160万人，受威胁人口在1亿人以上。经过半个多世纪的努力，至2004年末，全国血吸虫病患者数降至84.3万人（其中晚期血吸虫病患者2.8万人），宿主钉螺面积减少为原来的四分之一，感染人数和受威胁人数大大减少，中国血吸虫病防治工作取得了巨大成绩。这些成绩的获得与中国重视科学防治以及全民参与密不可分。中国的经验总结如下：

第一，统一领导，形成合力。新中国成立初期，毛泽东主席就提出了"全党动员，全民动员，消灭血吸虫病"的号召。在党的统一领导下，中国成立了血吸虫病防治领导小组，而不仅仅是卫生部门单独出力。该领导小组充分整合了卫生、农业、水利、化工、商业、教育、民政等部门，以及军队和共青团、妇联等方面的组织资源；广泛动员全民参与，当时参加灭螺工作的不仅有血吸虫病流行地区的群众，还有大量非流行地区的农民、学生和解放军。

第二，科学防治，中西医结合。中国坚持走科学防治的道路。在血吸虫病防治工作中，中共中央认真听取科学家和专业人员的意见，如对捕获的钉螺应采用火焚而非土埋的方法，同时支持和推动科学研究工作，坚持中西医结合，针对人群、牲畜以及宿主钉螺展开全方位监测。

第三，全民动员，因地因时制宜。中国把消灭血吸虫病作为政治任务，紧紧依靠群众，动员全民参与消灭钉螺、治疗患者、管理粪便、安全用水、个人防护等多环节，打响了防治血吸虫病的人民战争。例如，冬季农民较闲，水位低落，大部分钉螺暴露在地面上，防治重点是大规模治疗全劳动力患者，结合兴修水利来土埋和开垦灭螺，同时进行粪便管理。夏秋季农民下水割草、积肥、插秧、施肥等生产活动频繁，感染血吸虫病概率大，防治重点是粪便管理和个人防护，结合治疗半劳动力和儿童患者。

目前，中国正开展有计划、连续、系统的血吸虫病监测，这是继续有效开展血吸虫病防控工作的重要内容，主要包括以下几个方面：

第一，建立遍布全国的血吸虫监测网和监测点。建立健全县、乡、村和城市社区疫情监测体系，密切注视疫情态势、社会经济状况、人文和自然环境变化情况。完善患者监测和新发病例上报机制，同时建立综合监测点，开展人群外监测，如家畜、钉螺、可疑环境等方面的监测。

第二,及时开展疫情报告和个案调查。各级各类医疗机构、疾病预防控制机构(血防机构)、卫生检疫机构及其执行职务的医务人员,若发现血吸虫病病例,应区分急性或慢性,并在诊断后 24 小时内填写传染病报告卡进行网络直报。县级疾病预防控制机构(血防机构)负责对所报告的急性血吸虫病病例在 1 周内进行个案调查,填写个案调查表并及时录入数据库,通过血吸虫病信息专报系统网络上报。

第三,开展查螺行动和环境监测。中国血吸虫病防治工作的巨大成功在于全国广泛动员和开展的灭螺行动,切断了宿主传播途径。在防治取得成效的今天,中国政府依然每年春季进行 1 次查螺,调查范围包括现有钉螺环境(含易感环境和其他有螺环境)、可疑环境,并采用系统抽样和环境抽样方法,检查钉螺感染情况。

案例(二)　疟疾防治案例

据世界卫生组织资料显示,2022 年,全球 85 个国家估计有 2.49 亿例疟疾病例和 60.8 万例疟疾死亡。疟疾是一种通过某些类型的蚊子传播给人类的疾病,可危及生命。疟疾可防可治。2021 年 6 月 30 日,世界卫生组织宣布中国通过消除疟疾认证,称中国从 20 世纪 40 年代每年报告约 3 000 万疟疾病例、经过 70 年不懈努力到如今完全消除疟疾,是一项了不起的壮举。这是中国继天花、脊髓灰质炎、丝虫病、新生儿破伤风之后消除的又一个重大传染病,结束了疟疾在中国肆虐数千年的历史,在中国公共卫生史和全球消除疟疾史上具有重要的里程碑意义。

疟疾曾经是中国流行历史最久远、影响范围最广、危害最严重的传染病之一。新中国成立前,每年约有 3 000 万疟疾患者,其中 30 万人死亡,病死率高达 1‰。新中国成立后,中共中央、国务院领导中国人民抗击疟疾,经过了重点调查和防治(1949—1959 年)、控制严重流行(1960—1979 年)、降低发病率(1980—1999 年)、巩固防治成果(2000—2009 年)、消除疟疾(2010—2020 年)等 5 个阶段的艰苦历程。

2010 年,中国政府积极响应联合国全球根除疟疾倡议,确定了 2020 年实现消除疟疾的目标。经过不懈努力,中国将疟疾本地原发病例从每年 3 000 万降低至零,维护了人民身体健康和生命安全;建立了科学精准的疟疾防控策略和灵敏高效的报告、检测、治疗、监测和应急处置系统,具备了防止疟疾输入再传播的能力;研制了青蒿素等抗疟特效药和治疗方案,创新了 1 天内完成疟疾病例报告、3 天内完成病例复核和流行病学调查、7 天内完成疫点调查处置的消除疟疾"1-3-7"工作规范以及多部门和区域联防联控、边境地区防控合作等中国经验,为全球疟疾控制和消除贡献了中国智慧。2016 年 4 月,中国报告了最后一例本地原发疟疾病例,2017 年后连续 4 年未发现本地原发病例,2020 年 11 月向世界卫生组织提交了消除疟疾认证申请。经过世界卫生组织现场评估,中国于 2021 年 6 月 30 日通过了国家消除疟疾认证。

5 中国医疗保障体系

医疗保障体系是社会保障体系的重要组成部分,涉及社会保障体系中的大部分领域,如病伤、生育、养老等领域常见的医疗问题。建立医疗保障体系是一种社会责任,在国家事务和社会发展中发挥着越来越重要的作用。世界各国试图通过建立较为完善的医疗保障体系,进而完善其整个社会保障体系,来促进社会和谐发展与进步。中国已经建立了覆盖城乡全体居民的基本医疗保障体系。中国医疗保障体系对保障国民健康权与生存权、提高人群健康水平、促进医疗卫生事业发展、改善社会公平和维护社会稳定具有重要作用。

中国医疗保障体系包括基本医疗保险、医疗救助、补充医疗保险和商业医疗保险等多个层次(图5-1)。基本医疗保险、医疗救助、补充医疗保险属于社会医疗保障的范畴,由政府制定筹资和待遇政策,主要由政府所属的机构提供保障服务,而商业医疗保险则由保险公司通过市场化的机制来提供服务。基本医疗保险包括城镇职工基本医疗保险和城乡居民基本医疗保险,城镇职工必须参加城镇职工基本医疗保险,城镇非就业居民和农村居民以家庭为单位自愿参加城乡居民基本医疗保险。城乡医疗救助是中国多层次医疗保障体系的托底层次,包括城市医疗救助和农村医疗救助两种形式。城乡医疗救助体系通过政府拨款和社会捐助等多渠道筹集资金,主要是为城乡低保家庭成员、五保户和其他经济困难家庭人员提供资助,以确保贫困人口享有基本医疗服务。

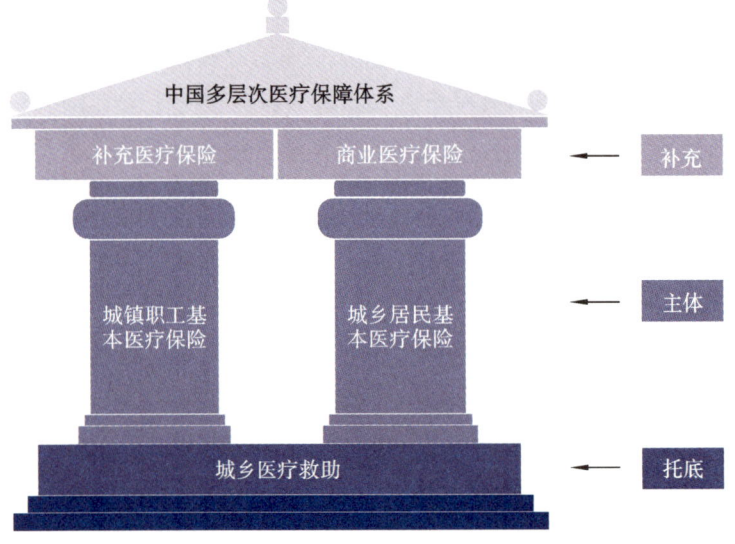

图 5-1 中国多层次医疗保障体系

下文将先详细介绍城镇职工基本医疗保险和城乡居民基本医疗保险,之后再介绍城乡医疗救助、商业医疗保险与补充医疗保险。

5.1　城镇职工基本医疗保险

5.1.1　制度背景

为保障城镇职工医疗权益,中国先后建立了公费医疗和劳保医疗制度(计划经济时期)、城镇职工基本医疗保险制度(在社会主义市场经济环境下成长起来)。从1994年国务院决定在江苏省镇江市和江西省九江市开展职工医疗保障综合改革试点(两江试点)开始,到1998年12月《国务院关于建立城镇职工基本医疗保险制度的决定》(简称《决定》)颁布,城镇职工基本医疗保险制度框架在中国基本确立。目前,中国城镇职工基本医疗保险制度已经在全国范围内普遍建立。

《决定》提出,医疗保险制度改革的主要任务是:适应社会主义市场经济体制,根据财政、企业和个人的承受能力,建立保障职工基本医疗需求的社会医疗保险制度。《决定》还提出,建立城镇职工基本医疗保险制度的原则是:基本医疗保险的水平要与社会主义初级阶段生产力发展水平相适应;城镇所有用人单位及其职工都要参加基本医疗保险,实行属地管理;基本医疗保险费由用人单位和职工双方共同负担;基本医疗保险基金实行社会统筹和个人账户相结合。

5.1.2　主要内容

5.1.2.1　覆盖范围

根据《决定》,城镇职工基本医疗保险制度应覆盖城镇所有用人单位,包括企业(国有企业、集体企业、外商投资企业、私营企业等)、机关、事业单位、社会团体、民办非企业单位及其职工,即所有的正规就业人群都要参加基本医疗保险,从而实现"广覆盖"。

随着中国经济体制改革的进一步深化和产业结构的调整,非全日制、临时性和弹性工作等灵活形式就业的人员逐步增加。为解决灵活就业人员的医疗保障问题,2003年中华人民共和国劳动和社会保障部(简称"劳社部")发布了《关于城镇灵活就业人员参加基本医疗保险的指导意见》,明确将灵活就业人员纳入基本医疗保险制度范围,鼓励灵活就业人员通过劳动保障事务代理机构或社区劳动保障服务机构等实现整体参保。

进入21世纪以来,中国农村劳动力向城市转移加速,民工潮进一步扩大,这部分人虽然在城市工作和生活,但是不能享受所在城市的保障和福利。为做好农民工医疗保障工作,劳社部于2006年开展了农民工参加医疗保险专项扩面行动。至此,所有的城镇劳动力都被职工基本医疗保险制度覆盖。截至2022年底,中国职工基本医疗保险参保人数达3.62亿人。

5.1.2.2　资金筹集

根据《决定》规定,职工基本医疗保险费由用人单位和职工共同缴纳。用人单位缴费率应控制在职工工资总额的6%左右,职工缴费率一般为本人工资收入的2%。随着经济发展,用人单位和职工缴费率可作相应调整。这个筹资水平是根据当时中国生产力水平比较低,财政和企业承受能力有限的实际情况制定的。该文件同时规定,退休人员参加基本医疗保险,个人不缴纳基本医疗保险费。目前中国用人单位缴费率平均为7.5%左右,职工个人缴费率平均为2%。为解决关闭破产国有企业退休人员的医疗保障问题,人力资源社会保障部等4部委于2009年5月联合发出了《关于妥善解决关闭破产国有企业退休人员等医疗保障有关问题的通知》。该通知明确,在企业实施关闭破产时,要按照《中华人民共和国企业破产法》相关规定,通过企业破产财产偿付退休人员参保所需费用。企业破产财产不足偿付的,可以通过未列入破产财产的土地出让所得、财政补助、医疗保险基金结余调剂等多渠道筹资解决。省级政府对困难市、县应给予帮助和支持。对地方依法破产国有企业退休人员参加城镇职工基本医疗保险,中央财政按照"奖补结合"原则给予一次性补助。

5.1.2.3 基金运行与管理

中国基本医疗保险基金由统筹基金和个人账户构成。根据《决定》,职工个人缴纳的基本医疗保险费,全部计入个人账户。用人单位缴纳的基本医疗保险费分为两部分,一部分用于建立统筹基金,一部分划入个人账户。划入个人账户的比例一般为用人单位缴费的 30% 左右。统筹基金和个人账户要划定各自的支付范围,分别核算,不得互相挤占。2021 年,为进一步健全互助共济、责任共担的职工基本医疗保险制度,国务院办公厅印发《国务院办公厅关于建立健全职工基本医疗保险门诊共济保障机制的指导意见》,改进了个人账户计入办法。个人账户计入标准原则上控制在本人参保缴费基数的 2%,单位缴纳的基本医疗保险费全部计入统筹基金。调整统筹基金和个人账户结构后,增加的统筹基金主要用于门诊共济保障,提高参保人员门诊待遇。

中国基本医疗保险基金实行财政专户管理。筹资工作由统筹地区的医疗保险经办机构负责,医疗保险基金先进入经办机构的基金收入账户,然后由经办机构交与当地财政部门管理的财政专户统一管理。根据医疗保险经办机构的支付计划,地方财政部门从财政专户上向医疗保险经办机构的基金支出账户拨付基金。最后,基金由医疗保险经办机构的基金支出账户流向医疗机构。

5.1.2.4 保障范围与待遇给付

中国基本医疗保险支付实行目录管理,这主要是为了保障参保人员依法享有基本医疗服务、规范医疗机构合理处方、合理控制医疗费用。支付目录包括药品目录、诊疗项目目录和医疗服务设施目录。其中,药品目录采用"准入法"管理,即所列药品为基本医疗保险准予支付的范围;诊疗项目目前主要采用"排除法"管理,但部分地区对诊疗项目目录实行"准入法"管理;医疗服务设施目录采用"排除法"管理。

城镇职工基本医疗保险的待遇给付包括三个方面:普通门诊、门诊大病和住院。城镇职工基本医疗保险基金实行社会统筹和个人账户相结合(统账结合),即个人账户保门诊小病,统筹基金保住院和门诊大病。城镇职工基本医疗保险设有起付线、共付比例、封顶线。按照《决定》的要求,起付标准原则上控制在当地职工年平均工资的 10% 左右,最高支付限额原则上控制在当地职工年平均工资的 4 倍左右。起付标准以下的医疗费用,从个人账户中支付或由个人自付。起付标准以上、最高支付限额以下的医疗费用,主要从统筹基金中支付,个人也要负担一定比例。

5.1.2.5 医疗服务管理

中国医疗保险机构进行医疗服务管理的目的是合理控制医疗费用、保证医疗服务质量。医疗服务管理的内容可以概括为"定点医疗、三个目录"。定点医疗是指医疗保险经办机构与医疗机构签订定点医疗协议,医疗机构接受医疗保险经办机构的考核与监督,参保人员只有在定点医疗机构就医才能获得医疗保险报销。定点医疗机构包括辖区内的综合医院、专科医院、社区卫生服务机构。随着医疗保险覆盖人群的扩大,定点医疗机构的数量也大大增加,一般辖区内的公立医疗机构和具有一定规模的民营医疗机构都被纳入了定点医疗机构的范围。

　　"三个目录"即上文提到的药品目录、诊疗项目目录、医疗服务设施目录。三个目录都按照临床必需、安全有效、价格适宜的原则制定。其中,药品目录由人力资源社会保障部制定,诊疗项目目录和医疗服务设施目录由各省人力资源和社会保障部门制定。药品目录分为甲类和乙类,甲类目录由国家统一制定,各地不得调整。乙类目录由国家制定,各省、自治区、直辖市可以根据当地实际情况,进行适当调整,增加和减少的品种数之和不得超过国家乙类目录药品总数的15%。各地级和县级统筹地区的人力资源和社会保障部门无权调整药品目录,但是可以适当调整报销比例。一般乙类目录药品要扣除20%左右的自付费用,剩余的才能进行报销。

5.1.2.6　医疗保险支付

　　2011年以来,中国医药卫生体制改革把医疗保险支付方式改革作为一项重要的任务。越来越多的地区从原来的按项目付费向混合型付费转变。

　　总额控制。规定医疗机构业务收入的增长速度不得超过议定的值,例如上海等地采用这种办法。

　　次均住院费用。规定医疗机构的次均住院费用不得超过议定的值,例如南京、镇江、广州、深圳等地采用这种办法。

　　按病种付费。对若干病种采用定额支付,例如北京市早在2011年就已在六家试点医院实行按病种付费,涉及108个病种,在全市则对阑尾炎、甲状腺肿、白内障、卵巢良性肿瘤、子宫肌瘤、拇外翻、胆囊结石等少数疾病实行按病种付费;而黑龙江省的牡丹江市则对绝大多数疾病实行单病种付费,2010年共有830个病种。

　　按人头付费。主要在门诊慢性病(如精神病)管理中实行。患者签约一家定点医疗机构,承诺一年内都在这家医疗机构首诊,医疗保险机构按人头向定点医疗机构支付患者一年的门诊费用。但患者就医时还需支付一定比例的自付费用。

　　按病种分值付费。按病种分值付费是中国原创的一种支付方式。它是以大数据为基础,在汇集大量真实世界病例的基础上,按照"诊断+操作"的分组规则对病例进行分组,并根据一定的结算规则进行医疗保险支付。

　　在中国的实践中,预付制与风险共担机制相配合,共同推动医疗保障服务的优化,即如果医疗机构的实际费用超过了预先确定的费用,医疗保险机构将分担一定的超支费用,具体的分担方式由医疗保险机构和医疗机构双方协商,并在定点医疗协议中体现。

5.1.2.7　医疗服务监管

　　在中国,医疗服务监管主要包括定点准入、实时监控、年度考核、奖惩机制等几个方面。

5.2　城乡居民基本医疗保险

案例　被誉为"中国模式"的中国农村合作医疗制度

　　20世纪80年代,世界卫生组织和世界银行在对中国的考察报告中指出,中国实行的农村合作医疗制度,是"发展中国家解决卫生经费的唯一典范"。时任世界卫生组织总干事马勒博士曾积极向发展中国家推荐中国的农村卫生工作经验。

中国农村合作医疗制度被世界卫生组织和世界银行誉为"以最少投入获得了最大健康收益"的"中国模式"。它最早可以追溯到20世纪30年代的保健药社和卫生合作社，先后经历了30—40年代的萌芽阶段、50年代的初创阶段、60—70年代的发展和鼎盛阶段、80年代的解体阶段、90年代以来的恢复和发展阶段（新农合制度在此阶段建立）。中国农村合作医疗制度的发展与完善是20世纪60年代至70年代中国用较少卫生费用解决8亿农民基本卫生问题的基础。1978年，中国农村合作医疗的覆盖率达到90％以上。中国农村合作医疗制度改善了中国农村医疗面貌，提高了广大人民群众的健康水平。实施农村合作医疗制度以后，2003年，中国婴儿死亡率由新中国成立初期的200‰下降至25.5‰，孕产妇死亡率由1 500/10万下降至51.3/10万，人口死亡率由17‰下降至6.4‰，人均预期寿命由35岁提高至72.4岁。

早期的中国农村合作医疗制度具有以下特点：第一，它是当时推动合作社经济发展并完善其社会服务功能的重要表现形式。中国农村合作医疗制度以保健药社的形式出现，并且坚持预防为主。第二，医务人员发挥重要作用。当时的医务人员不拿工资，平时忙于农活，有需要时当医生，被称为"赤脚医生"。他们是由"巡回医疗队"培养的。"巡回医疗队"是中国农村合作医疗制度得以巩固、发展的重要支柱。第三，中国农村合作医疗制度以农民自主集资为主。保健药社的日常经费由农民交纳的"保健费"、从农业社提取的15％～20％的公益金和医疗收入三方保障筹资。第四，中国农村合作医疗制度是一种低成本、广覆盖的农村卫生保障制度，使广大农民群众能就近享受基本的初级卫生服务，患病农民也能享受医疗卫生服务的公平性和可及性。

早期的中国农村合作医疗制度存在的问题：第一，缺乏相关的法律和组织保障，没有正式的法律文件，无法可依，管理缺乏科学性。第二，"文化大革命"时期急于求成，由于受到极左思潮的影响，过多地迎合政治的需要，在卫生决策和管理上不顾主客观条件和医疗卫生特性，破坏了医疗卫生体制健康发展，也阻碍了农村医学的健康发展。第三，卫生人员技术水平较低，农村合作医疗总体绩效较低。第四，筹资水平有限，抗风险能力差；农村集体经济解体后，农村合作医疗失去了主要的经济来源，这是农村合作医疗制度难以长期存在的根本原因之一。第五，农村合作医疗制度采取的保门诊、保小病的做法，提高了合作医疗的受益面，但保障水平低，难以满足多层次的需求。

城乡居民基本医疗保险制度由城镇居民基本医疗保险制度和新农合制度于2016年整合形成。本节首先将分别介绍城镇居民基本医疗保险和新农合的相关内容，之后再介绍城镇居民基本医疗保险制度和新农合制度的整合。

5.2.1　城镇居民基本医疗保险

5.2.1.1　制度背景

2007年，中国城镇居民基本医疗保险试点工作正式启动，88个城市被列入试点范围。2008年3月，国务院颁布《国务院关于开展城镇居民基本医疗保险试点的指导意见》（以下简称《指导意见》）。2010年，城镇居民基本医疗保险试点在中国全面推开。城镇居民基本医疗保险最鲜明的特点是政府对每一个参保居民实行普惠制补助。

和城镇职工基本医疗保险主要保障城镇地区就业人口基本医疗需求、建立统账结合的社会保险制度的目标不同,城镇居民基本医疗保险制度的目标是:建立覆盖全体城镇非从业居民,筹资机制合理、管理体制健全、运行机制规范的以大病统筹为主的社会保障制度。

城镇居民基本医疗保险试点工作的原则是:坚持低水平起步,根据经济发展水平和各方面承受能力,合理确定筹资水平和保障标准,重点保障城镇非从业居民的大病医疗需求,逐步提高保障水平;坚持自愿原则,充分尊重群众意愿;明确中央和地方政府的责任,中央确定基本原则和主要政策,地方制订具体办法,对参保居民实行属地管理;坚持统筹协调,做好各类医疗保障制度之间基本政策、标准和管理措施等的衔接。

5.2.1.2　主要内容

和城镇职工基本医疗保险一样,城镇居民基本医疗保险也多由各地社会保障管理部门制定相关政策,并由医疗保险经办机构进行管理。城镇居民基本医疗保险实行和城镇职工基本医疗保险类似的目录和管理政策,以下仅对其与城镇职工基本医疗保险不一致的规定进行阐述。

（1）覆盖范围

根据《指导意见》规定,城镇居民基本医疗保险制度的覆盖范围包括"不属于城镇职工基本医疗保险制度覆盖范围的中小学阶段的学生(包括职业高中、中专、技校学生)、少年儿童和其他非从业城镇居民"。它和覆盖全体就业人口的城镇职工基本医疗保险制度一起,实现了城镇居民医疗保险全覆盖。

（2）资金筹集

城镇居民基本医疗保险的筹资方式主要有财政补助和个人缴费两种。在2007年的试点工作启动时期,政府按每年不低于人均40元的标准给予补助。对属于低保对象、丧失劳动能力的重度残疾人等困难居民,政府给予额外补助。财政补助经费纳入了各级政府的财政预算。随着2009年3月《中共中央　国务院关于深化医药卫生体制改革的意见》的出台,各级政府对城镇居民基本医疗保险制度的支持逐步加强,城镇居民基本医疗保险人均财政补助标准也逐年提高,从2009年人均80元的补助水平,提高到2017年的人均450元,极大地提高了居民医疗健康保障水平。

对于个人缴费,目前中国并没有实施统一的标准,由各地根据当地的经济发展水平以及不同人群的基本医疗消费需求,并考虑当地居民家庭和财政的负担能力,恰当确定。2017年城镇居民基本医疗保险人均个人缴费标准达到180元。

（3）保障范围与待遇给付

城镇居民基本医疗保险基金实行社会统筹,不设个人账户,重点用于参保居民的住院和门诊大病医疗支出。在2007年试点工作启动之时,城镇居民基本医疗保险仅保住院和门诊大病,普通门诊不予报销。2009年,《人力资源和社会保障部　财政部　卫生部关于开展城镇居民基本医疗保险门诊统筹的指导意见》发布,要求各地在重点保障参保居民住院和门诊大病医疗支出的基础上,逐步将门诊小病医疗费用纳入基金支付范围。

城镇居民基本医疗保险保障住院和门诊大病时执行与城镇职工基本医疗保险相同的报销目录,但目前参保者享受的保障待遇普遍低于城镇职工基本医疗保险。各地具体的城镇居民基本医疗保险起付线、支付比例和封顶线由地方确定。在"十二五"期间,城镇居民基本医疗保险政策范围内的住院费用支付比例达到了75%。目前,中国已经开展了城镇居民基本医疗保险的普通门诊统筹,即把参保人员的门诊费用也纳入统筹基金报销的范围,有效地解决了城镇居民普通门诊医疗费用负担。普通门诊统筹一般要求参保人员在基层医疗卫生机构就医,封顶线一般仅为数百元。

5.2.2　新农合

5.2.2.1　新农合制度的建立

为了解决农民无医疗保障制度的问题以及农村居民日益突出的因病致贫、因病返贫问题,2002 年 10 月,中共中央、国务院下发《中共中央 国务院关于进一步加强农村卫生工作的决定》,提出逐步建立新农合制度。2003 年,国务院办公厅转发卫生部等部门《关于建立新型农村合作医疗制度的意见》,标志着建立新农合制度工作的正式开展。此后,一种新的医疗保障制度在全国范围内逐步实施。

新农合制度是由政府组织、引导和支持,农民自愿参加,个人、集体和政府多方筹资,以大病统筹为主的农民医疗互助共济制度。

5.2.2.2　新农合制度的目标与原则

(1)新农合制度的目标

新农合制度不同于以往任何一项医疗保障制度,具有明显的中国特色。其目标是建立一种满足广大农民卫生服务需求的基本医疗保障制度,解决农民因病致贫、因病返贫问题,减轻农民就医时的经济负担,提高卫生服务利用率,促进农村卫生服务体系的建设,提高人群健康水平。

(2)新农合制度的原则

新农合制度遵循不同于以往的合作医疗制度、符合中国农村发展理念和农民特性的独特原则。

第一,以家庭为单位自愿参加的原则。新农合最大的制度特点就是坚持"农民自愿参加"的基本原则,目的在于让农民自己认可这项利民的制度,自愿参加,因势利导,最终实现新农合全覆盖。

第二,以政府财政筹资为主的原则。以往的合作医疗制度以农民个人或者集体经济为筹资主体,但实践证明,其筹资金额较为有限,抗风险能力较低,且缺乏可持续性。而新农合制度从建立之初就明确了"以政府财政筹资为主"的原则,并规定中央和地方财政要对参合农民给予一定补助。

第三,保障范围以大病统筹为主,兼顾门诊的原则。新农合制度以住院费用补助为主,兼顾门诊费用补偿。

第四,以县级为统筹单位的原则。以往的合作医疗制度以乡镇为单位进行统筹,一方面管理能力较弱,另一方面抗风险能力较低。因此,新农合制度以县为单位进行统筹和组织实施,从而增强了抗风险能力和监管力度。

第五,采取"卫生系统经办,各部门协调配合"的原则。中国规定,由县级以上人民政府负责本行政区域内新农合工作的统一协调和指导,成立由财政、卫生、民政等相关部门组成的新农合管理委员会,明确监督管理机构和经办机构的职责与任务。

5.2.2.3　主要内容

（1）资金筹集

新农合的筹资方式主要有财政补助和个人缴费两种。2003年启动之初,新农合人均筹资水平仅有30元,其中中央政府和地方政府各自按照人均10元的标准安排补助资金,农民个人自付10元。近年来,新农合人均筹资标准逐年提高,政府财政承担起新农合制度筹资主体的责任。

（2）补偿模式

新农合基金主要补助参合农民的住院医疗费用和门诊大病费用（部分地区已开通普通门诊费用统筹服务）。各统筹地区根据筹资总额,结合当地实际确定基金的支付范围、支付标准和额度。新农合主管部门制定新农合报销药物目录（一般以省为单位）,用于约束药物补偿范围。新农合报销药物目录采用分级设计,包括村级、乡级和县级及以上层级。定点医疗机构级别越高,则允许使用和报销的药物品种越多。乡级新农合报销药物目录以国家基本药物目录（基层部分）为主体,可根据当地突出健康需求和新农合基金支付能力适当增加。村级新农合报销药物目录使用国家基本药物目录（基层部分）,如地方根据实际确需增加民族药或地方特殊疾病用药,可适当增加相应药物品种。新农合对国家基本药物目录内的药品报销比例要明显高于国家基本药物目录外药品。

（3）支付方式

新农合对定点医疗机构实施门诊总额付费,根据门诊总额预算结余的处理方法分为三种:门诊总额预付、门诊总额预算＋弹性结算、门诊总额限制等。新农合住院支付方式主要有按单病种付费、按床日付费、按总额付费及混合支付等。

5.2.3　城镇居民基本医疗保险制度和新农合制度的整合

2016年1月,国务院印发《国务院关于整合城乡居民基本医疗保险制度的意见》,将城镇居民基本医疗保险制度和新农合制度合并为统一的城乡居民基本医疗保险制度。整合城乡居民基本医疗保险制度是推进医药卫生体制改革、实现城乡居民公平享有基本医疗保险权益、促进社会公平正义、增进人民福祉的重大举措,对促进城乡经济社会协调发展、全面建成小康社会具有重要意义。

5.2.3.1　基本政策的整合

城乡居民基本医疗保险实现了"六统一":一是统一覆盖范围。城乡居民基本医疗保险制度覆盖范围包括城镇居民基本医疗保险和新农合所有应参保（合）人员,即覆盖除职工基本医疗保险应参保人员以外的其他所有城乡居民。二是统一筹资政策。城乡居民基本医疗保险继续实行个人缴费与政府补助相结合为主的筹资方式,鼓励集体、单位或其他社会经济组织给予扶持或资助。三是统一保障待遇。遵循保障适度、收支平衡的原则,均衡城乡保障待遇,逐步统一保障范围和支付标准。城乡居民基本医疗保险基金主要用于支付参保人员发生的住院和门诊医药费用,政策范围内住院费用支付比例保持在75%左右。四是统一医保目录,包括城乡居民基本医疗保险药品目录、诊疗项目目录、医疗服务设施目录。五是统一定点管理。统一城乡居民基本医疗保险定点机构管理办法,建立健全考核评价机制和动态的准入退出机制。六是统一基金管理。城乡居民基本医疗保险执行国家统一的基金财务制度、会计制度和基金预决算管理制度。城乡居民基本医疗保险基金纳入财政专户,实行

"收支两条线"管理。基金独立核算、专户管理。

5.2.3.2　管理体制的整合

一是鼓励有条件的地区理顺医保管理体制,统一基本医疗保险行政管理职能。整合城乡居民基本医疗保险经办机构、人员和信息系统,规范经办流程,提供一体化的经办服务。在整合经办机构的基础上,进一步完善管理运行机制,优化经办流程。二是鼓励有条件的地区创新经办服务模式,推进管办分开,引入竞争机制,在确保基金安全和有效监管的前提下,以政府购买服务的方式委托具有资质的商业保险机构等社会力量参与基本医疗保险的经办服务,激发经办活力。

5.3　城乡医疗救助、商业医疗保险与补充医疗保险

5.3.1　城乡医疗救助

医疗救助体系能够为广大贫困人群提供医疗保障,提高贫困人群的健康水平,帮助他们尽早摆脱贫病交加的处境。对于中国而言,医疗救助体系有着维护人民权益,实现政府职责,体现社会公平,促进国民经济更高质量、更有效率、更加公平的重要作用与意义。所以,为贫困人群构建医疗救助体系,对于中国经济社会的和谐发展具有重要的作用。医疗救助体系是医疗保障体系的重要组成部分,其构建在医疗保障体系建设中占有重要地位。

5.3.1.1　城乡医疗救助资金的筹集与管理

目前中国的城乡医疗救助资金通过多渠道筹集,包括财政拨款、彩票公益金、社会捐助、基金利息收入等。改善贫困人口的健康状况是政府义不容辞的责任,政府应为贫困人口提供必要的医疗救助资金支持。在中国,中央财政安排专项资金,对困难地区开展的城乡医疗救助工作给予补助,而地方各级财政特别是省级财政切实调整财政支出结构,增加投入,进一步扩大医疗救助资金规模。由于中国尚处于社会主义初级阶段,各地经济发展水平不同,政府对于医疗救助的财政拨款受当地经济发展水平的严重制约。除政府财政拨款外,社会捐助也是城乡医疗救助资金来源的重要组成部分。

中国医疗救助资金大多纳入财政专户,实行专账管理、专款专用(在这方面,中国尚没有通过一定资金运作形式实现保值增值的经验)。例如建立基金会,把财政资金和非财政资金(通过社会捐赠等渠道得到的资金)交由专门机构运营。基金会负责同医疗机构进行救助资金的结算,并严格执行资金使用程序,帮助受助对象恢复健康。

医疗救助资金要实现依法管理、规范管理,必须坚持做到以下几点:第一,实行专户储存和专项管理。民政部门是管理医疗救助资金的主体,而财政部门行使对资金的监管权力并承担相应责任;必须建立财政专户,对医疗救助资金实行预算化管理。县(市、区)民政、财政、审计等部门要对医疗救助资金的使用情况进行监督检查,发现问题应及时纠正并及时向当地人民政府报告。第二,实行封闭运行。封闭运行可简单地概括为钱账分离,即管钱者不管账,管账者不管钱,资金始终在政府财政专户和医疗机构的银行账户之间流动。第三,资金使用必须公开透明,要将医疗救助资金的筹集、管理和使用情况,以及救助对象、救助金额等情况通过张榜公布等方式定期向社会公布。第四,不断提高管理效率,使管理成本最小

化。涉及医疗救助资金管理的各相关部门应相互协调,不断提高资金管理效率、降低管理成本。

5.3.1.2 城乡医疗救助对象

在中国,城乡医疗救助是城镇职工基本医疗保险、城乡居民基本医疗保险以及商业医疗保险的补充形式,救助对象为低收入人群。

农村医疗救助的救助对象是农村五保户、农村贫困户家庭成员和地方政府规定的其他符合条件的农村贫困农民。城市医疗救助的救助对象主要是城市居民最低生活保障对象中未参加城镇职工基本医疗保险的人员、已参加城镇职工基本医疗保险但个人负担仍然较重的人员和其他特殊贫困人群。另外,中国也将患重特大疾病的低保家庭成员、低收入老年人、重度残疾人以及其他因患重特大疾病难以自付医疗费用且家庭贫困的人员纳入了中国城乡医疗救助的范围。

城乡医疗救助制度建立以来,救助对象不断扩展,在纳入传统困难群体的同时,逐步纳入了其他符合条件的救助对象。具体救助对象的界定标准,由地方民政部门会同财政等有关部门,根据本地经济条件和医疗救助基金筹集情况、贫困人群的支付能力以及基本医疗需求等因素制定,并报同级人民政府批准后执行。

5.3.1.3 城乡医疗救助办法及医疗救助服务

医疗救助可通过不同的途径开展,中国各地结合本地经济、社会发展水平及财政收入状况等因素,采取了多种医疗救助办法,主要是资助参保和补贴医疗费用。资助参保通过为没有能力缴纳医疗保险费用的人群缴纳部分或全部参保费用,使其获得参加医疗保险的资格。补贴医疗费用是指在扣除各项医疗保险可支付部分、单位应报销部分及社会互助帮困部分后,对救助对象个人负担超过一定金额的医疗费用或特殊疾病医疗费用给予一定比例或一定数额的补助。

目前,城乡医疗救助服务以住院救助为主,同时兼顾门诊救助。住院救助主要用于解决因病住院救助对象个人负担的医疗费用;门诊救助主要用于解决患有常见病、慢性病,需要长期药物维持治疗以及急诊、急救的个人负担的医疗费用。

5.3.1.4 城乡医疗救助工作的管理部门

医疗救助涉及多个部门,其管理由民政部门、财政部门、人力资源和社会保障部门、卫生部门及其他部门共同参与。

中国城乡医疗救助工作主要由民政部门管理,从中央到地方都设有专门机构,具体负责制定医疗救助制度,并协调参与其实施过程的各个部门间的关系以及救助资金的发放、使用等。财政部门主要负责编制医疗救助资金的年度预算,建立城乡医疗救助资金财政专户,进行专户管理、专账核算以及资金的使用监督。人力资源和社会保障部门负责配合医疗救助工作的组织和实施,做好医疗保险和医疗救助政策的衔接。卫生行政部门负责协调和监督医疗服务的提供,保证医疗救助工作的顺利开展。其他部门,如审计部门,以及总工会、红十字会等组织也会参与医疗救助工作的管理。

5.3.2 商业医疗保险

5.3.2.1 市场地位与规模

随着中国市场经济体制的进一步完善和居民收入的提高,居民的医疗卫生服务需求在不断增加,商业医疗保险在医疗保障体系中发挥的作用也越来越重要。新医改明确提出要加快建立和完善以基本医疗保障为主体,其他多种形式补充医疗保险和商业健康保险为补充,覆盖城乡居民的多层次医疗保障体系,从而明确了商业医疗保险在医疗保障体系中发挥补充作用的地位。当前商业医疗保险市场中,学生医疗保险、补充医疗保险以及包含医疗险、意外险、财产险及人寿险在内的综合保险较为常见。2012 年,《关于开展城乡居民大病保险工作的指导意见》又明确指出,支持商业保险机构承办大病保险,发挥市场机制作用,提高大病保险的运行效率、服务水平和质量。

5.3.2.2 市场结构

在中国,以企业为单位、集体参加商业医疗保险是比较常见的集体投保行为,企业在为员工提供福利的同时,提高了自身的劳动生产力。此类商业医疗保险往往是对基本医疗保险的补充。例如,部分商业医疗保险可以报销基本医疗保险报销目录外的一些药品,也可以为参保者提供患病后的营养费补贴。学生集体参保也较为常见,学生可以参加覆盖住院服务的城乡居民基本医疗保险,若同时参加商业医疗保险,则患病后可以获得更好的保障。基本医疗保险参保者也可以通过参加商业医疗保险来获得更高的报销比例或更广泛的报销范围。年龄、性别、经济状况、教育水平以及地域等因素对商业医疗保险的选择有一定影响,年龄、性别等因素也会成为购买商业医疗保险的限制条件。

2015 年,《国务院办公厅关于全面实施城乡居民大病保险的意见》印发,进一步明确支持商业保险机构承办大病保险。具体措施为:地方政府人力资源社会保障、卫生计生、财政、保险监管部门共同制定大病保险的筹资、支付范围、最低支付比例,以及就医、结算管理等基本政策,并通过适当方式征求意见。原则上通过政府招标选定承办大病保险的商业保险机构。招标主要包括具体支付比例、盈亏率、配备的承办和管理力量等内容。符合保险监管部门基本准入条件的商业保险机构自愿参加投标,中标后以签署保险合同的形式承办大病保险,承担经营风险,自负盈亏。

5.3.2.3 市场行为

中国鼓励用人单位和个人参加商业医疗保险。商业医疗保险的保费一般根据保险的定位、目标人群的支付能力,结合保险机构的运营成本等测算而来。对于个体参保者而言,参保前一般需要提供相关健康信息,以确定保费;如果以企业或者其他群体为单位参保,则可以享受群体参保的费率。

由于目前商业医疗保险的市场份额相对不高,对医疗机构难以形成谈判力,因此商业医疗保险的保障一般以医疗费用事后报销、住院等休工天数补贴形式为主。商业医疗保险可能会对参保者可选择的就诊机构做相应要求。

中国商业医疗保险的需求人群包括已经享受基本医疗保险的居民,此类参保者对基本医疗保险规定范围以外的特殊检查、治疗、用药的需求较大,商业医疗保险可以满足这部分非基本的医疗服务需求。

5.3.2.4 公共政策

在中国,商业医疗保险由国家金融监督管理总局进行规制。2006 年首次发布、经修订后 2019 年重新发布的《健康保险管理办法》,统一了健康保险业务经营的监管标准。为了加快发展健康服务业,国务院提出"商业健康保险产品更加丰富,参保人数大幅增加,商业健康保险支出占卫生总费用的比重大幅提高,形成较为完善的健康保险机制"的目标,为商业医疗保险的发展奠定了政策基础。此外,部分地区开展了商业医疗保险机构运营基本医疗保险模式的探索,在未来可能会为商业医疗保险提供更多发展机会。

5.3.3　补充医疗保险

5.3.3.1　补充医疗保险的发展概况

中国补充医疗保险是伴随医疗制度改革而产生的。1993 年,《中共中央关于建立社会主义市场经济体制若干问题的决定》中明确指出"建立多层次的社会保障体系"。1994 年,《关于职工医疗制度改革的试点意见》规定,发展职工医疗互助基金和商业性的医疗保险,作为社会医疗保险的补充,以满足国家规定的基本医疗保障之外的医疗需求,但要坚持个人自愿参加、自主选择的原则。

在国家宏观政策的指导下,各地对各种补充医疗保险进行了积极的探讨。许多地区和城市在建立城镇职工基本医疗保险制度的同时,纷纷积极筹建和制定多种形式的补充医疗保险,并制定有关政策和具体实施办法。

5.3.3.2　补充医疗保险的商业化运作

目前,中国补充医疗保险的管理方式主要是捆绑式经营和商业化运作两类。捆绑式经营是指政府社保机构仍以经营基本医疗保险的方式来经营补充医疗保险。其特点首先是管理困难、运作过程难以操作,其次是其带来的财政负担和企业负担都较为沉重。商业化运作是指社保机构借助商业保险机构实现补充医疗保险的经营管理。这种方式可减轻财政压力,节约人力资源,优化医疗资源的配置,加强对医疗机构的管理,进而促进基本医疗保险管理的规范化和科学化。补充医疗保险受到了广泛的关注。在中国,商业医疗保险常作为补充医疗保险来运作,所以实现补充医疗保险的商业化运作,将成为完善医疗保障体系的重要方面。

(1)补充医疗保险商业化运作的发展空间

商业保险机构自身独特的优势可以促进其占据医疗保险市场的潜力增加,若具备先进的管理手段和灵活的经营策略,还可以接受社保机构和其他补充型医疗保险机构的特定项目管理委托。总体来看,中国近年来的医疗保险需求增长迅速。由于商业医疗保险具有保健和投资的双重功能,各医疗保险机构的个人商业医疗保险产品不断增多。

(2)补充医疗保险商业化运作过程中应注意的问题

第一,合理界定补充医疗保险的性质。政府应只解决基本医疗问题,剩下的医疗问题要留给市场解决;应充分调动医疗保险机构的积极性。

第二,社保机构和医疗保险机构应加强对医疗服务供需双方的行为调控。要建立医院之间的竞争制度,以提高医疗服务效率。同时,要通过信息化管理和不定期抽查等形式防止医疗资源浪费或医患合谋欺诈等情况的发生。

第三,要不断加大补充医疗保险产品的开发力度,满足不同层次的补充医疗保险需求。

第四,提高补充医疗保险承办机构的专业化水平。

6 中国药品供应保障体系

药品在人民群众防病治病、康复保健、救灾防疫等方面发挥着不可替代的作用,在经济发展、国家安全中的重要作用也日益凸显。作为一种特殊商品,其研发创新难度大、生产与使用中的专业技术性强、正常使用也可能引发不良反应、质量低下和滥用误用对患者健康与社会稳定危害大。药品供应保障体系与公共卫生服务体系、医疗服务体系、医疗保障体系并列为中国基本医疗卫生制度四大支柱体系。同时,药品供应保障也是健康中国建设的重点任务之一。

6.1 中国药品供应保障组织体系

中国药品供应保障组织体系可分为:药品行政监督管理组织体系,药品技术监督管理组织体系,药学教育、科研组织和社团组织体系,药品生产与经营组织体系,医疗机构药学组织体系。

6.1.1 药品行政监督管理组织体系

中国药品监督管理行政机构共分四级,即国家药品监督管理局、省(自治区、直辖市)级药品监督管理局、市(州、盟)级和县(区)级市场监督管理机构。其基本框架见图6-1。

6.1.1.1 国家药品监督管理局

国家药品监督管理局是国家市场监督管理总局管理的国家局,为副部级,主要负责药品、医疗器械和化妆品的安全监督管理、标准管理、注册管理、质量管理、监督检查以及上市后的风险管理等。

6.1.1.2 省级及以下药品监督管理机构

中国省级药品监督管理局是省级人民政府的工作机构,在本辖区范围内履行法定的药品监督管理职能;设置的职能处室包括综合规划财务处、政策法规处、行政审批处、药品注册管理处、药品生产监督管理处、药品流通监督管理处、医疗器械监督管理处和化妆品监督管理处等。省级以下药品监督管理机构由地方政府分级管理,业务受上级主管部门的指导和监督。

6.1.1.3 其他药品监督管理相关机构

(1)市场监督管理机构

市场监督管理机构负责相关市场主体登记注册和营业执照核发,查处准入、生产、经营、交易中的有关违法行为,实施反垄断执法,价格监督检查和反不正当竞争执法,药品、保健食品、医疗器械、特殊医学用途配方食品广告审查和监测等工作。市场监督管理机构管理同级药品监督管理机构。市、县两级市场监督管理机构负责药品零售、医疗器械经营的许可、检查和处罚,以及化妆品经营和药品、医疗器械使用环节质量的检查和处罚等工作。

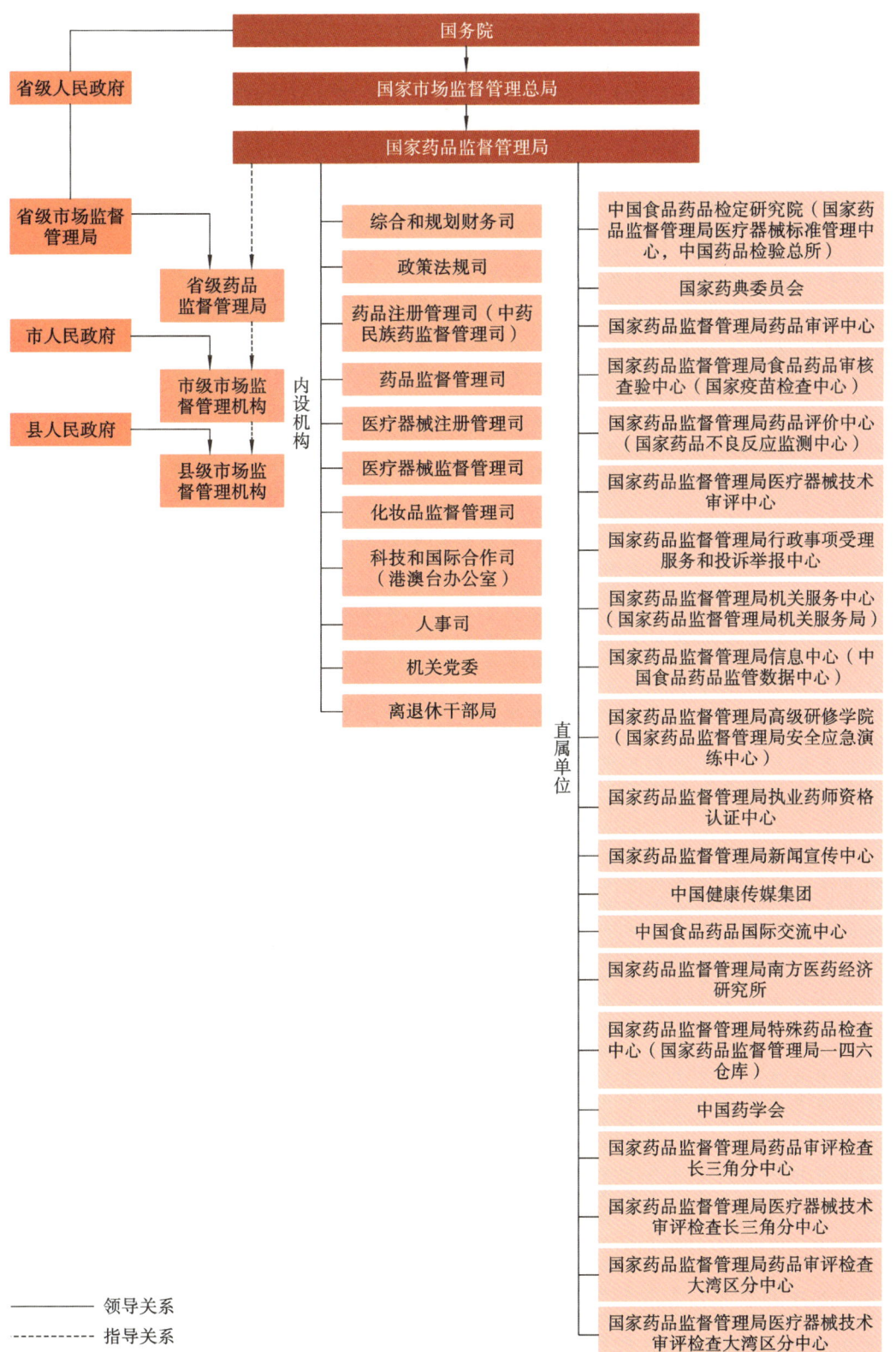

图 6-1　中国药品监督管理行政机构基本框架

（2）卫生健康行政机构

卫生健康行政机构是各级政府中负责医疗卫生行政工作的机构。中国最高卫生健康行政管理机构是国家卫生健康委。国家卫生健康委负责完善国家基本药物制度,组织拟订国家药物政策和基本药物目录,开展药品使用监测、临床综合评价和短缺药品预警,提出药品价格政策和国家基本药物目录内药品生产鼓励扶持政策的建议等工作。国家药品监督管理局会同国家卫生健康委组织国家药典委员会编制、修订和编译《中华人民共和国药典》,建立重大药品不良反应和医疗器械不良事件相互通报机制和联合处置机制。

（3）中医药管理机构

中医药管理机构负责拟订中医药和民族医药事业发展的战略、规划、政策和相关标准;指导民族医药的理论、医术、药物的发掘、整理、总结和提高;组织开展中药资源普查,促进中药资源的保护、开发和合理利用等工作。

（4）医疗保障管理机构

医疗保障管理机构负责拟订医疗保险、生育保险、医疗救助等医疗保障制度的政策、规划、标准并组织实施,监督管理相关医疗保障基金,完善就医费用结算平台,组织制定和调整药品、医疗服务价格和收费标准,制定药品和医用耗材的采购政策并监督实施,监督管理纳入医保范围内的医疗机构的相关服务行为和医疗费用等工作。

另外,中国发展和改革宏观调控部门、人力资源和社会保障部门、工业和信息化管理部门、中央网络安全和信息化委员会办公室、商务管理部门、海关以及公安部门等也承担各自职责范围内的药品监督管理职能。

6.1.2　药品技术监督管理组织体系

药品监督管理工作的技术性很强,在实施药品行政监督管理的过程中,必须有技术支撑。药品技术监督管理机构是药品监督管理的组成部分,为药品行政监督提供技术支撑与保障。中国药品技术监督管理机构包括药品检验机构和国家药品监督管理局直属的其他技术机构。

6.1.2.1　药品检验机构

药品检验机构是执行国家对药品质量监督、检验的法定专业检验机构,代表国家对药品进行监督检验,检验结果具有法律效力。中国的药品检验机构共分四级,即中国食品药品检定研究院(简称"中检院")、省(自治区、直辖市)级药品检验机构、市(州、盟)级药品检验机构和县级药品检验机构。

根据《中央编办关于国家药品监督管理局所属事业单位机构编制的批复》,中检院为国家药品监督管理局所属公益二类事业单位,是国家检验药品生物制品质量的法定机构和最高技术仲裁机构。中检院的主要职责有:承担食品、药品、医疗器械、化妆品及有关药用辅料、包装材料与容器的检验检测工作,承担相关产品严重不良反应、严重不良事件原因的实验研究工作,组织开展有关国家标准物质的规划、计划、研究、制备、标定、分发和管理工作,负责生产用菌毒种、细胞株的检定工作,承担医用标准菌毒种、细胞株的收集、鉴定、保存、分发和管理工作等。

6.1.2.2　国家药品监督管理局直属的其他技术机构

（1）国家药典委员会

国家药典委员会是中国最早成立的标准化机构,负责组织编制《中华人民共和国药典》

及制定、修订国家药品标准,是法定的国家药品标准工作专业管理机构。国家药典委员会的常设办事机构实行秘书长负责制,内设业务管理处(质量管理处)、信息管理处(编辑部)、中药处、化学药品处、生物制品处、办公室、人事党务处(纪律检查室)、财务处、通则辅料包材处等9个组织机构,下设《中国药品标准》杂志社等分支机构。

(2)国家药品监督管理局药品审评中心

国家药品监督管理局药品审评中心是药品注册技术审评机构,为药品注册提供技术支持;内设业务管理处、人事处(老干部服务与管理处)、质量管理处、合规处、临床试验管理处、数据管理处、办公室、财务处、党委办公室、纪律检查室、中药民族药药学部、中药民族药临床部、化药药学一部、化药药学二部、药理毒理学部、化药临床一部、化药临床二部、统计与临床药理学部、生物制品药学部和生物制品临床部等组织机构。

(3)国家药品监督管理局药品评价中心

国家药品监督管理局药品评价中心内设办公室、综合业务处、化学药品监测和评价部、生物制品监测和评价部、中药监测和评价部、医疗器械监测和评价部、化妆品监测和评价部、科研和信息管理处、党委纪律办公室(人事处)等9个机构。

(4)国家药品监督管理局食品药品审核查验中心

国家药品监督管理局食品药品审核查验中心为国家药品监督管理局所属公益二类事业单位(保留正局级);内设办公室、综合业务处(质量管理处)、信息管理处、检查一处、检查二处、检查三处、检查四处、检查五处、检查六处、人事处(党委办公室)、财务处等11个机构。

(5)国家药品监督管理局执业药师资格认证中心

国家药品监督管理局执业药师资格认证中心业务上受国家药品监督管理局人事司监督和指导,内设办公室(人事党务处)、考试处、注册管理处和信息处。

6.1.3　药学教育、科研组织和社团组织体系

药学教育、科研组织和社团组织都是中国药事组织的重要组成部分,其中药学社团组织包括中国药学会及经中国政府批准成立的各药学协会。政府机构改革以来,药学社团组织的行业管理职能有所强化。

6.1.3.1　药学教育组织

中国的药学教育经历了百余年发展,主要由高等药学教育、中等药学教育和药学继续教育三部分组成,已基本形成了多类型、多层次、多种办学形式的教育体系。

截至2016年底,中国设置涉药本科专业的普通高等院校共有458所,其中教育部主管35所,省、自治区、直辖市主管407所。2021年,中国具有药学学术学位授权单位143个,药学专业学位硕士招生单位46个,全国设置药学相关专业的普通高等院校已达498所。

药学继续教育主要由设有药学类专业的高等学校、中等学校和药学会提供。

6.1.3.2　药学科研组织

中国的药学科研组织主要包括独立的药物研究院(所)和附设在高等药学院校、大型制药企业、大型医院的药物研究所(室),其中独立的药物研究院(所)分别隶属于中国科学院、中国医学科学院、军事医学科学院等国家和地方科学院系统,以及中央和地方政府有关部门。

6.1.3.3 药学社团组织

药学社团组织是药事组织、药学人员与政府机构联系的纽带,发挥协助政府管理的作用。其功能包括进行行业或职业的社会管理,任务涵盖学术研究和行业、职业的技术管理,代表性组织有中国药学会、中国药师协会、中国医药企业管理协会等。

6.1.4 药品生产与经营组织体系

药品生产与经营组织是一种经济组织,主要包括药品生产企业及药品批发企业、药品零售企业等药品经营企业。药品生产企业是指生产药品的专营企业或兼营企业,是依法成立的、从事药品生产活动、给社会提供药品、具有法人资格的经济组织,习惯性地被称为药厂。药品经营企业是指经营药品的专营企业或兼营企业,可分为药品批发企业和药品零售企业;前者习惯性地被称为医药公司或中药材公司,后者习惯性地被称为零售药房(药店)。

6.1.5 医疗机构药学组织体系

医疗机构药学组织由医疗机构内提供合格药品,从事以患者为中心、临床药学为基础,促进合理用药的药学技术服务和相关药品管理工作的药学部门组成。为实现医药卫生体制改革下药事工作职能的转变,中国《医疗机构药事管理规定》提出,医疗机构应当根据本机构功能、任务、规模设置相应的药学部门,配备和提供与药学部门工作任务相适应的专业技术人员、设备和设施。药学部门下设的各部门基本上是按职能划分的。直接从事药品供应和药学服务的科室(如门诊、急诊药房,住院药房,中药房,静脉用药配制中心,临床药学室等)为基本的职能部门,保障药品供应和支撑药学服务的科室(如药品物流中心、制剂室、药品检验室、药学研究室等)为派生的职能部门。

中国《医疗机构药事管理规定》明确规定:二级以上医院应当设立药事管理与药物治疗学委员会,其他医疗机构应当成立药事管理与药物治疗学组。它们是医疗机构药品管理的监督机构,也是专门负责对医疗机构各项重要药事工作做出决定的专业技术组织。这些组织根据国家法律和政策制定医疗机构药品使用的方针政策,统一认识,协商解决各种用药问题;通过监督、指导其所属医疗机构科学管理药品和合理用药,加强医疗机构的药品管理,提高用药水平。

医疗机构药学组织在药事组织中占有重要地位和比重,在中国是药师人数最多的药事组织。图 6-2 为中国三级综合医院药学部门可设置的组织机构图。各医院可以参照并结合自身实际设置必需的部门。

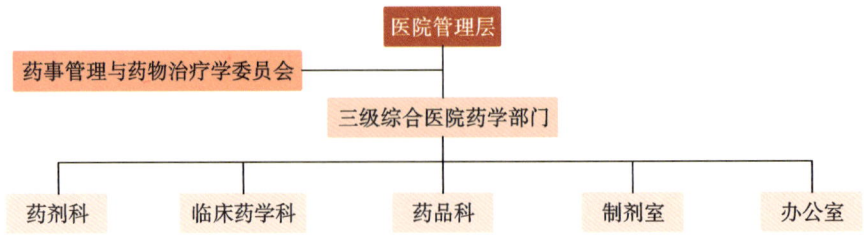

图 6-2 中国三级综合医院药学部门可设置的组织机构图

6.2　中国药品供应保障管理体系

《中华人民共和国药品管理法》明确指出,制定本法的目的是"加强药品管理,保证药品质量,保障公众用药安全和合法权益,保护和促进公众健康"。针对上述目的,中国药品供应保障管理体系主要有以下几个方面的核心内容。

6.2.1　新药研究质量管理与药品注册管理

从药品注册管理的角度来看,新药指在中国境内外均未上市的药品,分为创新药和改良型新药两类。新药开发研究需验证候选药物的安全性、有效性和质量稳定可控性,是一项需要多学科、多部门协作的复杂系统工程。研究过程主要包括临床前研究、临床研究和上市后监测,如图 6-3 所示。

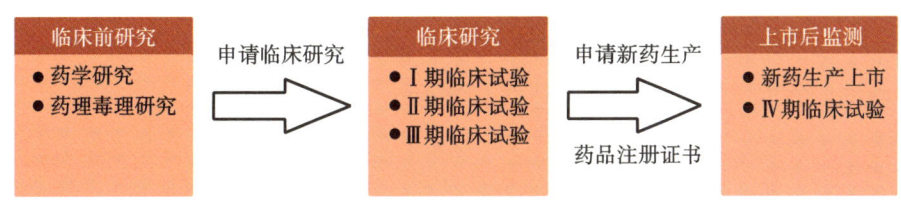

图 6-3　新药的研究过程

数据来源:《药品管理学》(第 2 版),张新平、刘兰茹,2023

药物临床前研究的安全性评价必须执行《药物非临床研究质量管理规范》。该规范是进行药效、毒性动物试验研究的准则,适用于为申请药品注册而进行的非临床研究,是指导科研机构研制安全、有效药物的指令性文件,旨在确保临床前研究的安全性和数据的可靠性。中国现行《药物非临床研究质量管理规范》于 2017 年 6 月 20 日经国家食品药品监督管理总局局务会议审议通过,自 2017 年 9 月 1 日起施行。

《药物临床试验质量管理规范》是规范药物临床试验全过程的质量标准,包括方案设计、组织实施、监查、稽查、记录、分析、总结和报告等内容;目的在于确保药物临床试验过程规范,数据和结果科学、真实、可靠,同时保护受试者和其他研究参与方的权益和安全。随着中国药品研发事业快速发展和药品审评审批制度改革深化,为了适应药品监管工作的需要,国家药品监督管理局会同国家卫生健康委,于 2020 年 4 月 23 日发布了新修订的《药物临床试验质量管理规范》。本规范自 2020 年 7 月 1 日起施行。

药品注册是指药品注册申请人依照法定程序和相关要求提出药物临床试验、药品上市许可、再注册等申请以及补充申请,药品监督管理部门基于法律法规和现有科学认知进行安全性、有效性和质量可控性等审查,决定是否同意其申请的活动。中国《药品注册管理办法》根据药品性质及中国临床用药实际种类,规定药品注册按照中药、化学药和生物制品等进行分类注册管理。各大类又分别按照不同类型药品研发的成熟程度,即对所研制药品的药学特性、药理毒理性质、临床特性的认知状况,该类药品在国内外的上市情况及是否已有国家药品标准,做进一步分类。

6.2.2 药品生产质量监督管理

《药品生产质量管理规范》是全球普遍采用的对药品生产全过程进行监督管理的法定技术规范。在中国,《药品生产质量管理规范》是药品生产企业管理生产和质量的基本准则,适用于药品制剂生产的全过程和原料药生产中影响成品质量的关键工序。中国现行《药品生产质量管理规范》自 2011 年 3 月 1 日起施行,对促进医药行业资源向优势企业集中、淘汰落后产能、调整医药经济结构、促进产业升级、培育具有国际竞争力的企业、加快医药产品进入国际市场发挥了积极作用。虽然 2019 年新修订的《中华人民共和国药品管理法》取消了《药品生产质量管理规范》强制认证。但取消《药品生产质量管理规范》强制认证,并不是取消《药品生产质量管理规范》制度。取而代之的是由省级药品监督管理机构开展的《药品生产质量管理规范》符合性检查,即由五年一次的认证检查改为《药品生产质量管理规范》符合性检查,而且是随机抽查,因此对企业持续符合《药品生产质量管理规范》的标准提出了更高要求。

6.2.3 药品经营质量监督管理

2019 年新修订的《中华人民共和国药品管理法》规定,药品经营企业从事药品经营活动,应当遵守《药品经营质量管理规范》,这一规定的根本目的就是要求药品经营企业进行任何经营活动时都必须以质量为核心,确保药品质量。

2000 年,中国国家药品监督管理局在《医药商品质量管理规范(试行)》的基础上修订形成了《药品经营质量管理规范》,同年又发布了《药品经营质量管理规范实施细则》和《药品经营质量管理规范(GSP)认证管理办法(试行)》。就中国实施药品经营质量管理而言,这是具有里程碑意义的一年。其后,受中国医药行业治理体制机制改革、配套法律法规变化等因素影响,《药品经营质量管理规范》在 2012 年、2015 年和 2016 年经历了 2 次修订和 1 次修正。《药品经营质量管理规范》及《药品经营质量管理规范实施细则》《药品经营质量管理规范现场检查指导原则》等配套文件共同构成了中国药品经营质量管理的规范体系。

6.2.4 医疗机构药事管理

医疗机构药事管理是指医疗机构以患者为中心,以临床药学为基础,对临床用药全过程进行有效的组织实施与管理,促进临床科学、合理用药的药学技术服务和相关的药品管理工作;具体包括药品供应管理、医疗机构制剂管理、调剂和处方管理、药物临床应用管理以及临床药学服务和药学保健等内容。以下主要介绍药品采购、处方点评和合理用药等方面的管理。

药品采购是保证医疗机构药品供应的重要工作,是为了满足医疗服务需要而获得必需药品的过程,其工作质量的优劣直接影响医疗机构医疗服务质量和经济效益的好坏。药品采购管理的主要目标是依法、适时购进质量优良、价格合适的药品。药品采购形式有集中招标采购、邀请招标采购、询价采购等。中国实施的药品带量采购是指在药品集中采购过程中开展招投标或谈判议价时,明确采购数量,让企业针对具体的数量进行报价及议价,价低者中标。其核心为"以量换价",可以理解为大型"团购"或"拼团"。2021 年 1 月《国务院办公厅关于推动药品集中带量采购工作常态化制度化开展的意见》的印发,标志着中国药品集中带量采购工作进入常态化、制度化、规范化的新阶段,该文件成为开展药品集中带量采购工作的纲领。

处方点评是根据相关法规、技术规范,对处方书写的规范性及药物临床使用的适宜性(用药适应证、药物选择、给药途径、用法用量、药物相互作用、配伍禁忌等)进行评价,发现存在或潜在的问题,制定并实施干预和改进措施,促进临床药物合理应用的过程。医院处方点评工作是在医院药事管理与药物治疗学委员会(组)和医疗质量管理委员会的领导下,由医院医疗管理部门和药学部门共同组织实施的。

合理用药是指将适当的药物,以适当的剂量,在适当的时间,经适当的途径,给适当的患者使用适当的疗程,达到适当的治疗目标。临床合理用药管理是指对医疗机构临床诊断、预防和治疗疾病用药全过程实施监督管理。医疗机构应当依据国家宏观管理规定,制定本机构基本药物临床应用管理办法,建立并落实抗菌药物临床应用分级管理制度;建立临床用药监测、评价和超常预警制度,对药物临床使用安全性、有效性和经济性进行监测、分析、评估,实施处方和用药医嘱点评与干预;建立药品不良反应、用药错误和药品损害事件监测报告制度,临床科室一旦发现上述事件应当积极救治患者,立即向药学部门报告,并做好观察与记录。医疗机构应当按照国家有关规定向相关部门报告药品不良反应,用药错误和药品损害事件应当立即向所在地县级卫生行政部门报告。

6.3　中国国家基本药物制度

基本药物是世界卫生组织于1977年提出的一个概念。2019年,《中华人民共和国基本医疗卫生与健康促进法》指出,基本药物是指满足疾病防治基本用药需求,适应现阶段基本国情和保障能力,剂型适宜,价格合理,能够保障供应,可公平获得的药品。

6.3.1　中国国家基本药物制度建设的目的与意义

作为深化医药卫生体制改革的核心政策之一,中国国家基本药物制度的根本目标是保证基本药物的可获得性、价格的可承受性、质量的高水平性和使用的合理性。中国国家基本药物制度建设涉及基本药物的遴选、生产、流通、使用、定价、报销、监测评价等各个环节,与公共卫生、医疗服务、医疗保障体系相衔接。自新医改以来,中国国家基本药物制度的建立和实施,对健全药品供应保障体系、适应群众的基本医疗卫生需求、保障群众基本用药、减轻患者用药负担起到了重要作用。

6.3.2　中国国家基本药物制度建设概况

1979年4月,中国政府积极响应并参与世界卫生组织基本药物行动计划,在卫生部、国家医药管理总局的组织下成立了"国家基本药物遴选小组",着手国家基本药物目录的制定工作。1982年,中国第一版《国家基本药物目录》正式颁布,包含278种药品,到2009年,目录中的药品数量已经增加到了307种,能够用于多数全球重点疾病,包括疟疾、艾滋病、结核病、生殖健康疾病,以及癌症和糖尿病等慢性病的治疗。

2009 年新医改的实施标志着中国国家基本药物制度正式开启新征程。《关于建立国家基本药物制度的实施意见》《国家基本药物目录管理办法（暂行）》《国家基本药物目录（基层医疗卫生机构配备使用部分）》(2009 版)、《国家基本药物临床应用指南（基层部分）》《国家基本药物处方集（基层部分）》以及《建立和规范政府办基层医疗卫生机构基本药物采购机制的指导意见》等政策文件，初步构成了以政府为主导、市场为助力、法律为依据的基本药物生产、流通、供应、使用和监管实施体系。

2014 年后的工作重点主要聚焦国家基本药物制度的巩固完善，重点解决制度的上下衔接和平衡、部分药物配送短缺、服务能力不足、基本药物供应保障、质量一致性评价和临床使用等问题。2018 年 10 月 25 日，中国《国家基本药物目录（2018 年版）》由国家卫生健康委正式发布。新版本目录进一步扩大了药品品种数，进一步优化了目录结构，规范了药品的剂型、规格，同时坚持中西药并重的原则。

6.3.3　中国国家基本药物制度的总体要求

中国国家基本药物制度坚持以人民健康为中心，强化基本药物"突出基本、防治必需、保障供应、优先使用、保证质量、降低负担"的功能定位，从基本药物的遴选、生产、流通、使用、支付、监测等环节完善政策，全面带动药品供应保障体系建设，着力保障药品安全有效、价格合理、供应充分，缓解"看病贵"问题；促进上下级医疗机构用药衔接，助力分级诊疗制度建设，推动医药产业转型升级和供给侧结构性改革。

6.3.4　中国国家基本药物制度的主要内容

中国国家基本药物制度是对基本药物的遴选、生产、流通、使用、支付、监测等诸多环节进行有效管理的制度。

6.3.4.1　基本药物遴选

基本药物的遴选原则包括防治必需、安全有效、价格合理、使用方便、中西药并重、基本保障、临床首选、基层能够配备。国家基本药物目录遴选调整应当坚持科学、公正、公开、透明；建立健全循证医学、药物经济学评价标准和工作机制，科学合理地制定目录；广泛听取社会各界的意见和建议，接受社会监督。

6.3.4.2　基本药物的生产供应

坚持集中采购方向，落实药品分类采购。做好上下级医疗机构用药衔接，推进市（县）域内公立医疗机构集中带量采购，推动降药价。对易短缺的基本药物，通过市场撮合确定合理采购价格、定点生产、统一配送或纳入储备等措施保证供应。

6.3.4.3　基本药物的采购管理

2019 年，国务院办公厅印发《国家组织药品集中采购和使用试点方案》，提出了"国家组织、联盟采购、平台操作"的总体思路和带量采购、以量换价、量价挂钩、招采合一、确保质量、保证回款等主要原则，以及成立试点工作小组及办公室（试点办）和联合采购办公室（联采办）的组织形式。联采办代表联盟地区开展集中采购，下设监督组、专家组、集中采购小组。

6.3.4.4　基本药物的使用管理

坚持基本药物主导地位，明确公立医疗机构基本药物使用比例。实施临床使用监测，开展药品临床综合评价。深化医保支付方式改革，制定药品医保支付标准，引导医疗机构和医务人员合理诊疗、合理用药。

6.3.4.5   基本药物的质量监管

对基本药物实施全品种覆盖抽检,加强对基本药物生产环节的监督检查,强化质量安全监管。推进仿制药质量和疗效一致性评价,对通过一致性评价的药品品种,按程序优先纳入基本药物目录;逐步将未通过一致性评价的基本药物品种调出目录。

6.3.4.6   国家基本药物制度绩效评估

将国家基本药物制度实施情况纳入各级政府绩效考核体系,加强督导评估,建立健全基本药物制度实施督导评估制度,充分发挥第三方评估作用,强化结果运用。

6.3.5   中国国家基本药物制度的调整优化

《"健康中国 2030"规划纲要》明确提出要巩固完善国家基本药物制度。2018 年 9 月,国务院办公厅印发《国务院办公厅关于完善国家基本药物制度的意见》(以下简称《意见》)。《意见》强化了基本药物"突出基本、防治必需、保障供应、优先使用、保证质量、降低负担"的功能定位,重点从基本药物的遴选、生产、流通、使用、支付、监测等环节对政策进行了完善。

一是在目录遴选方面,更加注重突出药品临床价值,坚持动态调整和调入调出并重。对新审批上市、疗效确切、价格合理、能够更好地满足疾病防治需求的药品,也可以考虑纳入目录。同时,考虑到国家基本药物制度已经在政府办基层医疗卫生机构实现全覆盖,允许地方增补药品是制度建设初期的过渡性措施。《意见》明确,原则上各地不增补药品,这也便于比较分析各地医疗机构基本药物使用情况。

二是在保障供应方面,更加注重发挥好政府和市场两方面的作用,总结借鉴近年来药品集中分类采购和解决药品短缺的有效经验做法,从鼓励企业技术改造、完善采购配送机制、加强短缺预警应对等方面做出系统安排,特别强调要提前预防药品短缺,通过监测预警及尽早应对药品短缺问题,多渠道、多方式保障基本药物不断档、不缺货。

三是在配备使用方面,更加注重基层与二级以上医疗机构用药的衔接,助力分级诊疗制度建设,强调各级医疗机构全面配备、优先使用基本药物,规范上下级医疗机构用药的品种、剂型、规格,实现上下联动,为基层首诊、双向转诊、小病在基层、康复回社区提供用药保障。同时,通过医保支付方式改革和财政补助等方式,建立医疗机构和医务人员合理诊疗、合理用药的激励约束机制。

四是在保证质量方面,更加注重与仿制药质量和疗效一致性评价联动,强调按程序将通过一致性评价的药品品种优先纳入基本药物目录,逐步将未通过一致性评价的基本药物仿制药品种调出目录,进一步强化基本药物是"安全药""放心药"的观念。

五是在降低负担方面,更加注重与医保支付报销政策做好衔接,兼顾公共卫生、疾病防治等方面的需要,明确基本药物目录内的治疗性药品,医保部门在调整医保目录时,按程序将符合条件的药品优先纳入目录范围或调整甲乙分类,逐步提高实际保障水平,最大限度减轻患者药费支出,增强公众获得感。

7　中医药服务与管理

中医药是中华文明的瑰宝,中医"治未病"的理念已融入健康中国行动中。目前,中国覆盖城乡,融预防保健、疾病治疗和康复于一体的中医药服务体系初步建成;中医药服务水平与效能不断增强。21世纪以来,中国经历了两场大规模的抗疫防疫战争,创造了人类文明史上人口大国成功走出疫情大流行的奇迹。中西医结合、中西药在这两场抗疫防疫战争中发挥了重大作用,成为中国疫情防控的特色和亮点。传承几千年的中医药经受住了多次实践考验,护佑了中国人民的健康,展现了中华民族瑰宝的时代价值,为全世界抗击传染病疫情和保障全体人民健康提供了方案。

7.1　中医药服务

7.1.1　中医药服务体系

7.1.1.1　中医预防保健服务体系

中医预防保健服务体系是以提供中医药服务为主的中医"治未病"服务体系。加强中医预防保健服务体系建设,是推动中国医改和中医药事业发展的重要方向之一。目前,中国已初步建立了区域性中医预防保健服务网络体系和系统化、全程化的中医预防保健服务内容体系,组建了中医特色鲜明、能独立开展中医预防保健工作的服务平台。中国中医预防保健服务体系包括中医预防保健服务提供体系、中医预防保健服务技术(产品)体系和中医预防保健服务支持体系三个部分。其中,中医预防保健服务由各级中医医院中医预防保健科、综合医院中医预防保健科,以及社区卫生服务中心和乡镇卫生院等城乡基层医疗卫生机构提供;中医预防保健服务技术(产品)体系包括用于个体人健康状态信息的采集、存储、整合与动态检测、监测等的方法和技术;中医预防保健服务支持体系建设包括创建科技创新机制和研发机构、培养专业技术人员、完善中医特色健康保障服务模式、建立相关管理制度和标准规范,以及传播中医健康文化等。

目前,中国中医预防保健服务正蓬勃发展。部分中医医疗机构开设预防保健科,有效整合现有资源,积极开展中医预防保健服务,如推拿、艾灸等。社会办中医养生保健机构如雨后春笋般涌现出来,服务内容日益丰富,成为中医预防保健服务体系的补充。人力资源社会保障部还专门设置了从事中医医疗保健工作的职业,同时制定了相应的标准规范,极大地促进了中医预防保健服务的发展。

7.1.1.2　中医医疗服务体系

中医医疗服务体系是中国医疗服务体系的重要组成部分。根据《国务院关于扶持和促进中医药事业发展的若干意见》，中医医疗服务体系由中医医疗机构和其他医疗机构的中医药卫生资源共同构成，是在提供中医医疗服务过程中所形成的各部分相互关联的一个系统，包括城市中医医疗服务网络和农村中医医疗服务网络。目前中国已基本建立起覆盖城乡的中医医疗服务体系；在城市，形成以中医（民族医、中西医结合）医院、中医类门诊部和诊所以及综合医院中医类临床科室、社区卫生服务机构为主的城市中医医疗服务网络；在农村，形成由县级中医医院、综合医院（专科医院、妇幼保健院）中医临床科室、乡镇卫生院中医科和村卫生室为主的农村中医医疗服务网络，提供基本中医医疗预防保健服务。详见图7-1。

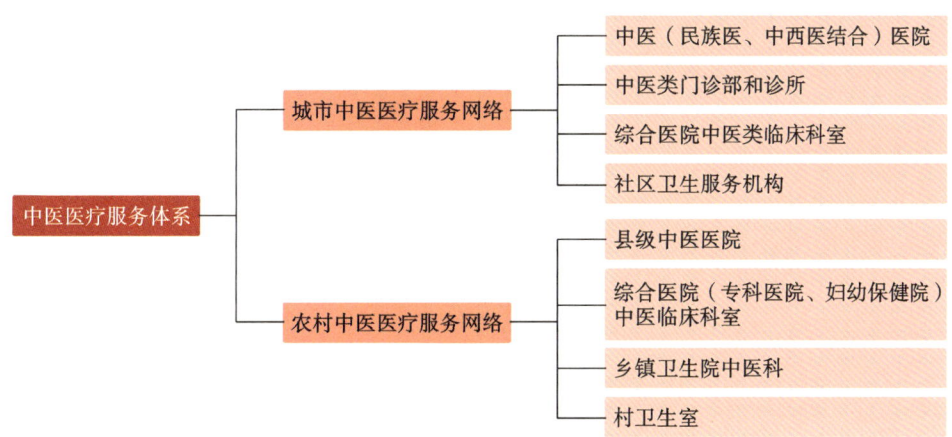

图7-1　中国中医医疗服务体系

中国大部分综合性医疗机构和基层医疗卫生机构都设有中医科，提供以草药、针灸、按摩等传统疗法为主的中医服务。这些服务都不同程度地被纳入城镇职工基本医疗保险及城乡居民基本医疗保险的补偿范围内。

截至2020年底，中国拥有中医类医院5 482个，其中公立中医医院2 332个，民营中医医院2 094个，三级、二级、一级中医医院分别为535个、1 926个与1 155个。在打造中医药服务高地方面，6个中医类医院纳入"辅导类"的国家医学中心创建范围，20个中医医院纳入了国家区域医疗中心输出医院的范围，8个中医项目被确定为国家区域医疗中心建设项目。

7.1.1.3　基层中医药服务体系

以县级中医医院为龙头，社区卫生服务中心、社区卫生服务站、乡镇卫生院、村卫生室为主体，县级综合医院、妇幼保健机构等非中医类医疗机构中医药科室为骨干，社会办中医医院、中医门诊部与诊所为补充的中国基层中医药服务网络已逐步完善。截至2020年底，中国99.0%的社区卫生服务中心、90.6%的社区卫生服务站、98.0%的乡镇卫生院、74.5%的村卫生室能够提供中医药服务，基层中医药服务能力提升工作效果显著，人民群众看中医的公平性、可及性和便利性得到明显改善。

7.1.2　中医药服务类型

7.1.2.1　中医"治未病"服务

中医"治未病"最早源自《黄帝内经》所载的"上工治未病，不治已病，此之谓也"。治未病的思想最早可见于《黄帝内经》,即不治已病治未病,这也是迄今为止中国卫生界普遍遵守的基本思想,可概括为未病先防、既病防变、瘥后防复。中医"治未病"要求不仅要治病,更要防止疾病的发生;不仅要防病,还要对疾病变化的趋势进行预测,在病变产生之前求得解救的办法,在疾病的治疗活动之中把握先机、掌握主动权。

在中国出台的多项文件中,中医"治未病"与中医预防保健等同。推行中医"治未病"健康工程,推动中医预防保健服务体系建设,是中国医改和中医药事业发展的重要方向之一。中医"治未病"服务以个人健康为中心,采取中医独特的预防保健技术来预防疾病发生。中国中医"治未病"健康工程已经历十余年的发展。随着中国新医改的不断深入,中医"治未病"在保障城乡居民健康、预防疾病发生等方面逐渐得到推广应用。据中国国家中医药管理局《全国中医药统计摘编》显示,2019—2021年中国中医类医院完成的健康检查及"治未病"人次数明显增加,年均增长率为8.8%,中医"治未病"预防保健服务体系构建取得了阶段性成效。

7.1.2.2　中医门诊服务

中医门诊服务是指在中医诊疗领域中,综合运用中医学的基本理论和临床经验,为患者提供全面、系统的中医诊疗服务。中国中医门诊服务的执业范围非常广泛,主要包括以下几个方面:第一,中医诊断,通过望、闻、问、切等中医诊断方法,对患者的病情进行诊断。第二,中医治疗,通过中药、针灸、推拿、拔罐等中医治疗方法,对患者进行治疗。第三,中医预防保健,通过中医养生保健理论和方法,指导患者进行预防保健。第四,中西医结合治疗,在中医综合门诊中,可以结合西医的检查和治疗方法,进行中西医结合治疗。第五,中医健康指导,通过中医健康相关理论和方法,对患者进行健康指导,帮助患者维持健康。

根据《医疗机构设置规划指导原则(2016—2020年)》的意见,中国各省基本确立了省级中医医院、市级中医医院、县级中医医院、乡镇卫生院、村卫生室在中医药工作中的功能定位,形成了一个层次分明、结构合理、功能齐全的中医药服务体系。随着中国社会经济的持续高速发展,中国人民生活水平不断提高、对医疗服务的需求不断增加,进而促使中国医疗服务工作不断发展,而中医门诊服务作为医疗服务工作的重要环节之一,也得到了长足发展。2020年,中国中医类医院诊疗量约59 699.2万人次,其中中医类门诊部约3 113.6万人次、中医类诊所15 738.2万人次。自2013年以来,中国中医类医疗机构诊疗量占总诊疗量的比重持续增长,到2020年中医类医疗机构诊疗量占总诊疗量的比例达到了16.8%。

7.1.2.3　中医住院服务

中医住院服务是指以中医类医疗机构为主体,中医技术人员秉承阴阳五行、脏腑经络、整体观念、辨证论治等核心理念,综合运用望、闻、问、切四诊法和辅助仪器,并以中药方剂为主要治疗手段,结合针灸、推拿、拔罐、冬病夏治等独特的治疗方法,向患者提供住院综合医疗服务的过程。

2019年4月,中国国家中医药管理局发布《三级公立中医医院绩效考核指标》,用于对全国三级公立中医医院进行全面、统一的数据采集和考核,其中对中医住院服务提出明确标准和要求。2020年,全国中医类医院出院人数约2 907.1万人,占全国中医类医疗机构出院总数的83%,中医类医院在提供住院服务方面的作用日益突出。

7.1.3　中医药服务理念、特色与优势

7.1.3.1　中医药服务理念

中医理念认为"天人合一"，早在 2 000 多年前自然哲学医学模式就已凸显，充分体现"以人为本"，并尊重人的自然、社会属性，关注心理、情绪、环境等主客观因素对身体健康的影响，并在长期临床实践中形成了"整体观念""辨证论治"等独特理论和治疗方法。随着疾病谱的改变，中医"辨证论治"的个体针对性疗法和中药对现在常见病、多发病的显著疗效越来越受到世界关注。中医从患者自身感受出发，在诊治身心疾病上有其独特的视角和方法，能够有效解决人群亚健康问题。

7.1.3.2　中医药服务特色

中医"形神兼备"的思维能够很好地体现中医药服务特色。中医药服务考虑"神"（即抽象的思维）和"形"（即具体的表现形式）两个方面。只有形神兼具，才能够身心健康。概括来说，中医药服务特色一方面体现于中医完整独特的理论上，即整体观念、辨证论治、恒动理论等；另一方面体现于其诊疗中应用的中医药技术上，如中医望、闻、问、切的四诊技术，以及中医针灸、推拿、拔罐等适宜技术。总而言之，中医药服务是在中医特色理论体系指导下进行的以中医诊疗技术为手段的服务。中医药被认为是除"四大发明"之外的"第五大发明"。2 000 多年来，中医之所以能够一直具有顽强生命力，并且服务水平得到不断提升，离不开其独特的诊疗方法、效果及特有的理论体系。

7.1.3.3　中医药服务优势

中医诊疗设备简易、技术简便，有助于为医疗机构减轻负担。中医药服务具有投入少、成本低的优势。中医"治未病"理论涵盖"未病先防""既病防变"，这与基层医疗卫生服务强调的预防、保健、医疗、康复、健康教育、计划生育、技术指导六位一体的综合服务要求类似。在该理念指导下将健康关口前移，对不同人群辨证论治，调节机体，预防疾病，能够为人类提供健康的生活环境，提高生活质量，为破除因病致贫、因病返贫的恶性循环提供新的解决思路。

中医理论体现出与西医还原论完全不同的健康理念。与现代西医所主张"治已病"的理念不同，中医主张"治未病"，以实现"未病先防、既病防变、瘥后防复"的目标。中国现存较早的医学典籍《黄帝内经》对"治未病"思想也有明确记载："上工治未病，不治已病，此之谓也"。从近些年中国颁布实施的《中医药发展"十三五"规划》《中医医院"治未病"科建设与管理指南(修订版)》等一系列政策文件来看，中国"治未病"导向比较突出，以"促进健康""预防为主""防治结合"等为特点的"治未病"理念逐渐得到人民重视。

7.1.4　中医药服务资源

7.1.4.1　中医类医疗卫生机构

根据中国卫生健康事业发展统计公报，中国医疗卫生机构的构成包括医院、基层医疗卫生机构、专业公共卫生机构以及其他机构。中医类医疗卫生机构包括中医类医院、中医类门诊部、中医类诊所、中医类研究机构、非中医类医疗机构中医类临床科室。中医类医疗卫生机构是提供中医医疗服务的主体。中国中医类医疗卫生机构数从 2015 年的 46 541 个增加到 2022 年的 80 319 个，以年均 8.1％的速度增长，较 2015 年增加 72.6％。

（1）中医类医院

根据中国卫生健康事业发展统计公报，中国中医类医院包括中医医院、中西医结合医院、民族医医院。至 2022 年末，中国中医类医院共 5 862 个，其中中医医院 4 779 个，占比 81.5%，中西医结合医院和民族医医院分别占 13% 和 5.5%。

（2）中医类门诊部与中医类诊所

根据中国卫生健康事业发展统计公报，中国中医类门诊部包括中医门诊部、中西医结合门诊部、民族医门诊部，中医类诊所包括中医诊所、中西医结合诊所、民族医诊所。中医类门诊部与中医类诊所是基层中医药服务网络的组成部分，大多数由社会力量举办。2015—2020 年中医类门诊部年均增速 16.6%，远高于中医类诊所。2022 年，中医类门诊部达 3 786 个，中医类诊所 70 631 个。

（3）中医类研究机构

根据中国卫生健康事业发展统计公报，中国中医类研究机构包括中医（药）研究院（所）、中西医结合研究所、民族医（药）学研究所。2020 年末，中国中医类研究机构共 43 个，其中中医（药）研究院（所）34 个、中西医结合研究所 2 个、民族医（药）学研究所 7 个。

（4）非中医类医疗机构中医类临床科室

根据中国相关标准要求，综合医院中医临床科室应设置为医院一级临床科室；应设立中医病床，床位数不低于医院标准床位数的 5%，具备一定规模的医院，可根据实际需要设立独立病区；应设置独立的中医门诊，三级综合医院开设中医专业不少于 3 个，二级综合医院不少于 2 个。2020 年末，中国综合医院中设有中医类临床科室的有 4 071 个，占同类机构的比重最高（86.7%），设有中医类临床科室的社区卫生服务中心和乡镇卫生院分别达 4 590 个、17 414 个，占同类机构的比重分别为 63.1%、50.1%。

7.1.4.2 中医床位数

中医床位指的是包括中医类医院、中医类门诊部及非中医类医疗机构中医类临床科室等在内的中医类医疗卫生机构所设的床位，其中中医类医院是主体。2020 年，中国医疗卫生机构床位约 910.1 万张，其中中医类医疗卫生机构床位约 143.3 万张，占比 15.7%；中医类医院床位约 114.8 万张（较 2015 年增加 40.1%），占全国医院床位总数的 16.1%，呈现稳步增长趋势。中医类医院床位中，中医医院床位约 98.1 万张（占比 85.5%），中西医结合医院共计约 12.5 万张（占比 10.9%），民族医医院达 42 379 张（占比 3.7%）。

7.1.4.3 中药资源

（1）中药资源的定义与分类

中药资源是自然生态资源的组成部分，是中医药事业发展的重要物质基础。中药资源是指在中医基础理论指导下，于特定范围或区域内散布的、可用于传统医药使用的药用动植物、矿物资源。中药资源并非仅仅是指狭义的传统中药资源，民间的中草药资源与壮药、苗药等民族药资源也同样包含在其中。随着人类对自然资源不断地开采和使用，一些自然资源逐渐稀缺，于是产生了通过生化技术进行人工种植、养殖、制造的人工中药资源。天然中药资源是相对人工中药资源而言的概念，可分为生物资源和非生物资源两大类，其中 99.4% 的资源为生物资源，包括药用动物与植物，可再生，而药用矿物资源为非生物资源，不可再生，约占总量的 0.6%。

（2）现有中药资源现状

中国中药资源的种类、分布、蕴藏量等相关信息主要是通过开展中药资源普查来获取的。中国自1960年起已经开展了4次中药资源普查工作。根据第四次全国中药资源普查数据,中国中药资源种类共有18 817种,其中药用菌物826种（约占4.39%）、药用植物15 227种（约占80.92%）、药用动物2 611种（约占13.88%）、药用矿物153种（约占0.81%）。此外,为了解国家中药资源的区域性变化特点,中国依据行政区域对中药资源的分布情况进行了细致划分。具体而言,海南省拥有近2 500种中药资源,云南省拥有8 875种中药资源,地区分布差异明显。

7.1.4.4　中医药人力资源

中医药人力资源包括中医类别执业（助理）医师（包括中医、中西医结合及各类民族医医师）、中药师（士）、见习中医师三类,从事中医药管理工作的相关人员不纳入统计。

（1）中医药人力资源总量

随着中国对中医药事业的重视及居民对中医药服务需求的增加,中国中医药人力资源总量迅速增长。2021年,全国医疗卫生机构中医药人力资源总量达884 815人。2017—2022年,全国执业（助理）医师数和中医类别执业（助理）医师数持续增长,分别从339万人、52.7万人增长到443.5万人、76.4万人,年均增长率分别为5.5%、7.7%。中药师（士）数从2017年的12万人增长到2022年的13.9万人,年均增长3%。可以看出,在中医药人力资源中,中医类别执业（助理）医师数增长速度较快,而中药师（士）数增长较缓。

（2）中医药人力资源配置及年龄结构

"十三五"期间,中国各地区每万人口中医药人力资源配置量稳步上升,最多从4.43人增长到5.87人;每万人口中药师（士）配置量最少从0.84人增长到0.93人。中部地区每万人口中医药卫生人员、中医类别执业（助理）医师、中药师（士）配置量整体低于全国平均水平,每万人口中医医院卫生技术人员配置量由"十二五"时期的居中,上升为"十三五"末期的领跑全国。在每万人口中医类别执业（助理）医师配置上,西部地区始终领先:西部地区人口相对较少,所以每万人口的配置量相对较高。在每万人口中药师（士）配置上,东部地区高于全国平均水平:东部地区中医药人力资源相对充足,在人口基数大的前提下,其依然领先。

与2017年相比,2021年中国中医药人力资源年龄结构有所变化。就公立中医医院中医执业（助理）医师而言,25岁以下人员占比上升0.5%,25～34岁人员占比上升7%,35～54岁人员占比下降6.3%,55～59岁人员占比上升1.3%,而60岁及以上人员占比下降2.5%。

7.2　中医药管理

7.2.1　中医药管理体系

新中国成立以来,为保障和促进中医药事业的发展,国家成立了专门的中医药管理组织,建立了从中央到地方的分层式中医药管理体系。在不断的实践探索中,中央层面的中医药管理机构先后经历了中医科、中医司、国家中医管理局、国家中医药管理局4次大的跨越。

随着中央层面中医药管理机构的不断升级,地方也陆续建立了相应的中医药管理机构。目前,中国中医药管理机构包含中央级、省级、市级、县级 4 个层级,管理内容涵盖医疗、教育、科研、文化传播等方面。

中国国家中医药管理局作为国家层面主管机构负责规划指导全国中医药管理事业。截至 2018 年,全国已有 31 个省级行政区域完成机构改革,省级层面普遍设立了中医药管理局(处、办),市级中医药管理体系得到进一步完善,而基层中医药管理体系则实现了"从无到有"的飞跃。全国设立相对独立的中医药管理局,并将其归入省卫生健康委管理的省份包括河北、吉林、四川等。省级中医药管理局多为副厅级,其中最典型的是吉林省,该省形成了较为完整的中医药管理体系。相对独立的中医药管理局模式赋予机构独立编制、人事权和专门财政经费,有助于中医药管理机构独立自主开展工作,一定程度上有利于中医药政策的落地。

中国中医药事业实行分部门、分级别监管,主要涉及国家发展改革委、农业农村部、国家卫生健康委、国家中医药管理局等多部委。国家层面设立国家中医药管理局统管中医药事务,省、市两个层面设立中医药管理机构,各县级卫生行政管理机构内设中医药管理部门,各级相关部门均对中医药工作予以配合,以确保中医药事业的政策法规得到有效落实。多部门协作管理体系为中国中医药事业发展提供了可靠的组织保障。

7.2.2 中医药法律体系

中医药事业的发展离不开法制保障。2003 年,《中华人民共和国中医药条例》的出台对于促进、规范中医药事业发展具有重要作用。然而,随着经济社会迅速发展,中国中医药事业发展出现了一系列问题,如中医药服务能力不足,中医药服务市场衰落,现行医师、诊所和药品管理制度难以适应中医药特点及发展需求等。为进一步保障和促进中医药事业发展,2008 年第十一届全国人大常委会将中医药法列入立法规划。《中华人民共和国中医药法》于 2016 年 12 月 25 日由第十二届全国人大常委会第二十五次会议正式通过,并于 2017 年 7 月 1 日起正式实施,这是中医药发展史上具有里程碑意义的大事。作为第一部全面、系统地体现中医药特点的综合性法律,《中华人民共和国中医药法》将中国管理中医药事业发展的方针政策用法律形式固定下来,从法律层面明确了中医药的重要地位,将人民群众对中医药的期望与要求以法律形式呈现出来。以宪法为立法依据的《中华人民共和国中医药法》,保障了中医药的法律地位,为中医药事业发展提供了基本遵循。

7.2.3 中药质量监管

7.2.3.1 全过程质量监管

传统中药包括中药材(涵盖植物、动物、矿物药)、中药饮片、中成药,是中药房里中药的主要形态,其中中药饮片、中成药等中药制剂由中药材经过特定环节加工炮制而成。优质药是治病的物质基础,优质的中药饮片、中成药能够确保中医临床疗效良好。因此,中药的质量监管应该从药材源头抓起。而中药材具备药品、商品、农副产品等多重属性,流通过程包括种植、采收、炮制、包装、储藏、运输、销售等多个环节,在每个环节都有可能出现质量问题,这也决定了相应质量管理的复杂性。

《中华人民共和国中医药法》第三章针对"中药保护与发展"做出了相关规定,其中第二十一条"国家制定中药材种植养殖、采集、贮存和初加工的技术规范、标准,加强对中药材生产流通全过程的质量监督管理,保障中药材质量安全"对中药材生产流通全过程监管总体要求做出了规定;第二十四条对中药材质量监测及中药材流通追溯体系建设做出了规定;第三十一条对医疗机构配制中药制剂做出了规定。

从法律层面而言,目前中国中药监管体系以《中华人民共和国药品管理法》为核心,并涵盖《中华人民共和国药品管理法实施条例》《药品生产质量管理规范》《药品经营质量管理规范》《中药材生产质量管理规范》等行政法规和部门规章。《中华人民共和国药品管理法实施条例》规定了包括中药在内的药品研发、生产、经营、使用和监督管理。《药品生产质量管理规范》《药品经营质量管理规范》《中药材生产质量管理规范》是有关药品生产、经营等的实施细则与操作规范。其他相关规范性文件也起着重要作用,如国家食品药品监督管理机构先后发布的《关于加强中药饮片监督管理的通知》《食品药品监管总局关于进一步加强中药饮片生产经营监管的通知》《食品药品监管总局关于进一步加强中药材专业市场质量监管的通知》等一系列文件,对中药饮片、中药材及中成药的生产、经营监管做出了明确的规定。总体来看,中国中药法律规范已初步形成体系。

在中药组织管理方面,改革开放以后,国务院设置国家医药管理局负责药品监管。而随着药品分散监管的出现,中药监管权改为归属于国家中医药管理局。在 1998 年的机构改革中,国务院整合卫生部药政管理局、国家医药管理局及国家中医药管理局相关职能,成立了国家药品监督管理局。其直属国务院,对药品从研发到销售进行全方位监管。2003 年增加食品、化妆品监管职能后,国家药品监督管理局更名为国家食品药品监督管理局,负责对药品(包括中药材、中药饮片、中成药)的研发、生产、流通、使用进行行政监督和技术监督。地方实行省级以下垂直管理。在 2008 年大部制改革背景下,国家食品药品监督管理局由国务院直属机构变为卫生部管理机构,省级以下药品监督管理机构由垂直管理变为地方管理。2013 年国家食品药品监督管理局更名为国家食品药品监督管理总局,2018 年又更名为国家药品监督管理局(由国家市场监督管理总局管理),对药品的生产、流通、消费等各个环节进行统一监管。

7.2.3.2　质量追溯体系建设

国际标准化组织将可追溯性解释为通过登记的识别码,对商品或行为的历史和使用或位置予以跟踪的能力。追溯体系建设是强化质量安全监管的重要举措。中药材质量可追溯体系概念最早于 2010 年在第三届中医药现代化国际科技大会上提出,以实现对中药材生产、使用全过程的质量监管。中药质量追溯体系采用现代物联网技术及区块链技术、云计算、大数据等其他信息技术,处理中药从种植、加工、生产、流通到使用等全过程的关键信息,进而实现中药"来源可知、去向可追、质量可查、责任可究",即实现"从农田到患者的过程追踪"或"从患者到农田的回溯监管"。中药质量追溯体系建设是保证中药安全、有效、质量可控的一项民生工程。

案例　药学家屠呦呦发现抗疟疾良药——青蒿素

自古以来,人类与疟疾开展了长期的斗争,中国远在公元前的《黄帝内经·素问》中即有记载。直到现在,疟疾仍在许多国家肆虐,威胁着人们的健康和生命。

　　2015年10月5日，瑞典卡罗琳医学院宣布将2015年的诺贝尔生理学或医学奖授予药学家屠呦呦与另外两位科学家，以表彰他们在疟疾等寄生虫病治疗研究方面的贡献，屠呦呦也成为首位获得诺贝尔科学奖项的中国本土科学家。

　　在青蒿素被发现之前，奎宁和氯喹是最主要使用的抗疟药。然而，奎宁和氯喹这类药物治疗疟疾的成效没有延续太久。20世纪60年代，全球许多地区开始出现具有抗药性的疟原虫，尤其是在东南亚和非洲地区，甚至已到无有效药物可用的地步。自此，研发新型抗疟药变得至关重要。到了1972年，屠呦呦及其课题组在筛选了2 000余种中草药方后发现，来自菊科植物青蒿的提取物对鼠疟原虫有一定的抑制效果，但最初由于提取方法不当，有效成分浓度过低。后来在受到中国东晋时期医药学家葛洪的启发，并改用低温乙醚提取法后，课题组成功提取了治疗疟疾的有效活性成分青蒿素，这种提取物对疟原虫的抑制率达到了100%。

　　与其他抗疟药相比，青蒿素类药物具有高效、快速清除疟原虫的作用，但因青蒿素类药物在人体内的半衰期较短，为达到彻底清除疟原虫并减缓抗性的目的，研究人员建议将青蒿素及其衍生物与其他抗疟药联合使用。2004年，《柳叶刀》（The Lancet）刊载论文表明，将青蒿琥酯与其他药物联合使用时恶性疟原虫的治愈率可达到80%以上，而且复燃率与配子体感染率也明显下降。截至2013年，全球87个恶性疟疾流行国家中有79个国家将以青蒿素为基础的联合用药作为恶性疟疾治疗的一线药物。

　　青蒿素为开发新一代抗疟药开创了道路。它来自中药，它的发现挽救了全球特别是发展中国家数百万人的生命。相信随着科研人员和医护人员的不断努力，全球疟疾一定会得到控制乃至消除。

8 中国卫生资源规划

编制卫生资源规划是落实健康中国行动的重要手段，也是推动中国医疗卫生服务体系建设的重要内容。中国卫生资源规划包括卫生人才规划、卫生设施规划、卫生药品规划、卫生资金规划等类型。本章将首先对中国卫生资源规划进行概述，包括卫生资源的定义、分类、配置方式，卫生资源规划的概念、类型、编制原则等内容；其次介绍中国的卫生资源规划指标，并在此基础上介绍中国卫生资源规划编制流程，包括确定卫生资源规划目标、制定卫生资源开发策略、编制预算等环节；最后通过中国卫生人才队伍建设规划案例帮助读者了解中国卫生资源规划的具体形式。

8.1 中国卫生资源规划概述

8.1.1 卫生资源规划相关概念

卫生资源是指社会在提供卫生服务的过程中占用或消耗的各种生产要素的总称，包括卫生人力、经费、设施、装备、药品、信息、知识和技术等，例如一个国家或地区拥有的卫生机构数、床位数、卫生人员数、卫生经费数及卫生经费占国民生产总值的百分比，是衡量一个国家或地区卫生状况的重要指标及卫生部门开展卫生保健活动的物质技术基础。

卫生资源可分为卫生人力资源、卫生物力资源、卫生财力资源、卫生信息和技术等，其中卫生人力资源是指能够提供卫生服务的人员，包括在岗的、在培训（将来准备从事卫生工作）的人员；卫生物力资源是指用于卫生服务的各类设施、器械、药品等实体资源；卫生财力资源是指为了提供卫生服务而支付的货币，包括政府、社会和个人的卫生投入，也称"卫生费用"；卫生信息和技术是指卫生相关的数据、专利、标准、流程等。

中国的卫生资源配置方式主要包括三种，分别是计划配置，即政府决定如何分配资源；市场配置，即价格、竞争等市场机制决定如何分配资源；计划和市场相结合，即政府和市场共同发挥资源配置功能。

卫生资源规划是指根据自然生态环境、社会经济发展、人群健康问题和卫生保健服务需求等因素，确定卫生资源的发展目标、规模和速度，统筹规划、合理配置卫生资源，改善和提高区域内卫生服务质量和数量，提高卫生资源使用效益和效率的科学计划方法。基于卫生资源规划提高资源配置效率是国际普遍做法，也是中国政府合理分配和利用卫生资源、满足人民卫生需求的重要手段。中国政府制定卫生资源规划时主要关注以下三组关系：宏观和微观的关系，即国家对全社会范围内的卫生资源进行调控和机构内部的卫生资源管理的关系;存量和增量的关系,即已有的和即将拥有的卫生资源的关系;公平和效率的关系,即卫生服务资源配置的两种主要价值导向的关系。

8.1.2　中国卫生资源规划的类型

中国卫生资源规划可以按照规划层面、规划主体、规划期限进行分类(图 8-1)。

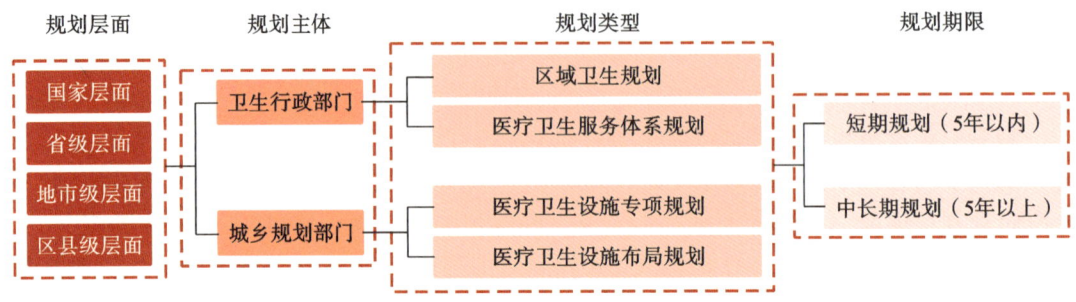

图 8-1　中国卫生资源规划的类型

从规划层面来看,中国卫生资源规划可以分为国家和区域层面的卫生资源规划,其中国家层面的规划主要包括制定国家卫生事业发展的目标、原则、战略蓝图等,具有指导性;区域层面的规划主要根据相应区域的特定经济社会发展和人群健康状况等因素,确定区域卫生发展方向、模式和目标,合理配置不同层次、功能、规模的医疗卫生机构,形成区域卫生的整体发展规划。在中国,往往由国家出台区域卫生规划指导意见,明确一段时期内卫生资源配置的要求,由省级卫生行政部门制定省域内的基本标准,地市级、区县级卫生行政部门再据此制定本区域的规划目标、资源配置标准、主要任务和保障措施,并负责实施。实施区域卫生规划是中国各级政府对卫生事业发展实行宏观调控的依据和手段,也是实现卫生全行业管理的途径。

从规划主体来看,中国卫生资源规划可以分为两类:一类包括区域卫生规划和医疗卫生服务体系规划等,主要由各级卫生行政部门编制和主导实施,主要涉及卫生系统内部的资源配置、服务供给和发展管理。另一类包括医疗卫生设施专项规划、医疗卫生设施布局规划等,由城乡规划部门编制,主要涉及医疗卫生设施用地安排、空间配置匹配度等。本章重点介绍前者,即由各级卫生行政部门编制和主导实施的规划。

从规划期限来看,中国卫生资源规划可以分为短期规划和中长期规划。短期规划主要是指各级政府按照国民经济和社会发展的五年规划来制定的规划,如《"十四五"国民健康规划》《"十四五"全民医疗保障规划》《"十四五"卫生健康标准化工作规划》等"十四五"时期的规划,这类规划的时间范围都是从 2021 年到 2025 年。中长期卫生规划则面向更长的时间范畴,如中共中央、国务院于 2016 年 10 月 25 日印发的《"健康中国 2030"规划纲要》,这是新中国成立以来首次在国家层面提出的健康领域中长期战略规划,主要内容包括提高人民健康水平、优化人口结构和健康素养、建设现代医疗卫生服务体系、构建全方位全周期健康服务模式、推进医药卫生体制改革、加强健康产业发展等六个方面。

8.1.3　中国卫生资源规划编制原则

为确保卫生资源规划的科学性、可行性,各国政府在编制卫生资源规划时往往遵循一系列原则。这些原则不仅符合卫生事业发展规律,而且与国家的政治体制紧密相连。国际常用的卫生资源规划编制原则主要有以下五个：一是目标性原则，明确可操作、可测量、可达成和可评价的具体目标；二是过程性原则，遵循科学的规划编制流程，包括背景分析、目标设定、目标修正、战略制定、战略实施和监测评价等步骤；三是协调性原则，协调好各级各类卫生机构和卫生人员的关系，对资源进行合理配置和有效利用，避免浪费；四是系统性原则，从整体和动态的角度考虑卫生系统内部和外部各种因素，分析其相互影响和作用，最终建立一个完整的卫生规划体系；五是可持续性原则，符合社会经济发展水平和人民健康需求，保证卫生事业长期发展，同时注重保护环境和资源。

中国根据本国国情，经过多年探索，逐渐形成了以下五个具体的卫生资源规划编制原则。

一是协调性原则。首先，中国卫生资源规划要与国民经济和社会发展相协调，政府应根据不同地区的情况，确定合适的卫生发展目标、规模和速度；要考虑社会经济对卫生事业发展和人群健康的影响，利用有利条件，抓住发展机遇，适应社会经济发展变化和要求，解决工业化、城镇化、人口老龄化等带来的健康问题；要以健康需求为导向，科学合理地确定各级各类医疗卫生机构的数量、规模和布局。其次，要协调各方的利益和诉求，充分听取各方意见，形成共识。卫生事业诸多问题的解决需要政府和社会各方共同努力。因此，要加强各方之间的互动和沟通协调。

二是系统性原则。系统性原则也称整体性原则，强调卫生规划工作者应将卫生事业及其各个组成部分视作相互联系的系统。卫生系统功能的实现不仅靠其自身，还受到社会其他系统的影响。卫生系统里的各个部分也是一样。编制卫生资源规划是为了提高卫生系统及其各个部分的服务效率，而不只是分配卫生资源。要让卫生资源更好地发挥作用，就要加强卫生系统内部和外部的合作，而这需要政府和市场一起发力。在这个过程中，中国政府需要落实其在制度、规划、筹资、服务、监管等方面的责任，保证公共医疗卫生的公益性，满足人民群众不同的医疗卫生服务需求。

三是可持续性原则。作为指导卫生系统运作的重要规划，卫生资源规划的编制尤其要强调可持续发展理念。编制卫生资源规划的目标之一是解决卫生问题。规划要考虑现在和将来的卫生需要，不仅要解决现有的卫生问题，还要预防和避免新的卫生问题的出现。有时，政府编制某项卫生资源规划是为了解决某个现有的具体卫生问题。由于政府高度重视，规划职能得以有效发挥，卫生问题便得以解决了。但问题解决后，规划往往就停止执行了，所以一段时间后，同样的卫生问题又出现了。

四是分类指导原则。中国人口众多，幅员辽阔，各地经济发展不平衡，卫生资源的数量和分布、卫生服务水平和人民的健康水平都有很大的差别。编制卫生资源规划时要根据不同地区、系统、机构、组织的具体情况，人民的健康需求，经济社会发展水平和卫生资源现状，合理统筹不同区域、类型、层级的卫生资源的数量和布局，分类制定配置标准。这一原则体现在确定目标、选择策略和配置资源上，如明确和落实各级各类医疗卫生机构的功能任务，根据人口数量、分布、年龄结构以及交通条件、诊疗需求等，实行"中心控制、周边发展"，合理配置各区域医疗卫生机构数量，推动各区域医疗资源均衡布局、同质化发展。

五是公平与效率兼顾原则。公平和效率是中国政府开展各项工作的基本原则。没有效率，卫生工作就不能持续开展；没有公平，就违背了卫生事业发展的目的。所以，编制卫生资源规划时要同时考虑公平和效率，既要将资源用好，也要保障社会各阶层，特别是弱势群体在获取卫生资源、卫生服务方面的机会公平。具体而言，首先，要保障基本医疗卫生服务的可及性，促进公平公正；其次，要注重卫生资源配置与使用的科学性和协调性，提高效率，降低成本，实现公平与效率的统一。

8.2　中国卫生资源规划的制定

8.2.1　卫生资源规划指标

卫生资源规划指标是定量或定性反映卫生资源规划实施效果的标准，具有指导区域卫生事业发展、优化卫生资源和活动、评价卫生资源规划实施效果、支撑卫生战略和政策、促进卫生服务水平提升和公共健康的作用。

中国的卫生资源规划指标可以分为两类：约束性指标和预期性指标。约束性指标是规划期结束时必须达到的指标，是政府的职责和承诺，也是上级政府对下级政府的要求；政府要利用公共资源和行政力量保证约束性指标的实现。预期性指标是规划期结束时希望达到的指标，是政府的意志；政府要用政策手段引导、调控、干预社会资源，使其达到或不偏离期望值。按照涉及卫生资源类型的不同，中国的卫生资源规划指标可以分为卫生人力资源配置指标、医疗卫生机构床位配置指标、卫生费用配置指标和其他卫生资源配置指标。

卫生人力资源配置指标包括数量指标及结构指标。常用指标包括以下五类：一是每千人口卫生技术人员数，反映当地的卫生技术人员总量（卫生技术人员是指在各种医疗卫生机构工作的卫生专业人员，包括执业医师、执业助理医师、注册护士、检验技师、卫生监督员等，不包括从事管理工作的卫生专业人员）；二是每千人口执业（助理）医师数，即每千人口中取得执业资格且实际从事医疗、预防保健工作的卫生人员数量，从事管理工作的执业资格获得者不包括在内；三是每千人口注册护士数，即每千人口中取得注册护士资格的卫生人员数量；四是其他卫生技术人员数，对于特殊的专科医师及公共卫生医师，一般以每万人口计算，如每万人口精神卫生医师数、每万人口儿科医师数等；五是卫生人力资源的结构及分布，反映卫生人力资源的质量及配置的合理性，在卫生资源规划中可以对卫生人力资源的专业结构、学历及职称结构等提出合理的要求。

医疗卫生机构床位配置指标也包括数量指标及结构指标。常用指标包括每千人口医疗卫生机构床位数（区域内医疗卫生机构床位总量配置指标）以及医疗卫生机构床位配置结构及分布——根据区域内医疗卫生机构床位分布现状及存在的问题，可以增加某些特殊床位的配置指标，以满足相应方面的特殊需要，如康复、精神卫生、儿科等，一般按每千人口配置，也可以根据某种特殊床位占总床位的比重来配置。例如，为大力发展社会办医，《"十三五"卫生与健康规划》制定了到 2020 年社会办医院床位占医院床位总数的比重超过 30％的预期目标。为促进基层卫生事业的发展，卫生资源规划中还可以明确各级医疗卫生机构床位规模（表 8-1）。

表 8-1　2025 年中国卫生资源规划相关指标水平

主要指标	2020 年现状	2025 年目标	指标性质
每千人口医疗卫生机构床位数（张）	6.46	7.40～7.50	指导性
其中：市办及以上公立医院（张）	1.78	1.90～2.00	指导性
县办公立医院及基层医疗卫生机构（张）	2.96	3.50	指导性

主要指标	2020 年现状	2025 年目标	指标性质
每千人口公立中医类医院床位(张)	0.68	0.85	指导性
每千人口执业(助理)医师数(人)	2.90	3.20	预期性
每千人口中医类别执业(助理)医师数(人)	0.48	0.62	预期性
每千人口注册护士数(人)	3.34	3.80	预期性
每千人口药师(士)数(人)	0.35	0.54	预期性
医护比	1∶1.15	1∶1.20	预期性
床人(卫生人员)比	1∶1.48	1∶1.62	预期性
二级及以上综合医院设置老年医学科的比例(%)	—	≥60.00	预期性
县办综合医院适宜床位规模(张)	—	600～1 000	指导性
市办综合医院适宜床位规模(张)	—	1 000～1 500	指导性
省办及以上综合医院适宜床位规模(张)	—	1 500～3 000	指导性

注:1.医院床位含同级妇幼保健院和专科疾病防治院(所)床位。

2."省办"包括省、自治区、直辖市举办;"市办及以上"包括省办及以上和市办,其中"市办"包括地级市、地区、州、盟举办;"县办"包括县、县级市、市辖区、旗举办。

3.适宜床位规模指综合医院单个执业点的床位规模。

数据来源:国家卫生健康委

卫生费用配置指标同样包括数量指标及结构指标。前者反映卫生费用的总量及其变化趋势,如卫生总费用;后者反映卫生费用的分配、使用情况及卫生服务的公平性,如卫生总费用中的政府卫生支出(表 8-2)。

表 8-2　中国"十四五"时期全民医疗保障发展主要指标

类别	主要指标	2020 年	2025 年	指标属性
参保覆盖	基本医疗保险参保率(%)	>95	>95[1]	约束性
基金安全	基本医疗保险(含生育保险)基金收入(万亿元)	2.5	收入规模与经济社会发展水平更加适应	预期性
	基本医疗保险(含生育保险)基金支出(万亿元)	2.1	支出规模与经济社会发展水平、群众基本医疗需求更加适应	预期性
保障程度	城镇职工基本医疗保险政策范围内住院费用基金支付比例(%)	85.2	保持稳定	预期性
	城乡居民基本医疗保险政策范围内住院费用基金支付比例(%)	70	保持稳定	预期性
	重点救助对象符合规定的住院医疗费用救助比例(%)	70	70	预期性
	个人卫生支出占卫生总费用的比例(%)	27.7	27	约束性

续表

类别	主要指标	2020 年	2025 年	指标属性
精细管理	实行按疾病诊断相关分组付费和按病种付费的住院费用占全部住院费用的比例(%)	—	70	预期性
	公立医疗机构通过省级集中采购平台采购药品金额占全部采购药品(不含中药饮片)金额的比例(%)	75 左右	90	预期性
	公立医疗机构通过省级集中采购平台采购高值医用耗材金额占全部采购高值医用耗材金额的比例(%)	—	80	预期性
	药品集中带量采购品种(个)	112	>500[2]	预期性
	高值医用耗材集中带量采购品种(类)	1	>5[3]	预期性
优质服务	住院费用跨省直接结算率[4](%)	>50	>70	预期性
	医疗保障政务服务事项线上可办率(%)	—	80	预期性
	医疗保障政务服务事项窗口可办率(%)	—	100	约束性

注:1 指"十四五"期间基本医疗保险参保率每年保持在 95% 以上。

2 指到 2025 年各省(自治区、直辖市)国家和省级药品集中带量采购品种达 500 个以上。

3 指到 2025 年各省(自治区、直辖市)国家和省级高值医用耗材集中带量采购品种达 5 类以上。

4 指住院费用跨省直接结算人次占全部住院跨省异地就医人次的比例。

数据来源:国务院办公厅

此外,卫生资源还包括房屋、设备、信息、技术等。中国各级政府通常会对大型医疗设备的配置量进行规划,如区域内电子计算机断层扫描仪、核磁共振成像仪等设备的每万人口配置量。2019 年,国家卫生健康委、国家中医药管理局发布了《全国基层医疗卫生机构信息化建设标准与规范(试行)》,为基层医疗卫生机构信息化制定了共计 4 个一级指标、58 个二级指标、212 个三级指标,其中包括基层医疗卫生机构要提供基于互联网的医疗健康服务,要具备预约、缴费、诊疗建议、医患沟通等 8 项功能。

8.2.2 中国卫生资源规划编制流程

中国各级政府在编制卫生资源规划时应综合考虑内外部影响因素,根据人群健康服务需要确定卫生资源配置目标,明确现实与目标的差距;应先认识问题,然后提出规划方案,等方案批准后,再组建领导小组和工作小组,明确分工,培训成员,并安排经费等事项。

第一步:卫生形势分析。编制卫生资源规划时要综合考虑政治、经济、社会发展、自然环境等多方面的因素,既要关注卫生系统自身情况,也要关注卫生事业的发展变化;不仅要关注现在的情况,还要关注过去和未来的情况。可以通过做调查、借鉴已有研究成果、查阅居民健康档案、开座谈会等方法收集资料,以便进行全面的动态分析。

中国各级卫生行政部门所做卫生形势分析的主要范围和内容有以下 4 个方面:一是现状分析,从自然、政治、社会、经济等方面分析,常用的方法有问题排列法、趋势外推法、标准分析法、专家评价法等；二是回顾性分析，针对人口、疾病、卫生服务需要与需求、卫生资源利用等方面进行分析；三是前瞻性分析，分析和预测经济、人口、疾病等方面的发展趋势；四是主要障碍分析，分析影响社会卫生问题解决和卫生事业发展的主要障碍，以制定有针对性的政策措施。

中国卫生资源规划中常用的卫生形势分析方法有以下 6 种：一是描述性分析方法，说明卫生服务或健康事件在社会人群中的分布状况和变化规律；二是因素分析法，明确人群健康和卫生服务方面存在的问题和影响因素，包括单因素分析法和多因素分析法；三是数学模型分析法，用数学模型从理论上说明卫生服务与有关因素变量间的函数关系；四是系统分析方法，即把要解决的卫生问题当作一个系统，对系统要素进行分析，诊断问题，揭示问题起因，提出解决问题的可行方案；五是投入产出分析，解释卫生服务投入（卫生资源）与产出（卫生服务利用）之间的关系，常用的方法是成本效益分析和成本效果分析；六是综合评价法，研究人群健康状况和医疗卫生需求、卫生资源、卫生服务利用三者之间的关系。

第二步：确定人群健康目标。卫生资源规划目标体现了卫生行政部门对卫生事业发展的规划及调控措施。制定目标时，卫生行政部门往往遵循以下 3 个步骤：明确规划主旨，也就是总体方向；确定优先发展和重点关注的领域，提出战略举措、具体措施；确定核心指标，根据基线水平设定定性、定量指标，为后期评估提供依据。因此，卫生资源规划目标具有层次性，是一个由总目标、具体目标和指标构成的目标体系。总目标明确长期导向和发展方向，反映了规划期内的人群健康预期。具体目标包括要达到的状况或条件的特征、质量、数量、时限以及涉及的人群和地区。指标是目标的具体体现，也是衡量目标实现的标准。

第三步：分析卫生资源需要，确定卫生资源规划目标。首先要分析需要哪些资源，需要多少，何时需要，如何分配等。在编制卫生资源规划过程中，通常要遵循以下几个方面的经验：根据效果定投入，根据经济水平定规模；先用好现有资源，再考虑增配资源；考虑投入成本和收益；尊重财务人员意见；制订弹性计划。其次，要根据上述分析确定卫生资源规划目标。常用计算方法包括卫生服务需求法、卫生健康需要法、服务目标法、卫生资源人口比值法 4 种方法。2020 年印发的《国家卫生健康委规划管理办法（试行）》明确指出，编制卫生健康规划应当做好现状调查、信息搜集、课题研究等基础性工作，深入研究重大问题，确定优先目标，研究提出重大项目和行动措施并进行充分论证。前期的基础性研究是编制规划的基础，而规划发展定位是规划思路的前提。

第四步：制定卫生资源开发策略及具体实施措施。卫生资源开发策略主要有 4 种：自力更生、动员社会资源、拓展筹资渠道、优化存量卫生资源配置。同时，制定具体实施措施时需要明确措施内容、措施实施原因、实施范围、实施主体以及实施时间。

第五步：监督和评价。主要包括以下 4 个步骤：建立规划执行与评价组织；明确分工及责任；制定详细的实施方案；制定实施情况的考核、监测办法，包括考核和监测的内容、方法、时间及负责人。

第六步：编制预算。中国编制卫生资源规划预算时主要考虑以下几个方面的问题：优先投入重点领域，保证重点目标和主要卫生策略；预算安排要适应当地经济发展水平，不超出财政和个人支付能力；进行成本效益和成本效果分析，把更多资金投向应对疾病的活动，并预留调整卫生资源分配所需资金；计算一次性投资预算时，要进行可行性论证，并考虑维修费用和人员工资增长等因素；考虑筹集卫生资金，包括单位自有资金的渠道；由于规划期较长,需要制定逐年滚动的年度预算。

第七步:可行性论证。区域卫生资源规划草案形成后,要组织区域内外有关部门和专家对草案进行审阅、研讨并提出意见,同时也要让公众了解规划的中心思想;要设置一套可行性论证评价指标体系,以便给参加论证评价的专家提供可以进行比较的资料。规划编制人员应尽可能不影响或诱导专家的意见。专家给出意见后,应根据专家意见,修改、补充和完善规划草案。条件允许的情况下,建议用电脑进行模拟,以检验草案的可行性,之后再做修改,形成送审稿。

第八步:上报审批。卫生资源规划必须经过必要的立法程序,草案要经过卫生资源规划领导小组通过、人民政府审定、人民代表大会常务委员会审议通过且颁布,才有法律效力。编制卫生资源规划的全过程都要体现政府负责、多部门配合、卫生部门管理、社会参与和法律保障的精神。

案例 中国卫生人才队伍建设"十四五"规划

"十三五"期间,中国卫生人员总量和人均数量都实现了增长。截至 2020 年末,中国共有 1 347.5 万卫生人员,包括 408.6 万执业(助理)医师、470.9 万注册护士。为进一步加强卫生人才队伍建设,为健康中国建设提供强有力的人才支撑,2022 年 8 月,国家卫生健康委印发了《"十四五"卫生健康人才发展规划》,提出"十四五"期间的总体目标是:促进人才服务能力提高与结构优化,完善人才管理制度机制,营造人才发展的良好环境。中国"十四五"期间卫生健康人才发展主要规划指标见表 8-3。

表 8-3 中国"十四五"期间卫生健康人才发展主要规划指标

主要指标	单位	2020 年	2025 年
人员总量	万人	1 347.5	1 600
执业(助理)医师	人/千人口	2.90	3.20
中医类别执业(助理)医师	人/千人口	0.48	0.62
注册护士	人/千人口	3.34	3.80
药师(士)	人/千人口	0.35	0.54
全科医生	人/万人口	2.90	3.93
专业公共卫生机构人员	万人	92.5	120

一、人才配备

加强卫生技术人才队伍建设。以医师和护士配置为重点,根据居民卫生服务需求量和医师标准工作量等因素确定人员数量和比例。扩大医师规模,到 2025 年全国执业(助理)医师达到 450 万人;壮大护士队伍,到 2025 年注册护士达到 550 万人;增加药师配置和培养培训,到 2025 年医疗卫生机构药师达到 77 万人;加强医学影像、检验、病理等技术人才建设,制定配置标准,明确岗位职责、能力素质要求及执业规范。

加强公共卫生人才队伍建设。到 2025 年,专业公共卫生机构人员数达到 120 万人,其中疾病预防控制机构人员数达到 25 万人。科学设置公共卫生岗位,调整公共卫生机构高、中、初级岗位结构,增加中、高级岗位比例,提高人员待遇。

加强基层卫生人才队伍建设。加快培养全科医生,到 2025 年全科医生数量达到 55 万人,每万人口全科医生数达到 3.93 人。加强村卫生室人才队伍建设,推动乡村医生向执业(助理)医师转变,到 2025 年乡村医生中执业(助理)医师比例达到 45% 左右。

加强中医药人才队伍建设。到 2025 年,每千人口中医类别执业(助理)医师达到 0.62 人,全国中药师达到 15 万人。构建符合中医药特点的人才培养模式,以重大项目促进中医药人才发展,实施中医药特色人才培养工程(岐黄工程)。

加强应对人口老龄化人才队伍建设。积极应对人口老龄化及人口政策变化,以适应老年人、孕产妇、婴幼儿等重点人群健康服务需求为导向,统筹预防、医疗、护理、康复、安宁疗护等各类人才资源配置,加强老年健康服务、托育服务、妇女儿童健康服务人才建设。

二、人才培养

构建以"5+3"为主体、"3+2"为补充的临床医学人才培养体系,健全在岗培训制度,鼓励乡村医生参加学历教育。加大对中西部地区高等医学院校的支持,缩小区域、院校和学科专业之间培养水平的差距。

实施医学高层次人才计划,重点培养一批在医疗卫生一线工作,医疗技术精湛,能成功诊治疑难、危重病症,具有重大科学价值、显著社会效益,社会影响较大、同行公认的临床医学领军人才。到 2025 年,卫生健康系统医学研发人员全时当量达到 18 万人年。以国家青年高层次人才计划、医学科技创新平台基地和科技计划项目为依托,开展高层次、创新型、复合型临床人才培养与优秀青年创新团队建设。继续做好突出贡献中青年专家等人才选拔工作,做好高层次人才分类统计。

适应疾病谱变化和医疗服务需求,重点加强重症、肿瘤、心脑血管等临床专(学)科人才培养和建设。以省域死亡率高、外转率高的疾病为重点,强化国家级高水平医院对省级医院的技术和人才支持,补齐专业专科短板,提升省域诊疗能力。加强县级医疗机构人才建设,重点加强肿瘤、心脑血管等专科人才队伍建设。

三、人才使用

健全事业单位用人机制,实行公开招聘和竞聘上岗。深化公立医院收入分配制度改革,实行多劳多得、优绩优酬。创新公立医疗卫生机构编制管理模式,合理核定医疗卫生机构人员编制总量,并进行动态调整,探索多种形式用人机制和政府购买服务方式。

完善院校教育、毕业后教育、继续教育三阶段有机衔接、标准规范的医学人才培养体系。以行业需求为导向,提高院校医学教育质量,促进医学人才供需平衡。

合理制定公立医疗卫生机构人员编制标准并建立动态核增机制,加强医院、基层医疗卫生机构、专业公共卫生机构之间的人才协作。完善职称评价标准,改进职称管理服务方式,坚持以用为本,完善岗位设置,明确岗位职责、任职资格条件、胜任能力要求等。扩大医疗卫生机构岗位设置和人员聘用自主权,优化医疗卫生机构岗位结构,提高中、高级专业技术岗位比例。

建立健全适应医疗卫生行业特点的薪酬制度。改善公立医院收支结构，提高人员经费支出占比。优化医务人员薪酬结构，提高保障性工资水平。允许公共卫生机构突破现行事业单位工资调控水平。落实基层医疗卫生机构绩效工资政策，提高基层卫生人员收入水平。

9 中国卫生筹资与卫生总费用

有限的卫生资源与居民日益增长的健康需求之间的矛盾永远存在。卫生筹资不仅涉及卫生资金的筹集，还包括如何对其进行有效分配和使用。筹集足够的资金并实现资金的有效分配和使用，是保证卫生服务体系有效运行以及其功能得以有效发挥的重要途径和手段。中国根据自身的发展历史和发展现状，采取了政府主导、多源协同的筹资策略和方法。根据《中国卫生健康统计年鉴（2022）》，2021 年中国卫生总费用为 76 844.99 亿元，占 GDP 的 6.72%，其中个人卫生支出占比为 27.60%，低于世界平均水平，人均卫生费用为 5 440.0 元。

本章涵盖中国卫生筹资、中国卫生资金的分配和使用、卫生总费用三部分内容。

9.1 中国卫生筹资

如前文所述，卫生资源是指社会在提供卫生服务的过程中占用或消耗的各种生产要素的总称，包括卫生人力资源和卫生物力资源等。卫生资金是卫生资源的货币表现。卫生资源首先以货币形式流入卫生领域，然后通过各种形式的卫生服务实现消耗和补偿，从而流出卫生领域、改善人群健康，这一过程被称为卫生资金运动。从某种意义来说，卫生筹资研究就是研究卫生领域的资金运动规律。

9.1.1 卫生筹资概述

9.1.1.1 卫生筹资概念

世界卫生组织把卫生筹资活动解释为实现足够的、公平的、有效率和效果的卫生资金的筹集、分配和使用活动的总和。它包括 4 个方面的内涵：如何为卫生服务筹集足够的资金、如何合理分配资金及组织服务、如何提高资金的使用效率、如何控制卫生费用不合理增长。卫生筹资是为提供卫生服务而进行的资金筹集活动，研究在一定时期和一定社会环境下卫生领域资金的筹集、合理分配和有效使用，具有资金筹集、风险分担和服务购买 3 项功能。对卫生筹资的评价，主要是对各种不同筹资方式的评价。

9.1.1.2 卫生筹资目标

1978 年，世界卫生组织和联合国儿童基金会在《阿拉木图宣言》中提出初级卫生保健策略，要求各国向居民提供最基本的、人人都能得到的、体现社会平等权利的、人民群众和政府都能负担得起的卫生保健服务。卫生筹资的目标包括中间目标和最终目标两类。卫生筹资的中间目标主要包括卫生筹资的公平、效率、风险共担及持续性。卫生筹资的最终目标包括改善健康状况、提供风险保障和提高患者满意度等。

9.1.2　中国卫生资金的筹集

9.1.2.1　中国卫生筹资来源

国际分类中，卫生筹资来源分为两大类：公共卫生支出和私人卫生支出。前者又被称为广义政府卫生支出，并且可以进一步被细分为政府预算（税收）和社会医疗保险支出，代表了政府组织和机构作为筹资主体在卫生筹资中所发挥的作用。私人卫生支出则是指由居民自行或者通过其雇主参加自愿医疗保险或社区保险（而非政府举办或强制保险）所支付的费用；这部分支出又被分为商业医疗保险支出以及个人卫生支出，非政府举办的卫生机构所发生的费用支出也计入私人卫生支出。

在中国，政府卫生支出、社会卫生支出以及个人卫生支出是卫生总费用的三个主要来源。政府卫生支出包括各级政府用于医疗卫生服务（包括医疗服务以及公共卫生服务）、医疗保险行政管理事务等领域的费用，其他用于医疗卫生领域的政府投入也纳入政府卫生支出。社会卫生支出指政府支出外的社会各界对卫生事业的资金投入，包括社会医疗保障支出（政府补贴除外）、商业医疗保险费、社会捐赠援助、社会办医支出和行政事业性收费收入等。个人卫生支出指居民在接受各类医疗卫生服务时的现金支付。中国卫生筹资来源与国际卫生筹资来源的比较见图 9-1，2000—2021 年中国卫生筹资结构变化情况见图 9-2。

国际卫生筹资来源	类别		具体内容	类别	中国卫生筹资来源
	公共卫生支出（广义政府卫生支出）	政府预算（税收）	政府用于医疗服务、公共卫生服务、卫生监督等的支出	政府卫生支出	
		社会医疗保险支出	政府提供的社会医疗保险[1]补助		
			个人（及其雇主）支付的社会医疗保险费	社会卫生支出	
	私人卫生支出	商业医疗保险支出	商业医疗保险费		
		其他非政府机构支出	非政府机构卫生支出及社会捐赠援助等		
		个人卫生支出	居民在接受各类医疗卫生服务时的现金支付	个人卫生支出	

图 9-1　中国卫生筹资来源与国际卫生筹资来源的比较

注：1 此处的社会医疗保险指城镇职工基本医疗保险及城乡居民基本医疗保险。

数据来源：《转型中的中国卫生体系》，孟庆跃等，2015

9.1.2.2　中国法定卫生筹资体系

中国法定卫生筹资体系覆盖基本医疗保险、医疗救助及疾病应急救助体系、公共卫生体系以及城乡居民大病保险等，其中基本医疗保险与医疗救助体系共同构成了覆盖城乡居民的基本医疗保障体系。具体而言，城镇地区职工参加城镇职工基本医疗保险，城镇地区非从业居民、农村地区居民则参加城乡居民基本医疗保险。医疗救助及疾病应急救助体系是城乡地区贫困人口的安全网，为贫困人口支付基本医疗保险费的同时对基本医疗保险报销后的费用提供进一步的补助。公共卫生体系主要由政府进行筹资，免费向全体居民提供基本

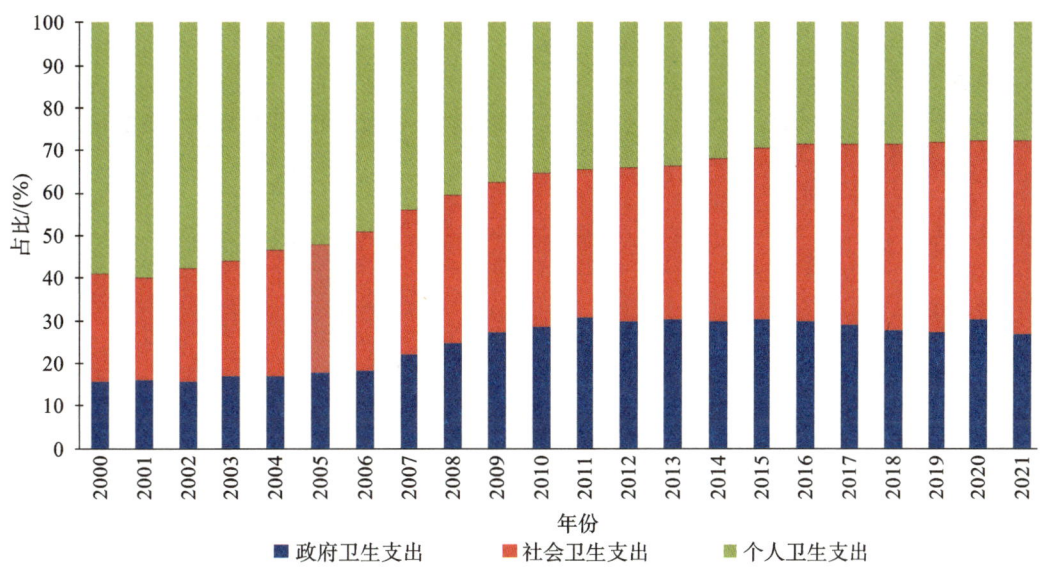

图 9-2　2000—2021 年中国卫生筹资结构变化情况

数据来源:《中国卫生健康统计年鉴(2022)》

公共卫生服务。城乡居民大病保险是在基本医疗保障的基础上,对大病患者发生的高额医疗费用给予进一步保障的一项制度性安排。中国法定卫生筹资体系概况见表 9-1。

表 9-1　中国法定卫生筹资体系概况

体系		覆盖			筹资		资金使用	
		宽度 (人口)	广度 (服务)[1]	深度 (费用)[1]	政府卫生支出	社会保险费	财政转移支付	医疗保险基金[1]
基本医疗保险	城镇职工基本医疗保险	城镇地区职工	定点机构的住院、门诊及零售药品费用	对于医疗保险药品/医疗服务/诊疗项目目录范围内费用设定起付标准、共付以及最高支付限额		个体与雇主共同承担,至少分别支出2%和6%的职工工资		个人医疗账户＋统筹基金
	城乡居民基本医疗保险[2]	城镇地区非从业居民(包括学生)及农村地区居民	住院为主,有条件地区覆盖门诊服务		√	个体缴纳保费＋政府补贴	√	统筹基金
医疗救助及疾病应急救助体系		贫困人口			√		√	

续表

体系	覆盖			筹资		资金使用	
	宽度（人口）	广度（服务）[1]	深度（费用）[1]	政府卫生支出	社会保险费	财政转移支付	医疗保险基金[1]
公共卫生体系	全体居民			√		√	
城乡居民大病保险					√		大病保险统筹基金

注：1 不同地区和医疗保险制度之间有差异。

2 城乡居民基本医疗保险由中央和地方财政进行管理并提供财政补助。因此，虽然城乡居民基本医疗保险具有自愿参保的特征，但其本质上属于公共或者社会保险，因而此项费用被列为社会卫生支出。

数据来源：《转型中的中国卫生体系》，孟庆跃等，2015

9.2 中国卫生资金的分配和使用

当筹集到卫生资金后，接下来需要考虑的是资金应怎样使用及为谁使用，这些都决定了谁能获得卫生服务、可获取何种类型的卫生服务，以及卫生服务的数量和质量如何。政府需要考虑将资金投向哪些机构以及哪些服务项目。如何发挥卫生筹资的功能，促进卫生服务体系有效落实、人群整体健康水平有效改善，不仅仅是一个经济领域的问题，很大程度上还是一个政治、社会和伦理领域的问题。

9.2.1 卫生资金的分配和使用概述

卫生资金的分配是指通过政府宏观调控和市场调节，科学合理地对卫生资金进行优化配置，最终使卫生资金流向卫生服务系统的各个领域的过程。卫生资金的分配结构描述了卫生资源将最终流向哪些机构、项目或地区。卫生资金的使用主体包括医院、社区卫生机构和公共卫生机构等，它们既是卫生资金的支付对象，也是卫生服务产品的提供者。资金支出的形式有诊疗费、检查费、医药费、健康教育费、预防保健费和突发公共卫生事件应急处理机构建设费等。

9.2.2 中国卫生资金的分配结构

9.2.2.1 中国卫生资金的统筹使用

（1）财政转移支付

中国在1994年建立分税制财政管理体制及相应的转移支付制度。转移支付有两种基本形式：一般性转移支付、专项转移支付。中共中央对教育、社会保障等部门下达一般性转移支付资金，以确保福利部门的资金投入。专项转移支付资金指中共中央为实现特定的政策及事业发展战略目标,以及对委托地方政府代理的一些事务进行补偿而设立的补助资金。地方财政需按用途使用资金。

(2)医疗保险基金

中国对两大基本医疗保险基金实行分开管理,在各个统筹区内与医疗机构分别结算,基本医疗保险基金由医疗保险经办机构集中管理,统一调剂,用于支付基本医疗保险参保人员发生的医药费、手术费、护理费、基本检查费等费用。统筹地区医疗保险管理部门按年度编制收支预算,编制收入预算时综合考虑当地经济发展水平、职工工资收入水平、医疗保险覆盖面、医疗保险筹资比例等因素,编制支出预算时综合考虑当地参保人员年龄结构、疾病谱、医疗费用增长、医疗保险受益面、保障水平和基金结余情况等因素。

城镇职工基本医疗保险实行定点医疗机构和定点零售药店管理。个人账户可用于支付本人的普通门诊费用、住院费用中个人自付部分以及在定点零售药店购药的费用,也可用于支付已绑定家庭共济关系的家庭成员的合规医疗费用。统筹基金用于支付符合规定的住院医疗费用、门诊大病医疗费用,以及逐步纳入的普通门诊费用等。起付标准以下的医疗费用,从个人账户中支付或由个人自付;起付标准以上、最高支付限额以下的医疗费用,主要由统筹基金支付,个人负担一定的比例。统筹基金的具体起付标准、最高支付限额以及在起付标准以上和最高支付限额以下医疗费用的个人负担比例,由统筹地区确定。在起付标准的设置上,中国一般对不同级别医疗机构有不同的规定,通常一级医院起付标准最低,二级医院次之,三级医院相对最高。在共付比例上也存在类似的趋势,一级医院共付率最低(报销比例最高),从而引导患者就诊下沉,合理利用卫生资源。

中国国家基本医疗保险药品目录、诊疗项目目录、医疗服务设施目录及相应的管理办法规定了基本医疗服务的范围和标准。国家基本医疗保险药品目录分为甲类和乙类两种。甲类药物全国基本统一,费用纳入基本医疗保险基金给付范围,并按基本医疗保险的给付标准支付费用。乙类药物是指基本医疗保险基金支付部分费用的药物,这类药物先由患者支付一定比例的费用,剩余部分再纳入基本医疗保险基金给付范围,并按基本医疗保险给付标准支付费用。《国家基本医疗保险、工伤保险和生育保险药品目录(2022年)》收录药品总数为2 967种,其中西药1 586种、中成药1 381种。

(3)医疗救助基金

医疗救助通过政府拨款和社会捐助等渠道筹资,根据救助对象的不同医疗需求,开展医疗救助服务。医疗救助采取以下方式:对救助对象参加城乡居民基本医疗保险的个人缴费部分给予补贴;对救助对象经基本医疗保险、大病保险和其他补充医疗保险支付后,个人及其家庭难以承担的符合规定的基本医疗自付费用给予补助。城乡低保家庭成员、五保户等在民政部门注册过的贫困居民自动成为医疗救助对象,凭相关证件或证明材料在定点医疗机构就医时,只需支付自付部分,其余由医疗救助基金支付,并与定点医疗机构即时结算。未在民政部门登记但属于医疗救助对象的参保者需全额垫付医疗费用并向民政部门申请报销。

(4)疾病应急救助基金

2013年,中国各省(自治区、直辖市)、市(地)政府组织开始设立本级疾病应急救助基金,并鼓励社会各界向疾病应急救助基金捐赠资金。疾病应急救助基金的救助对象是在中国境内发生急重危伤病、需要急救但身份不明确或无力支付相应费用的患者,对于符合上述条件的患者紧急救治所发生的费用，医疗机构可申请疾病应急救助基金补助。疾病应急救助基金实行直接支付。基金经办管理机构审核汇总医疗机构的支付申请后向同级财政部门提交用款申请，财政部门审核后将应急救助基金由社会保障基金财政专户直接支付给相应医疗机构。

9.2.2.2 中国卫生资金购买的服务

（1）基本医疗服务

根据基本医疗保险的规定，患者只有在医疗保险定点机构或者药店就诊才可以得到医疗保险基金的报销。患者通过其社会保障卡可以直接从医疗保险基金获得报销。在非定点医疗机构或药店，参保者可以通过自费获得医疗服务。

基本医疗保险均通过设立起付标准、共付比例以及最高支付限额，与患者共同分摊医疗费用。对服务供方，医疗保险机构通过事前审查、事中监督以及事后核查等方式，减少医疗机构提供的不必要服务；部分地区探索了按服务单元付费、按人头付费以及总额控制等支付方式，使医疗机构拥有更大的财务自主权。医疗保险经办机构对定点医疗机构、定点零售药店实施定点协议管理。定点协议管理指通过订立和履行定点服务协议，规范对定点医疗机构和定点零售药店的管理，明确医疗保险经办机构和定点医疗机构、定点零售药店的权利和义务。

（2）公共卫生服务

政府举办和社会力量举办的医疗卫生机构，只要符合相应的标准和要求，具备相应的服务能力，都可申请参与提供公共卫生服务。为了确保在同一范围内的社区居民享受到基本均等的公共卫生服务，地方政府及其相关部门结合当地经济社会发展水平、财政支付能力以及居民的基本公共卫生需求，确定本行政区域内公共卫生服务项目，作为政府购买服务的内容。针对个体的公共卫生服务项目（如免疫规划等），可以通过核算享受服务对象的人均成本确定单位项目补助定额。针对群体的公共卫生服务项目（如健康教育等），可通过核算综合成本确定综合项目补助定额，也可以将所有公共卫生服务项目打包，核定单一的综合项目补助定额。

中国卫生资金流向见图 9-3。

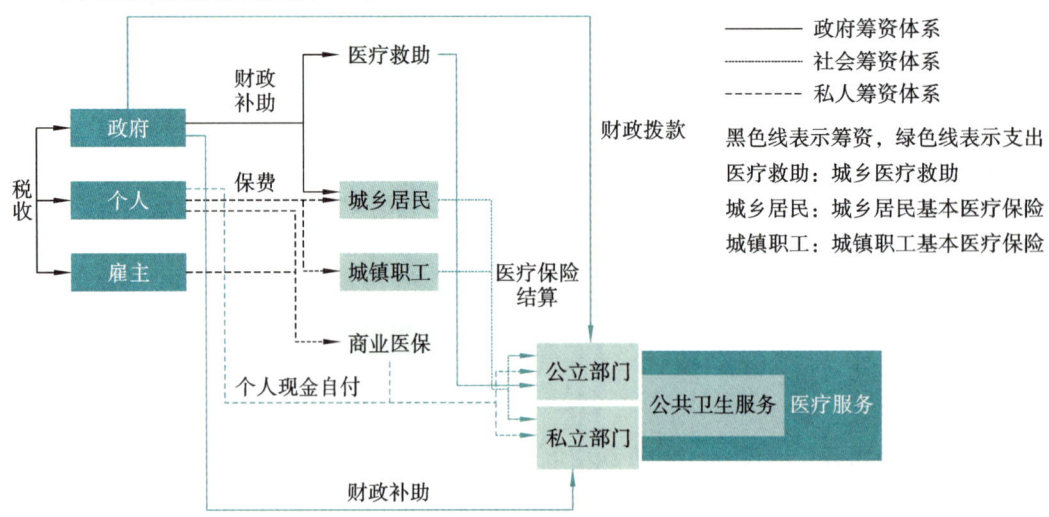

图 9-3 中国卫生资金流向

9.2.3 中国卫生资金的使用主体

9.2.3.1 医疗机构

在中国,公共卫生服务费用的筹资主要通过当地卫生部门财政拨款,按照人头经费予以拨付,另有部分有偿服务项目直接付费(例如流感疫苗未纳入国家基本公共卫生服务内容,因而使用者需要支付该服务的费用)。对于一些初级卫生保健服务以及急救服务,公立医疗机构可从当地卫生部门获得部分预算拨款,与患者按服务项目进行计费;如果是参保患者,当地医疗保险基金则以混合支付方式与机构进行结算。在医疗费用结算方面,服务接受方,即患者仍然按照服务项目进行付费,而医疗保险基金支付则在很长时间内也实施按项目付费,见表9-2。

表9-2 供方支付机制

提供者	支付者				
	当地政府	当地社会医疗保险基金[1]	私人/商业医疗保险	费用分摊	直接付费
基层公立医疗机构	补助	混合支付[2](总额预付、按人头、定额包干、按项目等)	按项目	按项目	按项目
二、三级公立医疗机构	补助	混合支付[2](总额预付、按项目等)	按项目	按项目	按项目
民营医疗机构	无	混合支付[2]/无	按项目	按项目	按项目
零售药店	无	按项目	无	按项目	按项目
提供预防服务的公共卫生服务机构或医疗机构	补助	无/按项目	无/按项目	无/按项目	有偿服务项目

注:1 通常为门诊服务按人头付费、住院服务按单元付费,总额预付和按项目付费则可以同时用于门诊和住院服务。

2 "混合支付"是指某种医疗保险制度对不同的服务类型采用混合的支付方式(例如门诊服务按人头付费,住院服务实行总额预付等)。

数据来源:《转型中的中国卫生体系》,孟庆跃等,2015

2011年,人力资源社会保障部发布《人力资源社会保障部关于进一步推进医疗保险付费方式改革的意见》,指出当前推进付费方式改革的任务目标是:结合基金收支预算管理加强总额控制,探索总额预付。在此基础上,结合门诊统筹的开展探索按人头付费,结合住院门诊大病的保障探索按病种付费。建立和完善医疗保险经办机构与医疗机构的谈判协商机制与风险分担机制,逐步形成与基本医疗保险制度发展相适应,激励与约束并重的支付制度。

9.2.3.2 医务人员

在中国,作为医疗机构的雇员,医务人员的工资水平、福利待遇等与医疗机构密切相关,人力成本主要通过服务收益获得补偿。在基本工资之外,工作量曾作为医务人员奖金收入的主要考核标准。理论上,绩效、患者满意度、医疗保险指标完成率等逐步纳入考核范围,对医务人员的奖金收入产生很大影响。随着卫生体制改革的推进,《中共中央 国务院关于深化医药卫生体制改革的意见》提出,实行以服务质量及岗位工作量为主的综合绩效考核和岗位绩效工资制度,有效调动医务人员的积极性。

从 2009 年 10 月 1 日起,中国公共卫生机构和基层医疗卫生事业单位开始实施绩效工资改革,2010 年全面实施绩效工资制度。中央与地方政府共同为绩效工资制度改革提供财政补助。绩效工资分为基础性绩效工资和奖励性绩效工资两部分。基础性绩效工资约占绩效工资总量的 60%～70%,主要体现地区经济发展、物价水平、岗位职责等因素,一般按月发放。奖励性绩效工资主要体现工作量和实际贡献等因素,根据考核结果发放,可采取灵活多样的分配方式和办法。根据实际情况,在绩效工资中可设立岗位津贴和综合目标考核奖励等项目。长期而言,绩效工资的设置有助于改善过度处方和其他不合理的医疗行为,提高效率、服务质量以及患者满意度。然而,绩效工资的负面效应也不容忽视,例如可能破坏员工之间的信任和团队精神。

9.3 卫生总费用

9.3.1 卫生总费用概述

卫生总费用以货币形式作为综合计量手段,全面反映一个国家或地区在一定时期内(通常指一年)从全社会筹集的用于医疗卫生服务的卫生资源的货币总额,包括经常性卫生费用和固定资本形成费用。经常性卫生费用是指核算期内居民最终消费的所有医疗卫生产品和服务的货币价值。固定资本形成费用是指核算期内卫生服务提供机构获得的资产(扣除同类资产的处置价值),即在卫生服务提供过程中重复使用或者使用期限在一年以上的资产的总价值。

卫生总费用是一个全社会的概念,反映全社会的卫生保健支出,包括卫生部门内部的资金支出以及其他单位和个人的医疗卫生支出,同时还包括社会各界、国际组织等对卫生事业的无偿援助和捐赠。卫生总费用是一种信息工具,能有效分析和评价国家或卫生系统的公平和效率,为政府卫生决策提供重要信息和客观依据。

9.3.2 卫生费用核算

卫生费用核算体系(System of Health Accounts,SHA),是按照国民经济核算的体系和原则,以整个卫生系统为核算对象,建立卫生费用核算指标和核算框架体系,专门研究卫生系统的资金运行过程。利用该核算体系可以核算一个国家或地区的卫生费用,并以此为指导进行卫生次账户核算,如疾病费用、不同年龄人群费用、公共卫生费用和药品费用等的核算。

卫生费用核算体系按照医疗卫生服务的筹资、生产和消费三个环节将卫生费用核算的维度划分为核心维度和扩展维度。核心维度包括服务功能、服务提供机构和筹资方案三个维度,主要回答三个基本问题:一是什么样的医疗卫生用品和服务被消费了,二是哪些卫生服务提供机构提供了这些医疗卫生用品和服务,三是什么筹资方案对这些医疗卫生用品和服务进行补偿。扩展维度中的筹资环节主要进一步回答筹资方案的资金是从哪里来的以及是如何进行筹资的,生产环节进一步回答卫生服务提供机构在生产医疗卫生用品和服务时所消耗的资源成本和资本投入有哪些,消费环节进一步回答医疗卫生用品和服务都被谁消费了,包括卫生费用的疾病别、年龄别、性别、地区及经济水平分布等。卫生费用核算方法包括来源法、机构法、功能法、支出法和矩阵平衡核算等,各国也会根据现行体制和卫生政策分析需要做出相应调整。卫生费用核算体系 2011(SHA2011)核算框架见图 9-4。

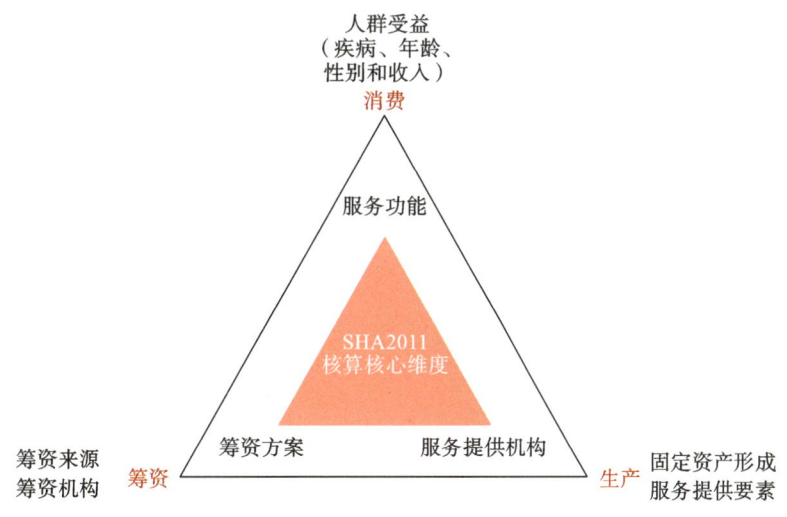

图 9-4　SHA2011 核算框架

9.3.3　中国卫生总费用

2021 年中国卫生费用筹资总额为 76 844.99 亿元,占 GDP 的 6.72%。人均卫生费用 5 440.0 元。按筹资分类来看,2021 年政府卫生支出 20 676.06 亿元,占卫生总费用的 26.91%;社会卫生支出 34 963.26 亿元,占卫生总费用的 45.50%;个人卫生支出 21 205.67 亿元,占卫生总费用的 27.60%。

1980—2021 年,中国卫生总费用的年均增长率为 16.57%;卫生总费用占 GDP 的比重从 3.15% 上升为 6.72%,年均增速为 1.87%。

1980—2021 年,政府卫生支出占卫生总费用的比重从 36.24% 下降到 26.91%,社会卫生支出占卫生总费用的比重从 42.57% 上升为 45.50%,个人卫生支出占卫生总费用的比重从 21.19% 上升为 27.60%。

1980—2021 年中国卫生总费用的基本情况见表 9-3。

表 9-3　中国卫生总费用(1980—2021 年)

年份	卫生总费用/亿元				卫生总费用构成/(%)			城乡卫生费用/亿元		人均卫生费用/元			卫生总费用占 GDP 比重/(%)
	合计	政府卫生支出	社会卫生支出	个人卫生支出	政府卫生支出	社会卫生支出	个人卫生支出	城市	农村	合计	城市	农村	
1980	143.23	51.91	60.97	30.35	36.24	42.57	21.19			14.5			3.15
1985	279.00	107.65	91.96	79.39	38.58	32.96	28.46			26.4			3.09
1990	747.39	187.28	293.10	267.01	25.06	39.22	35.73	396.00	351.39	65.4	158.8	38.8	3.96
1995	2 155.13	387.34	767.81	999.98	17.97	35.63	46.40	1 239.50	915.63	177.9	401.3	112.9	3.51
2000	4 586.63	709.52	1 171.94	2 705.17	15.47	25.55	58.98	2 624.24	1 962.39	361.9	813.7	214.7	4.57
2005	8 659.91	1 552.53	2 586.41	4 520.98	17.93	29.87	52.21	6 305.57	2 354.34	662.3	1 126.4	315.8	4.62
2006	9 843.34	1 778.86	3 210.92	4 853.56	18.07	32.62	49.31	7 174.73	2 668.61	748.8	1 248.3	361.9	4.49
2007	11 573.97	2 581.58	3 893.72	5 098.66	22.31	33.64	44.05	8 968.70	2 605.27	876.0	1 516.3	358.1	4.29
2008	14 535.40	3 593.94	5 065.60	5 875.86	24.73	34.85	40.42	11 251.90	3 283.50	1 094.5	1 861.8	455.2	4.55
2009	17 541.92	4 816.26	6 154.49	6 571.16	27.46	35.08	37.46	13 535.61	4 006.31	1 314.3	2 176.6	562.0	5.03
2010	19 980.39	5 732.49	7 196.61	7 051.29	28.69	36.02	35.29	15 508.62	4 471.77	1 490.1	2 315.5	666.3	4.85
2011	24 345.91	7 464.18	8 416.45	8 465.28	30.66	34.57	34.80	18 571.87	5 774.04	1 804.5	2 697.5	879.4	4.99
2012	28 119.00	8 431.98	10 030.70	9 656.32	29.99	35.67	34.34	21 280.46	6 838.54	2 068.8	2 999.3	1 064.8	5.22

续表

年份	卫生总费用/亿元				卫生总费用构成/(%)			城乡卫生费用/亿元		人均卫生费用/元			卫生总费用占GDP比重/(%)
	合计	政府卫生支出	社会卫生支出	个人卫生支出	政府卫生支出	社会卫生支出	个人卫生支出	城市	农村	合计	城市	农村	
2013	31 668.95	9 545.81	11 393.79	10 729.34	30.10	36.00	33.90	23 644.95	8 024.00	2 316.2	3 234.1	1 274.4	5.34
2014	35 312.40	10 579.23	13 437.75	11 295.41	29.96	38.05	31.99	26 575.60	8 736.80	2 565.5	3 558.3	1 412.2	5.49
2015	40 974.64	12 475.28	16 506.71	11 992.65	30.45	40.29	29.27	31 297.85	9 676.79	2 962.2	4 058.5	1 603.6	5.95
2016	46 344.88	13 910.31	19 096.68	13 337.90	30.01	41.21	28.78	35 458.01	10 886.87	3 328.6	4 471.5	1 846.1	6.21
2017	52 598.28	15 205.87	22 258.81	15 133.60	28.91	42.32	28.77			3 756.7			6.32
2018	59 121.91	16 399.13	25 810.78	16 911.99	27.74	43.66	28.61			4 206.7			6.43
2019	65 841.39	18 016.95	29 150.57	18 673.87	27.36	44.27	28.36			4 669.3			6.67
2020	72 175.00	21 941.90	30 273.67	19 959.43	30.40	41.94	27.65			5 111.1			7.12
2021	76 844.99	20 676.06	34 963.26	21 205.67	26.91	45.50	27.60			5 440.0			6.72

注：1. 本表系核算数，2021年为初步核算数。

2. 按当年价格计算。

3. 2001年起，卫生总费用不含高等医学教育经费，2006年起，包括城乡医疗救助经费。

数据来源：《中国卫生健康统计年鉴（2022）》

10 中国医药卫生法律制度与监督管理

医药卫生事业关系到亿万人民群众的健康,关系到千家万户的幸福,是重大民生问题。深化医药卫生体制改革,加快医药卫生事业发展,强化医药卫生法律制度和监督管理体系建设,适应人民群众日益增长的医药卫生需求,不断提高人民群众健康素质,是贯彻落实科学发展观、促进经济社会全面协调可持续发展的必然要求,是维护社会公平正义、提高人民生活质量的重要举措,是全面建成小康社会和构建社会主义和谐社会的一项重要课题。

10.1 中国医药卫生法律制度概述

10.1.1 中国医药卫生法律制度的概念与特征

中国医药卫生法律制度是调整公民因健康事务而产生的各种社会关系的法律规范的总称。作为中国法律体系的重要组成部分,其既有法律的一般属性,即规范性、国家强制性、国家意志性、普遍性、可诉性等,又有自己独有的特征。

10.1.1.1 中国医药卫生法律制度的立法特征

随着中国卫生法律体系的逐步完善,中国医药卫生法律制度逐渐成为社会主义法律制度的重要组成部分。首先,中国医药卫生法律制度围绕公民健康权益这一核心内容不断完善、细化,具有较强的专业性、科学性和技术性。其次,问题导向型制度完善成为中国医药卫生法律制度的新特征。在卫生法律、行政法规层面的制度趋于稳定的形势下,中国医药卫生法律制度的实施及因其实施引发的问题,实施效果反馈带动的修法乃至立法成为中国医药卫生法律制度建设的主要议题。此外,中国中医药法治建设也取得重大进展,传统中医药被提升到国家发展战略的层面并迈向现代化发展。

10.1.1.2 中国医药卫生法律制度的执法特征

第一,中国医药卫生法律制度的实施具有鲜明的政策性特征。各种具体措施以政策形式发布,总体规划和专项行动以政策方式落实。第二,中国医药卫生法律制度落实于标准体系上。作为中国医药卫生法律制度的重要组成部分,医疗卫生标准为医药卫生法律制度的落实提供指引。第三,中国药品监管系统法治建设稳步推进,药品监管系统法治建设的总体目标逐步落实。第四,中国医药领域反垄断不断升级。国家发展改革委逐步加大针对医疗健康领域价格横向垄断问题的执法力度。第五,积极构建药品行政执法与刑事司法衔接工作机制,打击药品违法犯罪。

10.1.1.3　中国医药卫生法律制度的司法特征

第一，司法解释让相关法律更具指引性。第二，司法机关严厉打击药品违法犯罪，创立制度化、常态化追责机制，加快建设医疗纠纷预警与应对机制。第三，司法机关重视典型案例判决的指导作用，通过公布指导性案例、典型案例等供相关案件参考，为医药卫生法律制度的执法监管提供司法引领。

10.1.2　中国医药卫生法律制度的基本原则

中国医药卫生法律制度的基本原则是统领卫生立法、执法、司法的元规则，指引和规范医药卫生法治的发展。即使法律未做出有关某些卫生事务的规定，在执行这些事务的过程中，法律也应当发挥指导、规范和制约等作用。中国医药卫生法律制度的基本原则包括以下三项。

10.1.2.1　保障公民健康原则

不同部门、不同位阶的医疗卫生法律规范，其目的均是保障公民健康。健康权是基本人权之一，受中国宪法的承认和保护。宪法上的健康权可以通过基本医疗卫生与健康促进法立法具体化为公民获得公共卫生服务资源以及基本医疗服务保障的权利，其表现形式包括基本医疗服务权、医疗保障权、医疗救助权、紧急救治权等。

10.1.2.2　政府主导原则

中国宪法明确规定了政府的基本医疗卫生服务供给义务。2019 年正式通过的《中华人民共和国基本医疗卫生与健康促进法》整体上比较完整地明确了政府主导责任，主要体现在政府投资兴办各级公立医院、开展医学教育、建立社会医疗保险制度、免费提供基本公共卫生服务和对困难人群提供医疗救助五个方面。但政府主导不等于政府包揽一切，中国坚持政府主导与发挥市场机制作用相结合原则。

10.1.2.3　预防为主原则

按照疾病发展规律，为提高医疗卫生资源利用效率，中国在卫生健康领域坚持预防为主、防治结合方针。其内涵包括在国家卫生健康投入方面向健康保健倾斜、重视健康风险的事前防控、建立灵敏的疾病风险预测与防控机制等。

10.1.3　中国医药卫生法律制度的产生与发展

通说认为，有文字记载的中国古代医药卫生法律最早可追溯至殷商时代。《韩非子》《周易》《春秋》《周礼》《左传》中都有古代重视繁衍健康后代的记载。《周礼》翔实记载了医事管理制度，包括司理医药的机构、病历书写和医生考核制度等。自唐宋以来，卫生立法更为细化。《唐律》中有许多涉及医药卫生的条文，对医师误伤、欺诈、调剂失误、以药害人等行为均有刑律规定，同时在饮食卫生、卫生管理等方面也有一些规定。宋代设立了管理宫廷内外的专门药政机构，开设了国家药局。在民国时期，卫生立法开始走向专门化、具体化，如《传染病预防条例》《医师法》等均为适例。新中国成立后，中国医药卫生法律制度的发展经历了四个阶段。

第一阶段：从 1949 年新中国成立到 1954 年新中国第一部宪法颁布。中国十分重视卫生事业和卫生法制建设，制定了大量卫生法规来促进医药卫生事业的发展和保障公民的身体健康。除起到临时宪法作用的《中国人民政治协商会议共同纲领》之外，先后颁布了《中央人民政府卫生组织条例》《种痘暂行办法》《管理麻醉药品暂行条例》《交通检疫暂行办法》等，此时为起步阶段。

第二阶段：1954年新中国第一部宪法颁布后至1978年改革开放前。在宪法指导下，中国先后颁布了大量医药卫生法律法规，例如1954年卫生部颁布的《卫生防疫站暂行办法和各级卫生防疫站组织编制规定》、1955年卫生部颁布的《传染病管理办法》、1956年国务院发布的《工厂安全卫生规程》、1957年全国人大常委会颁布的《中华人民共和国国境卫生检疫条例》、1963年卫生部等部委联合发布的《关于加强药政管理的若干规定》、1964年卫生部等部委联合发布的《管理毒药、限制性剧药暂行规定》等。

第三阶段：1978年改革开放开始至2013年。1982年《中华人民共和国宪法》明确指出"国家发展医疗卫生事业""保护人民健康"等内容，为完善医药卫生法律制度提供了宪法依据。此后，全国人大常委会先后通过了《中华人民共和国药品管理法》《中华人民共和国国境卫生检疫法》《中华人民共和国食品卫生法》等法律文件，同时国务院批准颁布了大量卫生行政法规，比如《麻醉药品管理办法》《精神药品管理办法》《医疗事故处理条例》等。此外，卫生行政部门制定和颁布了大量卫生规章和规范性文件。另外，地方卫生立法也较为普遍。

第四阶段：2014年至今。这一阶段的立法是第三阶段的深化发展，是在全面推进健康中国和法治中国建设的指导思想下做出的主动调整，立法的着眼点是在保障传统医疗卫生服务的基础上更侧重健康方面的法制构建，加强医疗器械领域的法制建设与监管。2019年，全国人大常委会通过了《中华人民共和国基本医疗卫生与健康促进法》，结束了发展医疗卫生与健康事业、保障公民享有基本医疗卫生服务无法可依的局面，使中国卫生领域正式拥有了自己的"基本法"。

10.2　中国医药卫生法律制度的主要构成

中国地域广阔，各地发展水平不一，加上卫生活动又具有广泛性与复杂性特征，因此卫生法律关系除了依靠法律来调整外，还需要由行政法规、部门规章、地方性法规等规范性文件来辅助调整，甚至在具体的实施层面，还需要大量的规范性文件作为补充。这些文件的位阶不同，各自具有不同的效力。中国医药卫生法律制度以健康权为核心，根据对象的不同，可以分为公共卫生法律制度、医事法律制度和医疗保障法律制度三个部分。这些法律法规及规范性文件基本涵盖了中国卫生事业发展所涉及的各个方面，包括公共卫生、疾病防治、医政与药政管理等各个领域。

10.2.1　公共卫生法律制度

10.2.1.1　传染病防治法律制度

传染病防治法是由国家制定并颁布，由国家强制力保障实施，调整国家、政府、社会组织、公民在预防、控制和消除传染病的发生与流行及保障人体健康和公共卫生活动中所产生的各种社会关系的法律规范的总称。1989年2月，中国颁布了《中华人民共和国传染病防治法》。该法于2004年8月得到修订，分别对传染病防治工作的方针、原则，传染病预防，疫情报告、通报与公布，疫情控制，医疗救治，监督管理，保障措施及法律责任等做出了明确、具体的规定。《中华人民共和国传染病防治法》是规范传染病防控工作,并使其制度化的重要法律依据和基本准绳。

10.2.1.2 突发公共卫生事件应急法律制度

突发公共卫生事件是指突然发生,造成或可能造成社会公众健康严重损害的重大传染病疫情、群体性不明原因疾病、重大食物中毒和职业中毒,以及其他严重影响公众身心健康的公共卫生事件。2003 年 5 月,国务院发布了《突发公共卫生事件应急条例》。这一条例总结了 SARS 防治工作的经验教训,对突发公共卫生事件的管理范围和具体内容进行了制度性建设,从法律角度进一步确立了应对突发公共卫生事件的快速处置机制,并强化了相应责任。2007 年 8 月,第十届全国人大常委会第二十九次会议通过了《中华人民共和国突发事件应对法》(简称《突发事件应对法》),对突发事件的预防与应急准备、监测与预警、应急处置与救援、事后恢复与重建等应对活动做出了明确规定。《突发事件应对法》与《突发公共卫生事件应急条例》以及相关部门规章,构成了较为完善的中国突发公共卫生事件立法体系。

10.2.1.3 精神卫生法律制度

在中国,精神卫生的定义有狭义和广义之分。狭义的精神卫生特指精神障碍的预防、诊断、治疗和康复活动,而广义的精神卫生除涵盖上述活动外,还包括心理健康促进以及相应的保障措施等。2012 年 10 月,第十一届全国人大常委会第二十九次会议通过了《中华人民共和国精神卫生法》(简称《精神卫生法》)。《精神卫生法》是一部规范精神障碍患者治疗、保障精神障碍患者合法权益和促进精神障碍患者康复的法律,是调整国家、政府、社会组织、公民在维护和增进心理健康、预防和治疗精神障碍、促进精神障碍患者康复、保障人体健康活动中所产生的各种社会关系的法律规范的总和,于 2013 年 5 月正式实施。

10.2.2 医事法律制度

10.2.2.1 医疗机构管理法律制度

目前,在医疗机构管理方面,中国立法主要有专项立法和综合立法两种模式。专项立法主要是制定行政法规、规章和其他规范性文件,如《医疗机构管理条例》和《医疗机构管理条例实施细则》对医疗机构的性质、宗旨、规划审批、登记、执业、监督管理等事项予以了明确规定,是有关医疗机构管理的核心法律文件。医疗机构管理规定不仅有专项立法文件支撑,还散见于其他综合立法文件之中,如《中华人民共和国药品管理法》《中华人民共和国职业病防治法》中,都有涉及医疗机构管理的相关法律制度规定。

10.2.2.2 医疗行为管理法律制度

医疗行为,即医务人员运用专业的医疗知识和技术,为患者提供的疾病诊断、治疗、护理、预防、康复以及其他以保障身体健康与生命安全为目的的服务。在医疗行为的管理方面,中国法律文件涵盖了从法律到行政法规,再到地方性法规与规章等多个层面,甚至还有相关的诊疗规范和诊疗指南作为补充,基本形成了完整的管理体系。从执业管理到机构管理,从药品、器械、急救到具体的诊疗行为,均有具体的管理规定。

10.2.2.3 卫生技术人员管理法律制度

执业医师法是调整医师资格考试、执业注册和执业活动中产生的各种社会关系的法律规范的总和。第九届全国人大常委会第三次会议于 1998 年 6 月通过了《中华人民共和国执业医师法》,该法自 1999 年 5 月施行,适用于在医疗、预防、保健机构中工作的,依法取得执业医师资格或者执业助理医师资格,经注册取得医师执业证书,从事相应的医疗、预防、保健业务的专业医务人员,包括计划生育技术服务机构中的医师以及来华短期行医的外国医师。

护士是指经执业注册取得护士执业证书,依照规定从事护理活动,履行保护生命、减轻痛苦、增进健康职责的卫生技术人员。目前,中国护理工作立法尚不完善,护士部分合法权益落实不足,一些基层医疗卫生机构护理质量欠佳。虽医护比例有所优化,但部分医疗卫生机构重医疗、轻护理,仍存在减少护士职数现象,给医疗安全带来很多隐患,完善护士管理立法势在必行。国务院有关部门、各级人民政府及其有关部门应当采取措施,改善护士的工作条件,保障护士待遇,加强护士队伍建设,促进护理事业健康发展。国务院有关部门和县级以上地方人民政府应当采取措施,鼓励护士到城乡基层医疗卫生机构工作。

乡村医生是指尚未取得执业医师或者执业助理医师资格,但已取得当地卫生行政机关颁发的乡村医生执业证书,并经注册后在村医疗卫生机构从事预防、保健和一般医疗服务的卫生人员。2003年8月,国务院颁布《乡村医生从业管理条例》(简称《乡医条例》),标志着乡村医生的准入、教育培训和管理步入法制化的轨道。《乡医条例》规定,国家实行乡村医生执业注册制度,县级人民政府卫生行政主管部门负责乡村医生执业注册工作。

执业药师是指经全国统一考试合格,取得执业药师职业资格证书并经注册登记,在药品生产、经营、使用等单位中执业的药学技术人员。目前,中国实行执业药师注册制度,只有注册才能执业,未经注册者,不得以执业药师身份执业。国家药品监督管理局是全国执业药师资格注册的管理机构,各省(自治区、直辖市)药品监督管理机构为本辖区执业药师注册机构。申请注册者,必须取得执业药师职业资格证书,遵纪守法、遵守药师职业道德,身体健康、能坚持在执业药师岗位工作,以及经所在单位考核同意。

10.2.2.4 医疗机构药事管理法律制度

中国药事管理相关法律法规以《中华人民共和国药品管理法》和《中华人民共和国药品管理法实施条例》为核心,它们分别从药品研发、生产、经营和使用等方面,对药品进行全过程、全周期监督管理,以此保证药品质量和用药安全。《中华人民共和国药品管理法》是为了加强药品管理,保证药品质量,保障公众用药安全和合法权益,保护和促进公众健康而制定的法律,在中国境内从事药品研制、生产、经营、使用和监督管理活动的单位或者个人必须遵守。

10.2.3 医疗保障法律制度

10.2.3.1 城镇职工基本医疗保险制度

城镇职工基本医疗保险制度是指国家立法实施的,面向所有用人单位及其职工以及灵活就业人员,以用人单位和在职职工双方共同缴费以及灵活就业人员个人缴费为主进行筹资,进而保障参保人基本医疗需求的社会医疗保险制度。城镇职工基本医疗保险制度是中国基本医疗保险制度的重要组成部分。1998年12月,在总结各地试点经验的基础上,国务院发布了《国务院关于建立城镇职工基本医疗保险制度的决定》,提出从1999年初开始,在全国范围内启动建立城镇职工基本医疗保险制度工作。这标志着中国城镇实施了近半个世纪的公费、劳保医疗制度,逐渐为新的职工医保制度所取代。2010年10月,中国第十一届全国人大常委会第十七次会议审议通过的《中华人民共和国社会保险法》将"职工基本医疗保险"列为基本医疗保险具体险种之一。

10.2.3.2　城乡居民基本医疗保险制度

城乡居民基本医疗保险制度是指城乡居民因疾病或非因工负伤需要治疗时,由国家为其提供基本医疗保障的一项社会保险法律制度。中国在坚持全覆盖、保基本、多层次、可持续等原则的基础上,通过政府补贴、个人缴费等多元化的筹资方式建立城乡居民基本医疗保险基金,实现社会互助共济,保障城乡居民的医疗保险权益。中国城乡居民基本医疗保险制度发端于城镇居民基本医疗保险制度和新农合制度:2016 年国务院整合城镇居民基本医疗保险和新农合两项制度,建立统一的城乡居民基本医疗保险制度。

长期以来,中国医疗健康领域涉及的部门非常多,部门之间协调不顺是阻碍医改深入进行的一个重要瓶颈。2018 年,国务院进行机构改革,组建了国家卫生健康委,树立了大卫生、大健康理念,开启了新一轮大部制改革。这种大部制改革理念与中国所呼吁的卫生领域法治观点不谋而合,既可以明确责任主体,减少医改的内部摩擦和阻力,让协调更顺畅,也有助于政府发挥强有力的领导作用,更加积极地推动改革。中国重视医疗卫生法治工作与深化改革工作之间的联系,积极推动法规和制度的修订完善;贯彻实施《中华人民共和国基本医疗卫生与健康促进法》,为医疗卫生事业发展保驾护航。

10.3　中国医药卫生监督管理

10.3.1　中国医药卫生监督概述

10.3.1.1　医药卫生监督概念、功能与作用

医药卫生监督是维护全体国民生命健康权益的重要保障,是指政府有关行政部门依据卫生法律、法规的规定对个人、法人和组织从事的与卫生有关的行政许可事项及其执行卫生法律法规的情况进行监督检查,并对其行为做出处理的行政执法活动。

医药卫生监督的功能就是卫生监督所具有或应发挥出的效能,包括规范功能、制约功能、预防功能和促进功能。规范功能是指医药卫生监督有规范人们行为导向的作用,它通过对守法者的认可和对违法者的惩罚指出什么行为是合法的或者是法律规定必须执行的。制约功能是指医药卫生监督主体的监督行为对相对人有关权利的限制和在具体行为上的牵制。预防功能是预防为主卫生方针的具体化,是强制和规范社会卫生事务或行为的一种制度,起到防患于未然的作用。医药卫生监督不是消极被动地监督,而是积极主动地参与或渗透于监督对象的整个运作过程,提前发现和排除可能发生危害健康的各种问题和潜在因素。促进功能是指医药卫生监督很大程度上能促进社会系统各方面、各环节、各领域,特别是涉及卫生活动的各方面不断完善,有效保护人民的健康和生产力水平不断提高。

医药卫生监督具有以下作用:一是推进国家治理体系和治理能力现代化。医疗卫生制度是现代国家制度的重要组成部分,对医药卫生领域的管理彰显了国家行政治理能力与治理水平。医药卫生监管制度作为医药卫生管理制度整体运行的基础和保障,能够有效保证卫生事业在法治轨道上科学发展,是规范和维护医疗卫生体系、推进国家治理体系和社会主义现代化建设的重要手段之一。二是保障人民健康权,维护全民健康战略地位。人民健康是民族昌盛和国家富强的重要标志。优化健康服务,打造健康生态,全方位、全周期保障人

民群众健康,为增进人民福祉和实现民族复兴提供坚实壁垒。医药卫生监督是国家行政部门监督管理卫生事业发展,保障国民健康的重要载体和实现手段。三是维护医药卫生行业环境。改革开放以来,中国医药卫生与健康服务供给市场的内外环境发生了巨大变化,市场手段不可避免地存在盲目、自发和趋利等固有弊端。医药卫生监督管理的目的在于纠正市场激励不当导致的市场失灵现象。规范医药行业中各主体行为不仅要依靠从业者的自我道德约束、行业规则和社会监督,更要采取市场调节和政府监管相结合的方式对医药卫生服务市场经济运行和资源配置进行干预,维护公共秩序,保证卫生服务质量。

10.3.1.2 医药卫生监督原则

在中国,医药卫生监督遵循"有法可依、有法必依、执法必严、违法必究"原则,除此以外,还遵循以下原则。

（1）合法性原则

合法性原则是现代法治国家、法治政府对执法的基本要求,主要包括医药卫生监督主体的设立必须合法、医药卫生监督职权的拥有应当合法、医药卫生监督职权的行使应当合法、违法行使监督职权应当承担法律责任等方面。

（2）合理性原则

合理性原则指医药卫生监督主体的设立、监督职权的拥有、监督职权的行使、对违法行为的追究和行政救济的实施等必须正当、客观、适度。具体而言,第一是公平公正原则,其基本要求是平等对待相对人,不歧视;第二是比例原则,指医药卫生监督主体实施监督行为时应当兼顾监督目标的实现和保护相对人的合法权益。

（3）正当法律程序原则

正当法律程序原则指医药卫生监督主体做出影响管理相对人权益的监督行为时必须遵循正当法律程序,包括事先告知相对人、向相对人说明行为的根据和理由、听取相对人的陈述和申辩、事后为相对人提供相应的救济途径等。

（4）信赖保护原则

信赖保护原则的基本内涵是医药卫生监督主体对自己做出的行为或承诺应守信用,不得随意变更,不得反复无常。

10.3.1.3 医药卫生监督主体

医药卫生监督主体是国家行使卫生监督管理职能、实现卫生立法目的的组织基础,指享有国家卫生监督权力,能以自己的名义从事卫生监督活动,并对行为后果独立承担法律责任的组织。根据中国医药卫生法律、法规,中国医药卫生监督主体由两大类组成,即卫生监督行政机关和法律法规授权组织。

卫生监督行政机关指的是依据国家法律的规定而设置的行使国家卫生监督管理职能的国家机关,包括各级人民政府的卫生行政部门、药品监督管理机关及其他卫生监督机关。卫生行政部门一般是指各级政府中负责医疗卫生行政工作的部门,主要负责医疗卫生方面的政策制定、环境保护工作,具体的执法、业务工作由下属事业单位等实施。下属事业单位包括负责行政执法的卫生监督局（所）,负责传染病、慢性病预防控制的疾病预防控制中心,负责妇幼卫生的妇幼保健院,还有各级医院、乡镇卫生院等。药品监督管理目前主要由国家药品监督管理局负责,其工作内容主要包括:第一,负责药品（含中药、民族药,下同）、医疗器械和化妆品安全监督管理。拟订监督管理政策规划,组织起草法律法规草案,拟订部门规章,并监督实施。研究拟订鼓励药品、医疗器械和化妆品新技术新产品的管理与服务政策。第二,负责药品、医疗器械和化妆品标准管理。组织制定、公布国家药典等药品、医疗器械标准,组织拟订化妆品标准,组织制定分类管理制度,并监督实施。参与制定国家基本药物目录,配合实施国家基本药物制度。第三,负责药品、医疗器械和化妆品注册管理。制定注册管理制度,严格上市审评审批,完善审评审批服务便利化措施,并组织实施。第四,负责药品、医疗器械和化妆品质量管理。制定研制质量管理规范并监督实施。制定生产质量管理规范并依职责监督实施。制定经营、使用质量管理规范并指导实施。第五,负责药品、医疗器械和化妆品上市后风险管理。组织开展药品不良反应、医疗器械不良事件和化妆品不良反应的监测、评价和处置工作。依法承担药品、医疗器械和化妆品安全应急管理工作。第六,负责执业药师资格准入管理。制定执业药师资格准入制度,指导监督执业药师注册工作。第七,负责组织指导药品、医疗器械和化妆品监督检查。制定检查制度,依法查处药品、医疗器械和化妆品注册环节的违法行为,依职责组织指导查处生产环节的违法行为。第八,负责药品、医疗器械和化妆品监督管理领域对外交流与合作,参与相关国际监管规则和标准的制定。第九,负责指导省、自治区、直辖市药品监督管理部门工作。第十,完成党中央、国务院交办的其他任务。

开展医药卫生监督管理工作的法律法规授权组织指的是经法律法规授权能够以自己的名义行使特定行政职能的行政机关以外的组织,包括社会组织、社会团体、企事业单位等。

10.3.2　中国医药卫生监督管理主要内容

10.3.2.1　医疗机构监督管理

医疗机构监督一般包括对医疗机构设置与执业的监督,指卫生监督主体依据相关法律法规,对医疗机构的设置审批、执业等级许可和执业活动是否合法进行监督检查,并对医疗机构设置与执业中的违法、违规行为进行处理的行政执法活动。为保证医疗质量安全、保障公民健康,中国持续加强对医疗机构的管理,规范医疗服务市场秩序。自 1994 年起中国颁布实施了多项医疗机构监督相关法律法规,如《医疗机构管理条例》《医疗机构管理条例实施细则》《医疗美容服务管理办法》《处方管理办法》等,现已形成较为完善的医疗机构监督法律法规体系。

医疗机构的设置与审批包括医疗机构设置规划、医疗机构设置审批、医疗机构执业登记及相关管理(如注销、变更登记及校验)三部分。首先,医疗机构设置规划主要负责部门为县级以上地方人民政府卫生行政部门,其规划依据为本行政区域内的人口、医疗资源、医疗需求和医疗机构的分布现状。其次,医疗机构设置审批以符合本行政区域内规划布局和医疗机构设置规划为前提;单位或者个人设置医疗机构,必须经所在地县级以上卫生行政部门审查批准,并取得《设置医疗机构批准书》后,方可向有关部门申请办理其他手续。最后,医疗机构执业登记主要审查申请执业的医疗机构是否具备法定的执业条件。

医疗机构执业监督一般指卫生行政部门针对医疗机构执业活动是否合法进行监督,包括执业许可监督,执业活动监督,执业规范、职责与义务监督三项内容。首先,执业许可监督包括执业准入监督和印章、名称使用监督,前者要求医疗机构必须取得《医疗机构执业许可证》方可执业,后者涉及医疗机构的印章、银行账户、牌匾以及医疗文件中使用的名称应当与核准登记的医疗机构名称相同等事项。其次,执业活动监督包括对诊疗范围、执业人员和诊疗活动的监督。最后，执业规范、职责与义务监督要求医疗机构按照相关临床诊疗规范执业，履行预防保健、突发卫生事件医疗支援等相关义务。

10.3.2.2　卫生技术人员监督管理

卫生技术人员监督指医药卫生监督主体依据卫生管理法律法规对卫生技术人员进行监督检查、追究违法行为人责任的行政执法活动。卫生技术人员即从事卫生技术工作的人员，是指通过高等或中等医药卫生教育或培训，掌握医药卫生知识，经卫生行政部门审查合格，从事医疗、预防、药剂、护理或其他卫生技术工作的专业技术人员。

卫生技术人员监督以从业资格监督、专项技术服务资格监督和诊疗行为监督为主要内容。

第一，卫生技术人员从业资格监督。卫生技术人员从业资格监督主要是对卫生技术人员获得相应从业资格的监督与管理。卫生技术人员从业资格是指为公众提供特定卫生技术服务的人员应具备的学识、技术、能力和身份资格。卫生技术人员往往需要通过一系列严格的审查程序才能获得相应从业资格。一般来说，从业资格的获得从考试或考核开始，例如执业医师资格考试、护士执业资格考试和执业药师职业资格考试等，以在卫生行政部门完成执业注册结束。

第二，卫生技术人员专项技术服务资格监督。卫生技术人员专项技术服务资格是指经执业注册或考核登记后，因某一领域内卫生技术服务项目众多且各项目危险性与复杂性不一，卫生技术人员在法定情况下进一步取得的实施特定专项卫生技术服务的资格。

第三，卫生技术人员诊疗行为监督。卫生技术人员诊疗行为直接关系到诊疗水平与患者健康水平，故各个国家和政府均实施严格监管手段来规范卫生技术人员诊疗行为。监管的主要手段是实施资质许可，即在行业准入方面严加管理，甚至细化到具体诊疗行为的准入。在卫生技术人员获得一般性的行业准入资格后，卫生监督的重点在于对卫生技术人员的具体行为，包括执业及从业范围等进行监督。

10.3.2.3　药品监督管理

药品监督管理是指药品监督管理机构依照法定职权，对药品的研发、生产、销售、使用、定价、广告等各个环节的监督检查活动。中国药品监督管理工作由国家药品监督管理局主管，进行药品监督管理的法律依据包括《中华人民共和国药品管理法》《药物非临床研究质量管理规范》《药物临床试验质量管理规范》《药品生产质量管理规范（2010年修订）》等。

药品监督管理的主要内容包括药品管理、执业药师管理和药品监督检验等，依据药品监督管理相关法律法规进行。药品监督管理相关法律法规是依法制定、发布的有关药品监督管理的规范性文件，涉及国家药品标准等事项。药品管理主要包括药品市场准入监督管理，药品生产、流通与使用监督管理，药品质量监督管理，非法药品查处及市场退出监督管理等。执业药师管理主要包括对在关键药学技术职业领域执业的药学技术人员的执业准入、执业行为及执业退出施行的监督管理。药品监督检验是指药品监督管理部门根据法律法规规定，对药品研制、生产、经营和药品使用单位使用药品等活动进行监督检验。

10.3.2.4　传染病防治监督

传染病防治监督是指政府卫生行政部门依据卫生法律法规对个人、法人和组织从事与传染病有关的事项许可，对执行传染病防治法律规范的情况进行监督检查，并对其行为做出处理的行政执法活动。进行传染病防治监督的目的在于有效预防、控制和消除传染病的发生和流行,保障人民健康,维护国家卫生法制的统一和尊严。

根据《中华人民共和国传染病防治法》,国务院卫生行政部门主管全国传染病防治及其监督管理工作,县级以上地方人民政府卫生行政部门负责本行政区域内的传染病防治及其监督管理工作。传染病防治监督一般包括预防监督、控制监督等环节。

案例 《中华人民共和国基本医疗卫生与健康促进法》出台

2019年12月28日,第十三届全国人大常委会第十五次会议通过《中华人民共和国基本医疗卫生与健康促进法》。该法基本上涵盖了国民健康立法所需要的基本要素,同时充分体现了"大卫生""大健康"以及"将健康融入所有政策"的新理念,自2020年6月1日起施行。

《中华人民共和国基本医疗卫生与健康促进法》的确立与中国医药卫生体制改革的不断深化相伴而行。随着中国特色基本医疗卫生制度的逐步建立,中国卫生事业发展中许多根本性、原则性的问题急需运用一部基础性、综合性的法律予以规范,同时将实践证明行之有效的经验做法和具体制度及时上升为法律的任务也应运而生。

在立法目的方面,该法主要着眼于以下内容:第一,落实《中华人民共和国宪法》中关于国家发展医疗卫生事业和保护人民健康的规定;第二,引领中国医药卫生事业改革发展的大局;第三,促进和保证健康中国建设的有效实施。在坚持政府主导,保基本、强基层、建机制的立法思路的指引下,该法在积极保障政府投入、动员全社会参与、全方位全周期保障人民健康、大幅提高人民健康水平、显著改善健康公平等方面做出宏观的法律规范和制度设计,充分发挥了法律在引领、推动医药卫生体制改革和保障健康中国建设方面的重要作用。

该法是中国医疗卫生领域第一部基础性、综合性法律,体现了从"以治病为中心"到"以人民健康为中心"的理念转变,为中国医疗卫生事业的改革与发展提供了法治保障。如今,卫生法治作为涉及多个传统法律部门的综合性法律领域,表现出各部分齐头并进的良好发展态势,由宪法相关条款、法律法规、规章文件、标准指南等共同组成的中国医药卫生法律制度体系已基本形成。

11　中国医药卫生信息体系

在当今信息化时代,医药卫生行业的信息化建设已经成为国家发展的重要战略之一。作为医药卫生行业信息化的核心,信息系统建设对于提高医疗服务的质量和效率、优化医疗资源的配置和利用、强化医药卫生管理与监督、提升公共卫生智能化治理能力等方面具有非常深远的影响。随着信息技术的不断进步和应用,中国医药卫生信息化建设已取得长足的发展,但仍需要不断加强信息系统建设和应用,提升信息技术和医药卫生行业的融合度和创新能力,促进医药卫生事业的持续健康发展。本章将从医药卫生信息系统的重要性、中国医药卫生信息化发展状况以及中国医药卫生信息管理体系等方面展开讨论,以期为深入了解中国医药卫生信息化建设的现状、问题和未来发展方向提供参考和启示。

11.1　医药卫生信息系统的重要性

11.1.1　宏观层面

随着社会主义市场经济体系的建立,医药卫生信息基础设施的建设对医药卫生事业的发展愈加重要。建设实用共享的医药卫生信息系统可以帮助职能部门和研究人员及时获取可靠信息,提供高效的医药卫生管理服务,全面提高医疗卫生服务质量、综合能力和管理水平。近年来,中国众多城市地区不断推进医药卫生信息系统建设,《“十四五”全民健康信息化规划》指出,“十三五”期间,卫生健康行业大力推进健康中国、数字中国两大战略融合落地,深入实施“十三五”全民健康信息化发展规划,加快健康医疗大数据规范应用和“互联网十医疗健康”创新发展,为支撑卫生健康事业高质量发展发挥了重要作用。从宏观层面来看,医药卫生信息系统建设对医药卫生事业发展的重要性主要体现在以下几个方面。

第一,促进卫生保健服务的普及和资源合理配置。在医改和信息化发展的推动下,中国卫生保健服务将迎来更深层次的变革。尽管公立医院仍是中国医疗卫生服务体系的主体,但促进医疗卫生服务升级的关键在于填补区域医疗资源的不平衡,通过实现分级诊疗和远程医疗等措施,形成“小病在基层,大病到医院,康复回社区”的就医新格局。其中,基于大数据、云计算、移动互联网和物联网的分级诊疗信息系统是非常重要的建设内容之一。该系统能够与各级医疗卫生机构信息系统互联互通,提供统一的转诊信息服务,优化医疗机构的就诊流程,引导居民养成良好的就医习惯,提高医疗服务的有序性、可及性、公平性和经济性,从而优化区域卫生资源的配置。

第二,促进医药卫生管理和监督的强化。根据国家卫生健康委发布的《卫生健康行政执法全过程记录工作规范》的要求,建立健全卫生监督体系,加快推进卫生监督领域"互联网＋阳光监管"新模式,着力打造"智慧卫监"综合管理服务平台,优化执法流程,提升执法效率,真正实现从传统执法模式向现代化执法模式的跨越式转变,对保障人民群众身体健康具有重要作用。对医疗机构、卫生人员行为的监督和评估,有助于促进医疗服务的规范化和标准化,提高患者满意度。实现以数据为驱动的公共卫生管理业务协同化、以数据为支撑的决策应用服务智慧化,可有力支撑卫生监督精细化管理,提升综合监管执法能力。随着互联网医疗需求的剧增,中国卫生监督的重点正在向全过程监督转变。利用大数据进行精细化分析,及时发现并查处违规行为,推动监督渠道由线下向线上转变,对实现全过程监督具有重要作用。

第三,提升公共卫生智能化治理能力。区块链、人工智能等前沿技术的应用,不仅可极大提高公共卫生信息系统的韧性,而且影响着健康治理的未来方向。公共卫生的本质是以"群体"为中心的社会治理过程,需要通过分布式的群体参与来实现信息系统的韧性。同时,公共卫生治理的智能化是公共卫生管理的一种创新形式,依托于机构编制与体制改革的信息化进程,并依靠专业独立的知识决策来实现公共卫生治理的科学高效,从而及时应对各种重大疾病与突发公共卫生事件。未来,公共卫生信息系统将成为智慧城市的重要组成部分,通过智慧城市指挥中心的协调,实现全城管理的智能化,为包括公共卫生在内的经济和民生各领域提供智能高效的服务。

第四,推动医药卫生行业的升级和转型。随着政府持续推进医药卫生体制改革和医疗数字化转型,医疗信息化行业正在经历重大的升级和转型,从以医疗服务信息化为中心,逐步过渡到医保信息化和医药信息化的快速发展阶段,再进一步升级到整个生命健康产业链的集成化和协同化发展阶段。在这个过程中,基于云计算和大数据技术并具有中台(middle platform)思维的数字化转型平台正在快速部署,支撑着医疗、医保和医药各业务核心系统的建设和运行,同时也支持各种创新医疗应用系统的建设和运行。数字化转型平台也在从服务于独立的医疗或医保部门向服务于整个产业链扩展。这些变化为医药卫生行业的升级和转型带来了机遇和挑战。

11.1.2　微观层面

2020年5月,国家卫生健康委办公厅发布了《国家卫生健康委办公厅关于进一步完善预约诊疗制度加强智慧医院建设的通知》,该通知要求加快建立完善预约诊疗制度、创新建设完善智慧医院系统、大力推动互联网诊疗与互联网医院发展。这促使许多医院重视自身信息系统建设,加快信息建设的进度。医院信息化建设已经成为医院实施精细化管理、降低运营成本、改革就诊流程的重要手段。在"十三五"期间,许多医院为配合国家医疗信息化建设"十三五"规划,开始利用第三方平台整合医疗数据,加强信息化管理水平,并推进各个职能科室信息化、无纸化进程。从微观层面来看,医药卫生信息系统建设对医院管理的重要性主要体现在以下几个方面。

第一,优化就医流程,节省就诊等候时间。自助挂号缴费系统和门诊排队叫号系统的使用,可以优化门诊就医流程,打破传统门诊中存在的"三长一短"(即挂号排队长、就诊排队长、缴费排队长和就诊时间短)问题。智能医疗设备,如自动检测设备、智能药柜等的引入,可以实现患者自行检测、取药,减轻医务人员的工作负担,提高就医效率。互联网医院的在线问诊、预约挂号等服务,可进一步方便患者就医,避免传统门诊中的人群聚集和交通拥堵问题,提升就医效率和患者的就医体验。

第二,建立和实施电子病历,提高病历质量。建立电子病历是整合医院内部各个功能系统(如医院信息系统、实验室信息系统、影像存储与传输系统等)数据的核心工作,电子病历处于医院信息化建设的核心位置。随着电子病历持续发展,医院信息化建设也从面向收费转为面向临床过程。电子病历成了实现医院临床数据结构化的重要手段,可以帮助后台更好地整合、分析数据,全面展现患者的诊疗流程,为人(人事管理、绩效考核)、财(预算管理、成本核算)、物(药品管理、物资管理)的管控提供重要数据支撑。建立和实施电子病历,不仅可以提高病历质量,更可以协助医生快速准确诊疗,帮助医院管理部门实现自动化、智能化管理,包括对医院病历质量、人员等方面的统一管理。

第三,推动临床信息化建设,提升诊疗质效。与医院信息化建设相比,临床信息化建设更侧重于患者。临床信息化建设的核心为建立以电子病历为中心的临床信息系统,该系统涵盖了护理、影像、检验等各个方面,其主要目的是协助医生快速准确地进行诊疗,提高工作效率,同时保证病历的质量和可追溯性。目前,中国三级医院的临床信息化建设程度最高,尤其是在临床检验信息管理和医学影像信息管理方面,渗透率最高。未来,临床信息系统将会结合大数据、人工智能等新技术,从信息化管理的提速增效向数据整合、智能分析迈进,进一步解决医疗资源短缺的核心问题。

随着中国对医药卫生事业发展越来越重视,扎实推进医保信息化建设已被写入《中华人民共和国国民经济和社会发展第十四个五年规划和2035年远景目标纲要》,这为加强信息系统建设和应用、提升信息技术和医药卫生行业的融合度和创新能力提供了更广阔的空间和更坚实的基础。在这一背景下,中国将继续推进信息技术应用和医疗服务的数字化转型,加强信息系统建设与医药卫生行业的深度融合,实现医药卫生事业的高质量发展,增进人民的健康福祉。

11.2　中国医药卫生信息化发展状况

11.2.1　中国医药卫生信息化政策规划及发展要求

11.2.1.1　政策规划

中国国家层面一直在不断推进信息产业的发展,并且逐步加强医疗卫生领域的信息化建设。自"十五"至"十四五"时期,中国明确了加强医疗卫生领域的信息系统建设,并陆续印发了支持、规范医疗信息化行业发展的政策。在多个政策实施方案中,《中共中央 国务院关于深化医药卫生体制改革的意见》以及《国民经济和社会发展第十二个五年规划纲要》都积极推进医药卫生信息化、远程医疗系统、公立医院信息化建设。近几年,中国医药卫生信息化布局加速推进。可以看出,中国政府高度重视医药卫生信息化发展,通过不断完善政策和加大投入力度,推动了医药卫生信息化的持续进步。

在政策层面,中国出台了一系列支持医药卫生信息化发展的指导性文件,包括《"十四五"国家信息化规划》等,见表11-1。这些文件明确了政府对医药卫生信息化发展的重视和

表 11-1　中国医药卫生信息化政策规划示例

发布时间	发布部门	文件名称	重点内容解读	政策性质
2020 年 9 月	国家卫生健康委、国家发展改革委、教育部、工业和信息化部、公安部、人力资源社会保障部、交通运输部、应急管理部、国家医保局	《关于进一步完善院前医疗急救服务的指导意见》	提高院前医疗急救基础设施、配套设施的信息化水平	规范类
2020 年 11 月	工业和信息化部办公厅、国家卫生健康委办公厅	《工业和信息化部办公厅 国家卫生健康委员会办公厅关于组织开展 5G＋医疗健康应用试点项目申报工作的通知》	试点推广：培育可复制、可推广的 5G 智慧医疗健康新产品、新业态、新模式	支持类
2021 年 9 月	国务院办公厅	《"十四五"全民医疗保障规划》	医疗保障信息化、标准化建设取得突破，医保信息业务编码标准和医保电子凭证推广应用	支持类
2021 年 9 月	国家卫生健康委、国家中医药管理局	《公立医院高质量发展促进行动（2021—2025 年）》	建设"三位一体"智慧医院，推进医院信息化建设标准化、规范化水平	支持类
2021 年 12 月	中央网络安全和信息化委员会	《"十四五"国家信息化规划》	积极探索运用信息化手段优化医疗服务流程；建设医疗重大基础平台，加快建设医疗专属云，推动各级医疗卫生机构信息系统数据共享互认和业务协同，建设权威统一、互通共享的各级全民健康信息平台	支持类

扶持力度，为行业的发展提供了政策支持。在实践层面，中国积极推进医药卫生信息化基础设施建设和应用推广，加强数据标准化建设和数据共享，促进医药卫生信息化与其他行业、领域的深度融合，如人工智能、大数据、云计算等。同时，中国也在加强法律法规建设，以保障医药卫生信息的安全性和有效性。

　　总体来说，从"十五"到"十四五"时期中国医药卫生信息化行业政策的落实取得了较好的成效，为医疗服务的现代化转型打下了坚实的基础；未来，还需要进一步加强技术创新和实践探索，提高医药卫生信息化的普及度和质量水平。

11.2.1.2　发展要求

中国医药卫生信息化发展要求可以从以下几个方面体现：

第一，医疗机构信息化建设。医疗机构信息化建设需要满足医疗质量管理、药品管理、病历管理、患者管理、医生排班等方面的需求，保证信息化平台的稳定与可靠运行。另外，医疗机构要落实信息安全管理要求，加强对数据备份和恢复的管理，确保数据的完整性、机密性和可用性。

第二，医药生产企业信息化建设。医药生产企业信息化建设需要建立全面、高效、数字化的信息化管理体系，为企业医药研发、生产、销售和质量管理等提供支撑。医药生产企业信息化平台需要满足准确性、实时性、安全性等要求，并与各级监管部门对接，确保企业合法合规运营。

第三，医药配送与零售企业信息化建设。医药配送与零售企业信息化建设需要建立端到端的信息化管理链路，以满足供应链、库存管理、业务处理等方面的需求。同时，需要建立电子商务门户网站并创建移动应用程序，以提供在线购买、在线支付等服务，进而满足消费者的多元化需求。

第四，医疗保险信息化建设。医疗保险信息化建设是指推进医疗保险管理、数据统计、资金结算、医保卡管理等业务信息化，建立全国性的医疗保障体系，实现信息化管理和统一监管。这就要求建立健全的医疗保险信息平台、保障患者的隐私安全和信息安全。

第五，医疗器械企业信息化建设。医疗器械企业信息化建设需要建立全面的信息化管理平台，对产品研发、生产、销售等各个环节进行数字化管理。同时，需要满足《医疗器械安全管理》的要求，保证产品的品质。

第六，医疗机构评审标准信息化建设。医疗机构评审标准信息化建设需要符合国家医疗机构评审标准及医疗质量管理、医疗事故管理等相关规范，保证信息系统的可用性、安全性和可靠性，提高医疗服务质量和患者满意度。

总的来说，医药卫生信息化发展要以提高信息化技术水平为核心，不断加强人才培养和技术创新，推动信息化技术在医药卫生领域的应用，建立健全的信息安全保障体系，引导医药卫生领域逐步形成科学、规范的信息化应用模式，提升医疗服务水平，改善医疗环境。同时，政府应制定符合国情的政策法规，为医药卫生信息化发展提供政策支持和保障，并推广和应用医药卫生信息化标准，为医药卫生信息系统的交互、互操作提供技术支持，促进医药卫生信息系统的集成和优化。

11.2.2　中国医药卫生信息化发展历程

中国医药卫生信息化发展历程可以追溯到 20 世纪 80 年代初期。当时，中国开始接触计算机技术，一些医院开始尝试利用计算机技术提高医疗服务质量和管理水平。但由于当时计算机技术和医疗服务的融合并不成熟，因此其应用范围较为有限。进入 20 世纪 90 年代后，随着信息技术的不断发展和普及，医药卫生信息化开始进入快速发展阶段。这一阶段以医院信息化建设为主要发展方向，各级医院开始建设医院信息系统和临床信息系统，并实现了信息系统在病历电子化、医疗质量控制、医疗资源管理、医疗保险管理等方面的应用。同时，中国也出台了一系列政策支持医药卫生信息化发展，促进医药卫生信息化普及和应用。随着移动互联网、云计算、人工智能等新技术的涌现，医药卫生信息化正朝着更加智能化、数字化、普及化的方向发展。目前,中国医药卫生信息化建设已经取得长足的进步,医院信息化、数字医疗、远程医疗等领域的信息技术正在不断发展和创新。未来,随着信息技术的进一步突破和其应用场景的拓展,医药卫生信息系统将成为医疗服务和医学研究的重要支撑。

11.2.3　中国医药卫生信息化现状

随着信息时代的到来,中国医疗卫生领域的信息化建设已成为重要议题。虽然中国已经建立了较为完善的医药卫生信息化基础设施,但新医改模式的应用仍然面临严峻考验。当前中国区域卫生信息化建设面临的主要问题包括信息孤岛、缺乏标准化工作流程和资金、人才不足等。在居民电子健康档案建设方面,中国已初具规模,近半数省份的居民电子健康档案建档率达90%以上,居民电子健康档案建设有望进一步推进。在临床信息化方面,中国正在积极推广电子病历的使用,同时也推进了医学影像、检验检查、远程会诊等领域的信息化应用。尽管产出与投入不协调现象较为普遍,但随着医疗卫生机构规模的扩大和国家政策的不断要求,电子病历系统的人员配置和资金投入已逐步增加,这对于提升医疗质量和效率具有重要意义。

11.3　中国医药卫生信息管理体系

11.3.1　中国医药卫生信息管理体系结构

2010年,卫生部提出了"十二五"期间卫生信息化总体框架"3521工程"。2013年,"3521工程"升级为"4631-2工程"。"4631-2工程"是中国医疗信息化发展的顶层设计规划,通过整合卫生资源,建立全方位、立体化的国家医药卫生信息管理体系,提高健康服务的质量和效率。"4631-2工程"具体包括四级人口健康信息平台、六项业务应用、三个基础数据库、一个覆盖各类医疗机构(包括中医机构)的融合网络和两个规范体系。图11-1展示了中国"4631-2工程"的总体框架。

11.3.1.1　区域人口健康信息平台

区域医疗信息化建设是指在一个特定的区域范围内,利用信息技术和平台,将各级医疗机构的信息系统进行集成,实现信息互联互通和协同工作。这是中国医药卫生信息化建设的重要组成部分,也是推进医药卫生体制改革、提高医疗服务质量和效率的重要措施之一。

为了推动区域医疗信息化建设,中国提出了建设区域人口健康信息平台的重要举措。根据《关于加快推进人口健康信息化建设的指导意见》的要求,应全面建成互联互通的四级人口健康信息平台,其中区域人口健康信息平台是实现中国卫生健康现代化的最重要、最基础的平台。区域人口健康信息平台的建设将有利于提高医疗服务质量和效率,促进医疗信息化的普及和应用,实现全民健康和医疗卫生现代化目标。

11.3.1.2　业务应用

"4631-2工程"共包含六项业务应用,分别是公共卫生、人口健康、医疗服务、医疗保障、药品供应保障和综合管理。这些业务应用是中国医药卫生信息化建设实施方案中所包含的

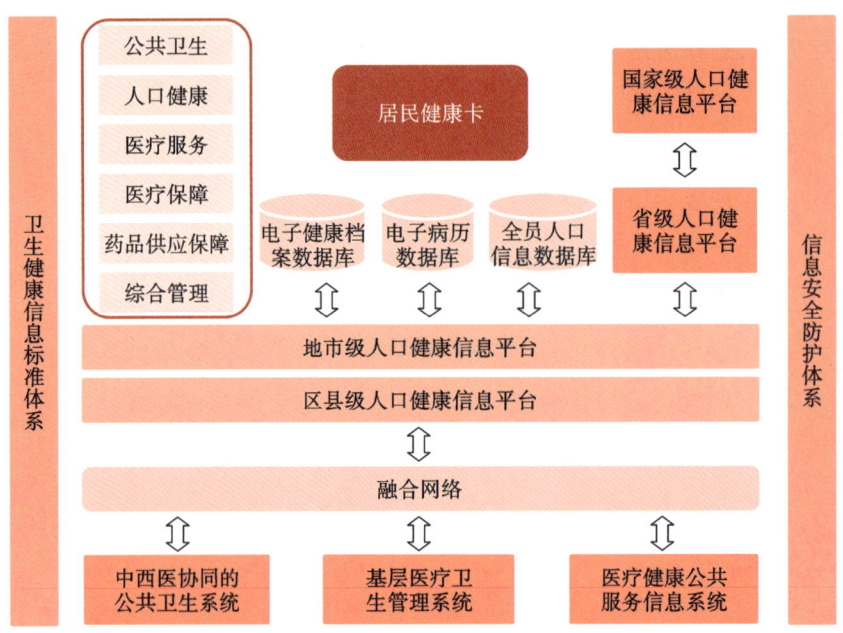

图 11-1　中国"4631-2 工程"的总体框架

内容,统筹建设和深化涵盖卫生各项业务领域的六大重点业务应用系统并实现各系统间互联互通,可提高医疗服务水平、促进医疗保障制度的完善、规范药品管理、加强人口健康工作管理、提高医疗管理水平。

11.3.1.3　基础数据库

三大基础数据库分别是电子健康档案数据库、电子病历数据库和全员人口信息数据库。电子健康档案数据库以电子健康档案为基础,内容主要来源于区域内各类医疗卫生机构运行的包括电子病历在内的相关业务应用系统。电子病历数据库以电子病历为基础,在按照业务规范要求把病历模板分段后,将有关患者健康和医护情况的终身电子信息,结构化存储在大量数据表中,从而实现数据的存储和查询。全员人口信息数据库为人口管理设计了户籍地、居住地和管理地(管理地是明确人口监测和家庭发展具体管理服务工作的单位)三个字段,用来分类登记户籍地信息、居住地信息和管理地等属性信息,分别用来统计户籍人口、常住人口和管理人口。

11.3.1.4　融合网络

按照区域卫生规划要求和属地管理原则,在地(市)区域公共卫生信息网络平台建设的基础上,区域内各级卫生行政部门、疾控部门及各级各类医疗卫生机构按照统一要求,依托国家公用数据网接入地(市)公共卫生信息网络平台,形成区域卫生信息网络。

11.3.1.5　规范体系

"4631-2 工程"总体框架中的规范体系包括卫生健康信息标准体系和信息安全防护体系。卫生健康信息标准体系是卫生健康信息化顶层设计的重要组成部分,当前中国卫生健康信息标准体系包含基础类、数据类、应用类、技术类、管理类、安全与隐私类等六类信息标准,具体见图 11-2。而信息安全防护体系是在信息产生、传输、集成等过程中确保医疗数据安全的一套防护体系,随着医疗信息安全标准缺失、医疗机构网络结构不合理、网络协同导

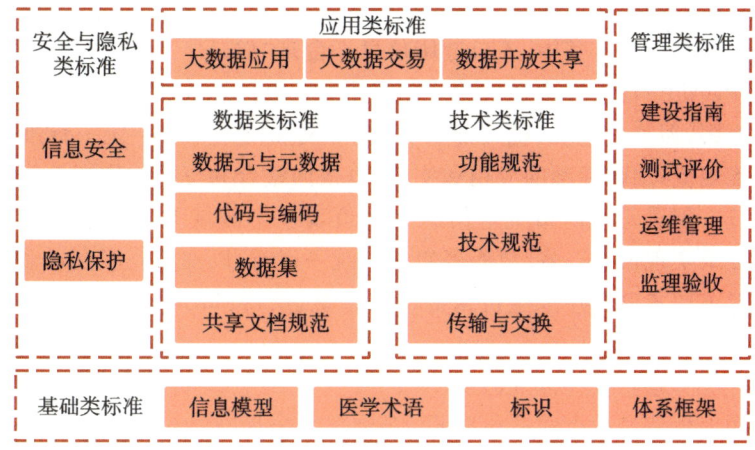

图 11-2　中国卫生健康信息标准体系框架

致信息外泄、患者隐私安全受到侵害等问题的出现而得以建立。

11.3.2　中国医药卫生信息管理体系运行机制

以"4631-2 工程"为基础,2021 年《"十四五"国家信息化规划》提出,积极探索运用信息化手段优化医疗服务流程,加快建设医疗专属云,推动各级医疗卫生机构信息系统数据共享互认和业务协同,建设权威统一、互通共享的各级全民健康信息平台。基于以上要求,可以将中国医药卫生信息管理体系运行机制划分为以下几个方面。

11.3.2.1　卫生数据治理

卫生数据治理是卫生信息管理的核心部分,也是最复杂的部分,涉及卫生健康信息标准体系建设、数据采集与整合、数据安全与隐私保护等多个方面。

卫生健康信息标准体系建设是卫生数据治理的基础。中国已初步建立卫生健康信息标准体系,包含基础类、数据类、应用类、技术类、管理类、安全与隐私类等六类信息标准,其中基础类标准具有指导性和全局性,数据类标准是保证语义层无歧义的重要基础,应用类标准为规范数据提供方式、数据应用方式提供指引,技术类标准对业务应用系统的技术水平、信息网络安全和隐私保护技术水平等进行约束,管理类标准用于指导业务应用系统合理应用相关标准并对标准应用情况进行评价与监督管理,安全与隐私类标准则对健康相关应用及服务提供过程中的数据安全与隐私问题予以规范约束。数据采集与整合也是卫生数据治理的关键环节;卫生信息管理体系通过各种信息系统,如电子病历、居民健康档案等信息系统,收集和整合卫生健康领域的相关数据。中国已建立标准化的居民健康档案,包括个人基本信息、健康体检记录、重点人群健康管理记录和其他医疗卫生服务记录。数据安全与隐私保护也是卫生数据治理的重要方面;卫生信息管理体系应建立健全的数据安全与隐私保护机制,以保护患者和卫生健康服务提供者的个人隐私和数据安全。中国高度重视网络安全,在信息安全方面,能够以相关法律文件为指导,实现信息共享与网络安全同步发展。对区域卫生信息平台的安全等级进行划分,并对卫生信息平台进行整改,有助于保障个人隐私和数据安全。

11.3.2.2　卫生信息平台建设

卫生信息管理体系需要一个开放的数据共享和交流平台,用于实现各类卫生健康机构和服务提供者之间的数据互通和共享，提升卫生健康服务的效率和质量，进而为决策者提供更全面和准确的数据支持。其中，人口健康信息平台是"4631-2 工程"的核心，而地市级人口健康信息平台在四级平台中扮演着"承上启下"的重要角色。区域卫生信息平台建设需遵循"四个统一"的原则，即统一标准、统一部署、统一专网和统一平台。统一标准是指遵循国家设定的信息标准规范，加强标准的应用和实施，以横向整合共享模式实现上下级单位的数据交换和共享。统一部署是指由市卫生信息中心负责全市区域卫生信息平台项目的统筹管理。统一专网要求实现市、县、乡、村等各级专网统一运行，以实现互联互通和信息共享。统一平台则要求对下属各种医疗卫生机构的信息系统进行接口开发，从而实现区域卫生信息互通共享。

11.3.2.3　卫生信息化人才队伍建设

为大力推动卫生信息化人才队伍建设，卫生部办公厅在 2011 年和 2012 年陆续发布了《全国卫生统计与信息化人才发展实施意见》《关于加强卫生统计与信息化人才队伍建设的意见》，明确规定了各级卫生行政部门、二级以上医院、公共卫生机构卫生信息化人员的配备标准。2022 年 8 月，国家卫生健康委印发了《"十四五"卫生健康人才发展规划》，提出完善人才管理制度机制、营造人才发展的良好环境的目标。卫生信息管理相关方包括需方（卫生行政部门、医疗卫生机构）、供方（信息科技企业）及运行维护方等，各方对于卫生信息化人才的特定需求不同。因此，目前中国首先采取以需求为导向的卫生信息化人才培养和利用机制，明确培养目标，制定人才培养顶层规划；其次建设统一的课程体系，以拓宽卫生信息化人才的视野；最后构建多层次、多角度的综合实践培养体系，以满足对复合型、应用型人才的培养需求。

11.3.2.4　卫生信息化应用普及

卫生信息化应用的普及和推广，是提高卫生服务质量和效率的重要途径。在硬件设施方面，应该注重基层医疗机构的建设，提高其信息化水平，从而实现基层卫生服务全覆盖。中国在 2017 年出台了《国务院办公厅关于推进医疗联合体建设和发展的指导意见》，要求县域主要组建医疗共同体，并推进省、市、县各级基层卫生数据中心的集约化建设，以实现卫生信息互联互通。这些措施可以提高信息系统的可用性和可靠性，从而为卫生信息化的推广提供更加有力的支持。除了硬件设施，人才队伍的不平衡性也是影响卫生信息化应用普及的一大障碍。为此，中国各地区采取了多种措施，例如针对卫生信息管理人才培训和晋升机制改革制定指导意见、推动卫生信息化人才转岗等。这些措施有利于提升卫生信息化人才的能力，从而推进卫生信息化的建设和普及。

在中国，卫生信息化应用已经广泛普及，湖北省推出的"健康湖北"公众服务平台是一个成功案例。该平台旨在打造全省统一的线上健康公众服务平台，将全省各级医院资源集中整合到一个平台上，包括预约挂号、门诊缴费、报告查询、在线问诊、健康监测等功能。用户可以通过一个平台便捷地享受到一站式医疗健康服务。该平台经过几年的升级更新，在原"问诊一点通"的基础上，依托湖北省健康医疗大数据中心，不断整合全省医疗卫生机构优势资源，构建以人为本的智慧健康服务体系，实现全生命周期的健康便民惠民服务和精细化管理，深入推进"一网式、一站式"医疗健康服务，旨在打造全省一体化、统一入口的健康公众服务平台。截至 2022 年 12 月，该平台已经汇集了全省数百家二级以上医疗机构和上千名注册医生，注册用户近 500 万人，提供各类服务逾 2 000 万次（包括抗疫服务逾 1 300 万次），通过平台申领电子健康卡数达 500 多万张。

1 Overview of China's Health System

China's basic political systems include the system of multi-party cooperation and political consultation under the leadership of the Communist Party of China (CPC), the system of regional ethnic autonomy, and the system of community-level self-governance. China's administrative organs are composed of the State Council of the People's Republic of China and local people's governments at all levels under its leadership. Local health administrative departments are under the leadership of the people's governments at the same level and accept the guidance of the health administrative departments at higher levels. Since the early 1980s, with the rapid growth of China's economy, the rapid advancement of urbanization, the rapid development of industrialization, the large-scale flow of population, and the deepening of the aging of the population, diseases related to lifestyle and aging have become one of the most important health problems in China.

1.1 Background of China's Health System

1.1.1 Geographical and Demographic Background

The People's Republic of China was founded on October 1,1949, with a total land area of about 9.6 million square kilometers, ranking third in the world, and a total sea area of about 4.73 million square kilometers. As of 2022, China has a total of 34 provincial-level administrative units, including 4 municipalities directly under the central government (Beijing, Shanghai, Tianjin, Chongqing), 23 provinces (including Taiwan), 5 autonomous regions and 2 special administrative regions (Hong Kong Special Administrative Region and Macao Special Administrative Region). At the sub-provincial level, there are 333 prefecture-level administrative units, 2 843 county-level administrative units, and 38 602 township-level administrative units.

China has a large population. In 2020, the Chinese population (excluding Hong Kong, Macao, and Taiwan) reached 1.41 billion, accounting for about 18% of the world's total population; 48.8% of the population was female; from 2010 to 2020, the average annual population growth rate was about 0.5%. According to the standards of the World Health Organization, China has entered an aging society in 1999, and the population aged 65 and above accounted for 14.2% of the total population in 2021. In recent decades, the education level of the Chinese population has increased significantly. The proportion of the Chinese population with high school (including technical secondary school) education or above increased from 9.4% in 1990 to 30.6% in 2020, while the illiteracy rate decreased from 15.9% in 1990 to 2.7% in 2020.

Since the mid-1980s, China's urbanization has been advancing rapidly, and the population flow has become more active. In 2011, China's urban population reached 691 million, surpassing the rural population for the first time. In 2020, China's urban population reached 902 million, accounting for 63.9% of the country's population. In the same year, China's floating population reached 376 million, accounting for 26.6% of the country's population, and the direction of population flow was mainly from rural areas to cities. The distribution of the Chinese population is very uneven, with dense populations in the eastern and central regions and sparse populations in the western plateaus. In 2020, the density of the Chinese population was 147 people per square kilometer.

1.1.2　Health Status of the Population

Like most other countries in the world, China's population and disease patterns have shifted from one dominated by high birth rates, high mortality rates, infectious diseases and malnutrition to one dominated by low birth rates, low mortality rates and chronic diseases. This is highlighted in the following aspects.

Average life expectancy. The average life expectancy of Chinese residents has increased significantly, from 35 years in 1949 to 70.8 years in 1996 and 78.2 years in 2021.

Child mortality rate. The infant mortality rate decreased from 46.9‰ in 1980 to 5.0‰ in 2021, and the mortality rate of children under five decreased from 62.7‰ in 1980 to 7.1‰ in 2021. The gap between urban and rural child mortality rates is narrowing, but it still exists. In 1995, the rural infant mortality rate was 2.9 times higher than the urban infant mortality rate, while in 2021 it was 0.8 times higher; the mortality rate of children under five in rural areas was 3.1 times higher than that in urban areas in 1995 and 1.1 times higher in 2021.

Maternal mortality rate. China's maternal mortality rate dropped from 88.8 per 100 000 in 1990 to 16.1 per 100 000 in 2021. The gap between urban and rural maternal mortality rates has gradually narrowed. In 1990, the maternal mortality rate in rural areas of China was 2.5 times higher than that in urban areas, while in 2021, the two were basically equal, with the maternal mortality rate in rural areas (16.5 per 100 000) slightly higher than that in urban areas (15.4 per 100 000).

Composition of the causes of death. Since the 1990s, the biggest change in the composition of the causes of death in the Chinese population is that the proportion of malignant tumors, cerebrovascular diseases and heart diseases has been increasing, while the proportion of infectious diseases, chronic respiratory diseases and digestive diseases has been decreasing. Along with this shift, non-communicable chronic diseases have become the major disease burden in China. Among the deaths caused by various diseases each year, malignant tumors, heart diseases, and cerebrovascular diseases are the top three contributors, and the number of deaths caused by them accounts for nearly 70% of the total deaths.

Infectious diseases. Infectious diseases, including cholera, leprosy, tuberculosis, schistosomiasis and malaria, used to be the most important diseases affecting the health of Chinese residents. Through the establishment of a disease prevention and control system and the implementation of vaccination programs and patriotic health campaigns, China has successfully reduced the incidence of infectious diseases and effectively controlled key infectious diseases, such as severe acute respiratory syndrome (SARS), human infection with highly pathogenic avian influenza, hand, foot and mouth disease, imported polio, and human infection with H7N9 avian influenza. In 2019, China reported a total of 21 cases of Class A infectious diseases with 1 death. Among these, there were 5 cases of plague with 1 death and 16 cases of cholera with no death. At present, the main infectious diseases in China include viral hepatitis, tuberculosis, acquired immunodeficiency syndrome (AIDS), etc. In 2021, the incidence of viral hepatitis in China was 87 per 100 000, the incidence of tuberculosis was 45.4 per 100 000, and the incidence of AIDS was 4.27 per 100 000. In 2021, the number of deaths due to AIDS, tuberculosis, and viral hepatitis in China were 19 623, 1 763 and 520, respectively.

1.2　The Basic Composition of China's Health System

In 2009, the "Opinions of the Central Committee of the Communist Party of China and the State Council on Deepening the Reform of the Medical and Health System" was promulgated. It is a programmatic document for a new round of medical and health system reform (referred to as the new medical reform) in China. Under the guidance of this document, China has built a framework for China's health system in recent years based on the principle of "one goal, four beams and eight pillars" (Figure 1-1). Among them, "one goal" is to establish a basic medical and health service system. The "four beams" refers to the public health service system, medical service system, medical security system, and drug supply guarantee system that cover both urban and rural residents. The "eight pillars" refer to the medical and health management system, the operation mechanism of medical and health institutions, the mechanism of diversified health investment, the mechanism of pharmaceutical price formation, the medical and health supervision system, the mechanism of medical and health science and technology innovation and talent guarantee, the medical and health information system, and the medical and health legal system.

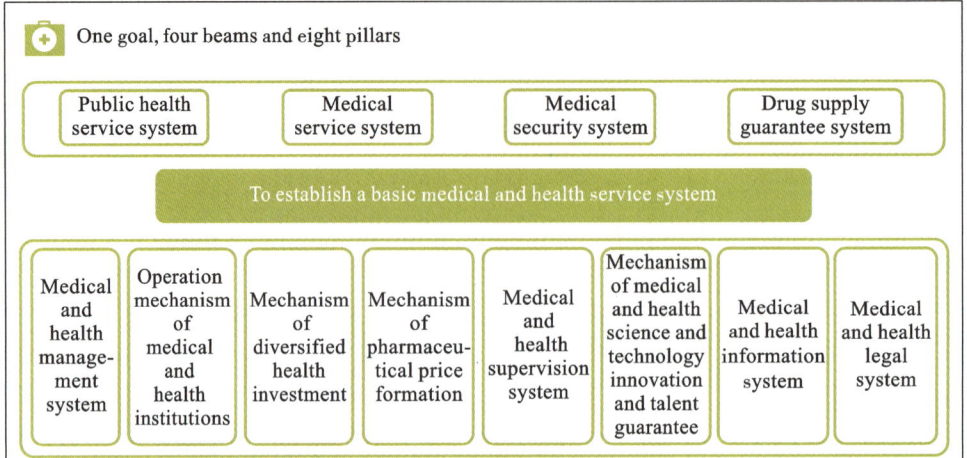

Figure 1-1 "One goal, four beams and eight pillars" in the construction of China's health system

1.2.1 Main Component Systems

1.2.1.1 The Public Health Service System

In China, public health services are mainly provided by primary medical and health institutions and professional public health institutions. China has established a public health service system based on community health service centers (stations), township health centers, village clinics, and other urban and rural primary medical and health service networks, with disease control and prevention, health education, maternal and child health care, mental health, emergency treatment, blood collection and supply, health supervision and other professional public health institutions responsible for specific professional guidance. The National Health Commission of the People's Republic of China has 19 internal institutions, including the Department of Medical Administration, the Department of Primary Health and the Department of Medical Emergency Response, as well as the CPC Committee and the Bureau of Retired Officials. It is mainly responsible for the supervision and administration of public health, medical services, health emergencies, etc. Local health administrative departments set up relevant institutions to take charge of local public health management.

1.2.1.2 The Medical Service System

In China, the medical service system consists of medical and health institutions such as second-level and third-level general hospitals, specialized hospitals and primary medical and health institutions. Among them, the second-level and third-level general hospitals mainly provide outpatient and inpatient medical services, specialized hospitals can provide medical services related to mental diseases and oral diseases, and community health service centers (stations), township health centers, village clinics and other primary medical and health institutions are responsible for providing basic medical services for residents in their jurisdictions. Both urban and rural residents can choose to go to various medical and health institutions.

1.2.1.3 The Medical Security System

China implements a multi-level medical security system with basic medical insurance as the mainstay, medical assistance as the foundation, and supplementary medical insurance, commercial medical insurance, charitable donations, mutual medical assistance and other forms of support developing together. Among them, the basic medical insurance includes the basic medical insurance for urban employees and the basic medical insurance for rural and non-working urban residents. The former covers the urban employed population, while the latter covers the urban non-employed population and the rural population. In recent years, the basic medical insurance has basically achieved population coverage (the coverage rate is stable at more than 95%), but its reimbursement ratio for expenses still needs to be improved.

Medical assistance is the foundation of China's multi-level medical security system. The medical assistance system raises funds through various channels such as government appropriations and social donations, mainly to provide financial assistance to urban and rural households eligible for subsistence allowances, households enjoying five guarantees (the elderly people, disabled individuals, and minors under the age of 16 in rural areas who are unable to work, have no means of livelihood, no legal guardians or supporters, or whose legal guardians or supporters are incapable of fulfilling their duties are guaranteed by the government to provide food, clothing, medical care, housing and burial) and other families with financial difficulties. This ensures that impoverished populations have access to basic medical services. Medical assistance primarily focuses on inpatient assistance while also considering outpatient assistance.

Critical illness insurance for urban and rural residents is an institutional arrangement that further guarantee the high medical expenses incurred by seriously ill patients on the basis of basic medical security, and is an expansion and extension of the basic medical security system. In order to avoid catastrophic family medical expenses for urban and rural residents, it is stipulated that the actual payment ratio of the critical illness insurance compensation policy shall not be less than 50%. The payment ratio is determined according to the level of medical expenses, and in principle, the higher the medical expenses, the higher the payment ratio.

With the further improvement of China's socialist market economy system and the increase of residents' income, the demand for medical and health services of residents is increasing, and the role of commercial medical insurance in the medical security system is becoming more and more important. In the current commercial medical insurance market, student medical insurance, supplementary medical insurance, and comprehensive insurance including medical insurance, accident insurance, property insurance, and life insurance are more common.

1.2.1.4 The Drug Supply Guarantee System

Since the 1980s, after more than 40 years of legal construction, China has established a relatively complete legal and regulatory system for drug management consisting of laws and regulations, departmental rules and other normative documents, including the Drug Administration Law of the People's Republic of China, the Law of the People's Republic of China on Traditional Chinese Medicine, the "Provisions for Drug Registration," the "Good Manufacturing Practice" (GMP), and the "Good Supply Practice" (GSP). Since 1995, China has successively implemented certification systems such as GMP, GSP and "Good Agricultural Practice for Chinese Crude Drugs" (GAP), and in 2006, the unannounced inspection system was implemented to strengthen the supervision and management of the quality of pharmaceutical production and operation. In addition, the National Medical Products Administration (NMPA) is the administrative institution for drug supervision and management in China. The drug regulatory departments of the people's governments of provinces, autonomous regions and municipalities directly under the central government are responsible for the drug supervision and management within their respective administrative regions. They implement unified supervision and management of drugs and their production, circulation and consumption. The National Administration of Traditional Chinese Medicine is responsible for the supervision and control of Chinese crude drugs.

In the process of solving the problem of drug accessibility, China has taken a series of measures to establish and improve the pharmaceutical management system and medical security system, which have reduced drug prices, stimulated the research and development of new drugs, and improved drug accessibility to a certain extent. In recent years, China has taken major measures to ensure access to drugs, including the establishment of a national essential medicine system, the improvement of the selection and adjustment mechanism of the National Essential Medicine List, the reform of the drug procurement mechanism, and the promotion of government-run primary medical and health institutions to implement zero-margin sales of essential medicines at purchase prices. As of 2013, all provinces in China had achieved full coverage of the essential medicine system in government-run primary medical and health institutions. In order to solve the problem of insufficient or unstable supply in the market, the implementation of fixed-point production of essential medicine varieties with small dosage and clinical necessity also ensures the supply of drugs to a certain extent.

Traditionally, the circulation of drugs in China has mainly flowed from manufacturers to wholesale enterprises, then to hospital pharmacies or retail enterprises, and finally to consumers. However, since the establishment of a national essential medicine system was officially implemented in 2009, China has begun to implement centralized bidding and procurement of essential medicines at the provincial level, which has changed the original drug circulation mode of primary medical and health institutions. In addition, since the pilot program of state-organized centralized procurement and use of drugs (also known as the "4+7" pilot program) was launched at the end of 2018, China has carried out 10 batches of state-organized centralized drug procurement. At the same time, various localities have also actively carried out centralized drug procurement in the form of provincial or inter-provincial alliances. In China, almost all medical institutions have pharmacies, which are responsible for the sale of drugs; hospitals are the main channel for drug sales.

1. 2. 2　Support Systems

1. 2. 2. 1　The Medical and Health Management System

The National People's Congress (NPC) of the People's Republic of China is the highest organ of state power in China, and its permanent organ is the Standing Committee of the NPC (NPCSC). The main functions and powers exercised by the NPC include amending the Constitution, supervising the implementation of the Constitution, formulating and amending fundamental laws in criminal, civil, state institutional and other areas, etc. The Education, Science, Culture and Health Committee of the NPC was established in 1983. It is mainly responsible for deliberating bills, draft laws and interrogatories on education, science, culture and health assigned by the Presidium of the NPC session or the NPC, submitting to the Presidium of the NPC session or the NPCSC proposals related to the Education, Science, Culture and Health Committee within the scope of the NPC's powers, participating in the legislative work of education, science, culture, health, sports, and population, and inspecting and supervising laws in the fields of education, science, culture, and health in accordance with the law under the leadership of the NPCSC, and so on.

The National Health Commission is subordinate to the State Council and is the highest health administrative organ in China. The National Health Commission and the National Administration of Traditional Chinese Medicine and the National Disease Control and Prevention Administration are the most important health administrative agencies in China. According to the division of responsibilities, among the other departments of the State Council, the National Development and Reform Commission, the Ministry of Civil Affairs, the Ministry of Finance, the Ministry of Human Resources and Social Security and other departments of the People's Republic of China also assume corresponding responsibilities in China's health governance, such as planning, financing, and insurance management. Among the national bureaus managed by the ministries and commissions of the State Council, the NMPA and other institutions are also involved in China's health governance.

In health governance, the specific responsibilities of administrative institutions at various levels in China differ, forming a top-down hierarchical management system. Each work department of a local government is under the unified leadership of the people's government at the same level, and is subject to the operational guidance or leadership of the competent department at the level above in accordance with the provisions of laws or administrative regulations. The health administrative organs at the provincial, municipal and county levels are the health administrative functional departments of the people's governments at the same level. Under the direct leadership of the people's governments at the same level, they are responsible for the health administration and management within their respective administrative areas, and accept the operational guidance of the health administrative organs at the higher levels. China's health management organization system is divided into four levels: national, provincial, municipal, and county. Townships (towns) generally do not have independent health administrative departments.

In China, non-governmental organizations (NGOs) are also involved in various areas of the health system, including philanthropic organizations, foundations, and professional associations. Professional associations, such as the Chinese Medical Association, the China Association of Chinese Medicine, the Chinese Preventive Medicine Association, the Chinese Medical Doctor Association, and the Chinese Nursing Association, play a certain role in health governance. Their main responsibilities include organizing on-the-job training or continuing education, reflecting the opinions, suggestions and requirements of medical workers to the government and relevant departments, and organizing experts to assist the government in demonstrating relevant laws and policies, etc.

1.2.2.2 The Operation Mechanism of Medical and Health Institutions

This section primarily introduces two key components: hospitals and primary medical and health institutions. Among them, public hospitals account for the vast majority of health resources, providing major outpatient and inpatient services. As early as over a decade ago, China began implementing pilot hospital reforms and gradually established corresponding institutional operating mechanisms. In 2010, China launched a pilot project to carry out a comprehensive reform of public hospitals, including exploring the separation of medical services from pharmaceuticals, eliminating the hospital compensation mechanism of "using drug sales to supplement medical income," and the updating of the wage distribution system for medical staff and the drug procurement system, etc. In 2012, China began to promote a pilot comprehensive reform of county-level public hospitals. The main content of it include reforming the compensation mechanism, such as changing the compensation of public hospitals from three channels of service charges, drug markup income and government subsidies to two channels of service charges and government subsidies, and eliminating the practice of "using drug sales to supplement medical income." After 2012, in order to accelerate the formation of a diversified medical pattern, China further proposed to vigorously promote the development of non-public medical institutions. Specific policies include requiring local governments to issue implementation rules to encourage social capital to run medical institutions, and encouraging areas with abundant public hospital resources to use social capital to participate in the transformation of some public hospitals. China is also further exploring and establishing mechanisms for the operation of hospitals. At present, there is a lack of objective evaluation of the impact of these operating mechanisms on hospital behavior.

In addition, in 2009, China began to reform the operational system of primary medical and health institutions, and implement systems such as the two-way referral system and the primary care first diagnosis system, as well as mechanisms such as the performance appraisal mechanism of primary medical and health institutions and personnel, and the income distribution mechanism of primary medical and health institutions. In 2012, it was clearly proposed that the income distribution of personnel in primary medical and health institutions should be based on the quantity and quality of services and be tilted in favor of the core and backbone health technicians.

In recent years, the facilities of primary medical and health institutions in China have been improved, but there are still problems of shortage and insufficient capacity of health technicians at the primary level. To this end, China has implemented strategies such as building a primary medical and health team, training health personnel for rural primary medical and health institutions, and introduced measures such as establishing a general practitioner system.

1.2.2.3 The Mechanism of Diversified Health Investment

In China, government health expenditure, social health expenditure, and personal health expenditure are the main sources of health financing and input. In terms of the sources of financing for total health expenditure, the proportion of government health expenditure to GDP decreased from 1980 to 1995 and nearly doubled from 2005 to 2012. However, the share of government health expenditure in the total government expenditure declined from 5.7% in 1995 to 4.5% in 2000, and although it began to rise slowly to 4.6% in 2005 and further to 6.7% in 2012, it remained at a low level. China's personal health expenditure as a proportion of total health expenditure is relatively high, reaching a peak of 60% in 2001 and then begin to decline gradually, falling to 34.3% in 2012, the lowest level since 1990. Personal health expenditure is also one of the main components of private health expenditure, and its share has declined year by year, from 95.6% in 2000 to 78.0% in 2012.

1.2.2.4 The Mechanism of Pharmaceutical Price Formation

In China, there are three forms of drug price management: government pricing, government-guided pricing and market-regulated pricing. Drugs included in the national drug catalog for basic medical insurance and drugs with monopoly production and operation characteristics outside the national drug catalog for basic medical insurance are subject to government pricing or government-guided pricing. Other drugs are subject to market-regulated pricing. The Drug Administration Law of the People's Republic of China has formulated a more detailed pricing method for the above three pricing forms. The drug pricing authority of the State Council and the drug pricing authorities of the provincial government formulate and publish the drug pricing catalog at the same level respectively in accordance with the central and local pricing catalogs. The government drug pricing department is responsible for monitoring the changes in the actual purchase and sale price and distribution price differential rate of drugs that are subject to government-guided pricing and market-regulated pricing. In 2009, the new medical reform began to study the abolition of drug markups, improve the public welfare of medical institutions, and reduce the burden of drug costs. The "Interim Measures for the Management of Prices in Drug Circulation," which came into effect in July 2012, controls the price differential rate (amount) at the wholesale stage and the sales stage of non-profit medical institutions, stipulates that the actual price difference in the wholesale stage shall be controlled in accordance with the method of "low price with high differential rate, high price with low differential rate," and gradually abolish the markups of drug sales by medical institutions.

In addition, medical institutions can apply to the health administrative department for practice registration of for-profit or non-profit medical institutions, and non-profit medical institutions enjoy certain preferential policies in terms of taxes and fees. China implements government-guided pricing for basic medical services provided by non-profit medical institutions and market-regulated pricing for for-profit medical institutions. For non-profit medical institutions, the National Development and Reform Commission, the Ministry of Health and the National Administration of Traditional Chinese Medicine issued the "Notice on Regulating the Management of Medical Service Prices and Related Issues," and officially promulgated the "National Medical Service Price Items Specification (2012 Edition)" to comprehensively regulate the management of medical service prices in 2012.

1.2.2.5　The Medical and Health Supervision System

China's medical and health supervision system usually includes three forms: first, set standards and enforce them; second, provide advice and policy guidance; third, set up prohibited matters. Health supervision is mainly carried out by the restrictions (regulations) set up (promulgated) by the government, that is, the specific regulatory activities are carried out by the relevant government departments, and their subordinate institutions can also undertake some regulatory activities, but they needs government authorization. The Central People's Government is mainly responsible for the overall design and arrangement of the development of public health undertakings at the national level, and local governments at all levels exercise the health supervision functions conferred by laws and regulations within their jurisdictions. The National Health Commission, the Ministry of Finance, the Ministry of Human Resources and Social Security, the Ministry of Civil Affairs, the National Development and Reform Commission, and the NMPA are the main state agencies involved in health supervision. Local governments have also set up corresponding departments. These agencies and departments carry out corresponding health supervision activities according to their respective functions, which provide guarantees for clarifying the scope and level of medical security, standardizing medical and health service behaviors, and ensuring the quality and safety of medical services.

For the supervision function with high professional and technical requirements, the Chinese government will also entrust relevant professional and technical associations and industry associations to formulate standards, participate in the implementation of the standards, and supervise the implementation of the standards. For example, in addition to carrying out relevant technical training for physicians, the Chinese Medical Doctor Association will also organize regular examinations of physicians, promote professional self-discipline and rights protection, and provide relevant information for the government to formulate policies, laws and regulations. These industry associations have also set up branches in various places to ensure coordination and joint interaction between the top and bottom of the work. Each industry association formulates the relevant articles, membership management regulations and other regulations within the association. All organizations or individuals participating in the work of the association must abide by relevant regulations, which also play a monitoring role in industry supervision.

1.2.2.6 The Mechanism of Medical and Health Science and Technology Innovation and Talent Guarantee

The Chinese government attaches great importance to the progress of medical and health science and technology, regards medical and health science and technology innovation as the focus of the country's scientific and technological development, strives to overcome difficulties in medical and health science and technology, and provides technical support for the people's health. In recent years, China has continuously increased its investment in medical scientific research, integrated superior medical research resources, implemented major special programs for medical and health science and technology, encouraged independent innovation, and strengthened research on major disease prevention and treatment technologies and key technologies for the development of new drugs. There have been significant breakthroughs in areas such as basic and applied medical research, high-tech research, traditional Chinese medicine (TCM) and integrated traditional Chinese and Western medicine research.

In terms of talent security, since 1949, China has gradually established a continuous and unified medical education system, including medical school education, post-graduation medical education and continuing medical education.

In China, medical school education includes undergraduate education, junior college education and other levels of education. After taking the national college entrance exam, the high school graduates will enter different levels of schools to receive different medical education according to their test scores. In addition to training clinicians, medical education also trains other types of health technicians, including nurses, health administrators, pharmacists, and medical laboratory personnel. Medical school education in China also includes postgraduate education. Undergraduate graduates are qualified for postgraduate studies by recommendation or by taking the national graduate school entrance examination. The duration of master's and doctoral studies ranges from 2 to 4 years, and they are awarded master's and doctoral degrees respectively after graduation.

Standardized training for residents belongs to post-graduation medical education, which refers to the systematic and standardized training that medical students receive as residents at recognized training centers with a focus on improving their clinical skills after completing their medical school education. Standardized training for residents is a unique and necessary educational stage of clinician training, which is of irreplaceable significance for improving medical quality and ensuring medical safety.

Continuing medical education refers to on-the-job continuing education after completing medical school education and post-graduation medical education. It aims to ensure that working health professionals keep abreast of new knowledge and technologies related to their profession and the development of medical science. Continuing medical education in China is subject to a credit system. Working health professionals are required to participate in continuing education activities each year and complete a certain number of credits.

In 1998, China promulgated the Law of the People's Republic of China on Medical Practitioners, announcing the implementation of a medical practice registration system. Health technicians need to pass the national unified physician qualification examination, and obtain the physician qualification certificate issued by the National Health Commission. Only those who have obtained the physician qualification certificate and have been registered to obtain the physician practice license are qualified to engage in medical activities independently. Institutions entrusted by the administrative departments of health of the people's governments at or above the county level shall, in accordance with the practice standards of physicians, conduct regular evaluations of physicians' professional level, work performance, and professional ethics. Currently, physicians can only practice medicine in the medical institutions where they are registered, but China is developing and implementing a multi-site practice system for physicians. There are three levels of health technician titles in China: junior, intermediate and senior.

1.2.2.7 The Medical and Health Information System

The medical and health information system is an important part of the health system, and China's new medical reform regards health informatization as an important task and an important support and guarantee. From the perspective of business fields, China's medical and health information system mainly includes hospital information system, public health information system, medical security information system, comprehensive health management information platform and regional health information platform. Among the above-mentioned medical and health information systems, except for the basic medical insurance information system for urban employees and urban residents in the medical security information system, which is mainly managed by the human resources and social security departments, all of the rest are mainly managed by the health administrative departments.

The management of China's medical and health information system mainly includes the formulation of medical and health information management policies and regulations and the development plan of medical and health information, the establishment of a comprehensive and systematic information resource development and sharing mechanism, the promotion of the standardization and unification of medical and health information standards, the strengthening of medical and health information infrastructure and network construction, and the enhancing of medical and health information security. At present, China's business application-based information system has played an important role in improving business efficiency and decision-making. With the popularization of information technology, the development of extended networks and advanced data mining technology, more and more data and information are rapidly accumulating.

1.2.2.8　The Medical and Health Legal System

The socialist legal system with Chinese characteristics is an organic and unified whole composed of multiple legal laws such as Constitution and related laws, civil and commercial law, administrative law, economic law, social law, criminal law, litigation and non-litigation procedure law, with the Constitution as the commander, the laws as the backbone, and the administrative regulations and local regulations as important components.

The Constitution of the People's Republic of China clearly stipulates the health rights and interests of residents: "Citizens of the People's Republic of China have the right to receive material assistance from the state and society in the event of old age, illness or loss of ability to work. The state develops social insurance, social assistance and medical and health services for citizens to enjoy these rights. " According to the adjustment object of the health law, China's medical and health legal system is divided into the legal system of medical and health institutions, the legal system of medical and health professions, the legal system of medical and health services and so on. These systems mainly regulate and guide a specific field. China currently lacks a comprehensive law that can govern the health legal system and link the Constitution with specific health laws and regulations.

At present, China does not have a specific health law, and has only a relatively complete system of health laws and regulations composed of individual laws and regulations focusing on public health and medical administration. In terms of medical aspects, it mainly includes the Law of the People's Republic of China on Basic Medical and Health Care and the Promotion of Health, the "Implementation Measures of the Law of the People's Republic of China on Prevention and Treatment of Infectious Diseases," the Mental Health Law of the People's Republic of China, the Drug Administration Law of the People's Republic of China and others. In addition, there are a large number of local regulations, ministerial and local government rules and normative documents, etc.

1.3　Development of China's Health System

Since the founding of the People's Republic of China in 1949, China's health system has gone through different stages of development, culminating in the formation of the current health system. The establishment and development of China's health system, especially the reform of organizational and governance models, is closely related to the reform of China's political, economic, and administrative systems. China's socio-economic development and reform can be divided into different stages, and the development of the health system presents different characteristics at different stages. From the founding of the People's Republic of China to the period before the reform and opening-up, China's health system was based on a planned economy and mainly relied on public financing for development. During this period, there were prominent issues such as a shortage of health services and insufficient service providing capacity. From the beginning of the reform and opening-up to 2002, China's health system gradually transitioned to being primarily based on a market economy. Governments at all levels mobilized all sectors of society to raise funds for the development of health services, health resources continued to increase, and the ability to provide health services was rapidly improved, but in the same period, the government's investment responsibility was weakened, and the personal health expenditure accounted for nearly 60% of the total health expenditure around 2000. Since 2003, China has continuously strengthened the responsibility of governments at all levels to invest in health. By 2021, the proportion of personal health expenditure in total health expenditure dropped to 27.6%.

1.3.1　The First Stage: From the Founding of the People's Republic of China to the Period before the Reform and Opening-Up (1949-1978)

At the beginning of the founding of the People's Republic of China, China's economic development level was low. The government took the realization of social equity as one of its core values and ran social equity through the design process of the socialist political system, economic system, and distribution system, gradually forming a planned economic system characterized by a high degree of centralization with the administrative management as the main means. The state managed social and economic affairs through administrative means, and in terms of income distribution, a system of "distribution according to work" was implemented. Under the strong unified planning and organization of the government, the top-down health administrative organization system had been formed, and the health system had also been established and developed rapidly: a relatively complete health system including medical treatment, prevention, health care, rehabilitation, teaching, and scientific research had been formed, especially the rural health service system represented by the rural cooperative medical care and the rural three-level medical and health service network, which had been highly praised by the World Health Organization. The basic framework of China's medical and health service system was largely formed during this period. Due to the constraints of the level of socio-economic development at the time, China's health system was characterized by "low level, wide coverage," the financing and reimbursement levels were low, and the overall planning unit was usually a city or county. Overall, health workers had a low level of education, poor capacity to provide health services, and provided poor quality of services. Publicly-financed health insurance covered the majority of urban dwellers, but the level of compensation was very low, especially in the case of rural cooperative health care. At that time, the situation of "lack of medical care and medicine" was more serious. It was partly because there was an overall shortage of health personnel at that time, and partly because although a large number of primary health personnel (such as barefoot doctors) could be trained through short-term training and other means, their service capacity was relatively low, and there was a shortage of high-quality health personnel. At the same time, since there was no direct relationship between the income of health technicians and the quality of medical service under the conditions of planned economy, the enthusiasm of health technicians to provide medical and health services was low, and the service efficiency was not high. In the period leading up to the reform and opening-up, various contradictions within China's health system became increasingly prominent.

1.3.2 The Second Stage: The Initial Stage of the Reform and Opening-Up (1979-2002)

The Third Plenary Session of the 11th Central Committee of the Communist Party of China held in 1978 ushered in China's transition from a planned economy to a socialist market economy, and made a historic decision to shift the emphasis in the work of the party and the country to economic construction and to carry out reform and opening-up. During this period, China's political, administrative, economic, and fiscal systems underwent tremendous changes, which had a profound impact on the health system.

First, reform of the political system. The Constitution of the People's Republic of China promulgated in 1982 established the program for China's political system and economic development in the new period, and the 13th National Congress of the Communist Party of China held in 1987 proposed establishing a highly democratic, well-regulated, efficient, and dynamic socialist political system as the long-term goal of political system reform. From 1979 to 2002, the reform of China's political system was mainly based on the separation of the functions of the party and the government, decentralization, and streamlining of institutions.

Second, reform of the administrative system. The reform of China's administrative system was carried out simultaneously with the transformation of the planned economic system to the socialist market economic system. With the development of China's economic and social undertakings, the Chinese government had begun to streamline administration and delegate powers. Local governments had begun to take on more health responsibilities, which was reflected in the fact that most medical institutions had begun to become independent operating entities that "operate independently and are responsible for their own profits and losses."

Third, reform of the economic system. From 1979 to 2002, the core of China's economic system reform was the gradual transition of resource allocation from administrative allocation to the basic role of the market. In the field of medical and health services, many health elements had been becoming more and more market-oriented, mainly regulated by the market, but the price of medical services was mainly in the form of government pricing.

Fourth, reform of the fiscal system. In 1994, China initiated the tax-sharing system reform, and the concentration of financial resources of the central government increased, while local government revenues declined, and the pressure on fiscal expenditure increased significantly. There was a contradiction between the continuous upward transfer of government financial power and the decentralization of government power in the field of health, and the government's investment in health had been greatly affected.

In order to solve the contradiction between the people's health needs and the efficiency of medical and health services during the period of planned economy, after the reform and opening-up, with reference to the practice of economic system reform, the health field has also begun to introduce more market mechanisms, including changing the income distribution method of medical institutions, adjusting the drug price policy and charging standards, etc. Medical and health services mainly focus on the needs of residents. In addition, private capital began to be allowed to open clinics and other medical institutions and provide medical and health services. At the same time, some public medical institutions were privatized. From 1979 to 2002, China's health service developed rapidly, with a rapid increase in the number of health institutions, health personnel, medical beds and equipment, and a significant increase in the capacity of health service delivery. However, due to the lack of institutional reform, the tendency of medical institutions to seek profits was becoming more and more serious, resulting in problems such as the rapid rise of medical costs and the escalation of the conflict between doctors and patients. In 2001, the proportion of the personal health expenditure in total health expenditure reached 60%, hitting a record high, while the proportion of government health expenditure was less than 16%. At the same time, the problems such as the lack of government investment in public health and the lag in the construction of rural health service system and medical security system were becoming more and more prominent. The emergence of these problems had made the reform of the medical and health system and the development of health undertakings included in the important agenda of the Central People's Government.

1.3.3　The Third Stage: The Deepening Stage of the Reform and Opening-Up (2003 to Present)

During this period, China's political, economic, and fiscal reforms entered a critical stage, and the economy continued to maintain a relatively high growth rate, but it faced some uncoordinated problems, such as the gap between the rich and the poor, the dual system between urban and rural areas, and the low social security coverage rate. In 2003, the Third Plenary Session of the 16th Central Committee of the Communist Party of China put forward the Scientific Outlook on Development, emphasizing people-oriented and balanced economic and social development. In 2007, the 17th National Congress of the Communist Party of China proposed to "continue to emancipate the mind, persist in reform and opening-up, pursue development in a scientific way, promote social harmony, and strive for new victories in building a moderately prosperous society in an all-round way,"of which the promotion of health development is one of the most important elements.

In 2003, the SARS epidemic spread throughout China, and China's health system experienced severe challenges. After the outbreak of SARS, the Chinese government began to reflect on the problems existing in China's health system, make efforts to solve the shortcomings of "emphasizing medical treatment over prevention" and "emphasizing urban areas over rural areas" in health work, strengthen the construction of public health service system, and vigorously promote the construction of rural health and urban community health. After 2003, the new rural cooperative medical care system has entered a period of accelerated development, but the positioning of the market and government functions in the medical and health system has not been fully clarified. There are still problems such as medical institutions relying too much on market competition to maintain their own development and the prominent situation of "difficult and expensive medical treatment", and the multi-level needs of the masses have not been well met.

In order to solve the contradictions and problems in the field of health and achieve the goal of everyone enjoying basic medical and health services, the new medical reform was officially launched in 2009, and the long-term goal was clarified: by 2020, a medical and health system covering urban and rural residents will be basically established. The new medical reform further clarified the responsibilities of the government in the field of health, and clearly proposed that the growth rate of government health investment should be higher than that of recurrent fiscal expenditure. For example, the per capita expenditure standard for basic public health services should be no less than 15 yuan in 2009 and no less than 20 yuan by 2011. Besides, the pilot reform of public hospitals has been implemented in some cities and the level of financing and compensation for basic medical insurance has continued to increase. In 2021, the per capita financial subsidy standard for basic medical insurance for rural and non-working urban residents reached no less than 580 yuan per person per year, 7. 25 times that of 2009. In 2021, the proportion of government health expenditure in total health expenditure reached 26. 91%. In addition, China has also stepped up efforts to encourage private capital to run medical institutions, relaxed the access scope for medical institutions run by social capital, and improved the practice environment for medical institutions run by private capital, resulting in an increase in the number of private hospitals from 6 240 in 2009 to 24 766 in 2021. Compared with the second stage of reform (1979-2002), which encourages social capital, the third stage mainly emphasizes encouraging social capital and private capital to enter the medical and health field on the premise of ensuring the public welfare and non-profit nature of government-run medical institutions, so as to meet the multi-level needs of the masses, and at the same time pays more attention to the improvement of the policy environment.

In 2018, the State Council embarked on its eighth institutional reform since the reform and opening-up, integrating the responsibilities of the National Health and Family Planning Commission and other institutions to form the National Health Commission. The National Working Commission on Ageing would be retained, and its daily work would be undertaken by the National Health Commission. The China National Committee on Ageing, which was managed by the Ministry of Civil Affairs, was transferred to the National Health Commission. The National Administration of Traditional Chinese Medicine would be managed by the National Health Commission.

Case Study   Rural Three-Level Medical and Health Service Network

From the 1950s to the 1970s, China established a relatively systematic rural three-level medical and health service network through the construction of three-level medical and health institutions with county-level medical and health institutions as the leader, township health centers as the main body, and village clinics as the basis, which effectively guaranteed the health level of farmers. This measure was praised by the World Health Organization as a model for developing countries to solve medical and health problems. The rural three-level medical and health service network mainly undertakes the tasks of preventive health care, basic medical care, health supervision, health education, etc., providing guarantee for farmers to obtain basic medical and health services, alleviating the problem of "difficult and expensive medical treatment," promoting the realization of rural medical and health development goals, and allowing farmers to receive treatment for minor illnesses within their villages, for common illnesses within their townships, and for major illnesses within their counties.

At present, the rural three-level medical and health service network in China is basically sound. By the end of 2021, China had established 17 000 county-level hospitals, 35 000 township health centers, and 599 000 village clinics across counties (districts, cities), townships, and administrative villages nationwide. Improving the rural medical and health system is the "first line of defense" to ensure the health of hundreds of millions of farmers, and it is the due meaning of comprehensively promoting rural revitalization. At present, China requires further deepening reforms to promote the healthy development of the rural medical and health system, including upholding and strengthening the overall leadership of the Communist Party of China over rural medical and health work, strengthening the overall planning and optimization of medical and health resources in counties, developing and expanding the rural medical and health workforce, and improving the level of medical and health security in rural areas. The goal is to achieve the following objectives by 2025: the functional layout of rural medical and health institutions will be more balanced and reasonable, the infrastructure conditions will be significantly improved, the rural medical and health personnel team will be developed and expanded, the personnel quality and structure will be significantly optimized, the operation mechanism of the rural medical and health system will be further improved, the reform and development of the rural medical and health system will make significant progress and so on.

2 China's Health Work Guidelines and the Healthy China Initiative

In China, health work guidelines serve as the guiding ideology for the development of health undertakings, possessing a comprehensive and overarching nature. They represent the fundamental guidelines for the Communist Party of China and the Central People's Government in leading health work. The Healthy China Initiative is a key task under China's health work guidelines during specific periods, aiming to promote public health and comprehensive development. Understanding and mastering the basic content of health work guidelines and the Healthy China Initiative, as well as the fundamental principles of formulating health work guidelines and health development strategies, are of paramount importance for guiding the reform and development of the health system.

2.1 China's Health Work Guidelines

A work guideline is a program that guides a job or career forward. Health work guidelines are the basic principles for the development of China's health undertakings. They are also the main basis for formulating various health systems and health policies.

2.1.1 Development and Content of China's Health Work Guidelines

Since the founding of the People's Republic of China, the Chinese government has formulated health work guidelines for different periods based on the country's fundamental conditions, the basic laws of the development of health undertakings, and the health needs of the people. These health work guidelines have been proven to adapt to the health development situation of specific periods, guide the development direction and path of health undertakings in different historical periods, and promote the sound development of China's health undertakings.

2.1.1.1 The Four Major Health Work Guidelines in the Early Years of the People's Republic of China (1949-1977)

(1) Formation of the Four Major Health Work Guidelines

From September to October 1949, the National Health Administration Conference was held. Given the severe shortage of medical resources, extremely poor medical and health conditions, and the prevalence of infectious diseases at the time, a preliminary health construction guideline was established, which is "putting disease prevention first, focusing on ensuring production and national defense construction, serving rural areas, factories, and mines, relying on the masses, and developing health care work." In August 1950, the Ministry of Health of the Central People's Government and the Ministry of Health of People's Revolutionary Military Commission of the Central People's Government jointly held the first National Health Conference, discussing and determining the general policy and tasks of China's health work. They established three major principles of health work: serving workers, peasants, and soldiers, putting disease prevention first, and uniting TCM and Western medicine. In September 1950, the 49th Executive Meeting of the Government Administration Council of the Central People's Government officially approved these three major principles. In December 1952, the second National Health Conference included "integrating health work with mass movements" into the principles, forming the four major principles of health work. These four principles are also known as the four major health work guidelines.

(2) Basic Content of the Four Major Health Work Guidelines

Serving workers, peasants, and soldiers. This guideline clarified the direction and service objects of health work, emphasizing that the health work must serve the people, which is a major issue of principle. Workers and peasants, as the main population of China, formed the foundation of the people's democratic regime and were the backbone of production construction in the People's Republic of China. The health challenges they face were particularly acute, yet the support they receive in terms of health security was relatively limited. Soldiers, as the core members of the national armed forces under the leadership of the Communist Party of China, were the cornerstone of national defense construction. Without the participation of the military, China's construction and development and the peaceful life of its people would not be fully guaranteed.

Putting disease prevention first. This guideline represented an economical, humane, proactive, and effective disease prevention and treatment strategy aligned with the fundamental interests of the masses. All medical, preventive and health care institutions, as well as all practitioners, should make prevention one of their primary responsibilities to ensure that the goals of disease prevention and health promotion are achieved.

Uniting TCM and Western medicine. This guideline aimed to unite practitioners of TCM and Western medicine to jointly provide health services. By giving full play to the respective professional advantages of TCM and Western medicine and promoting mutual learning and common development between them, the optimal allocation of medical resources and the overall improvement of the quality of medical services will be realized.

Integrating health work with mass movements. This guideline emphasized relying on and mobilizing the masses to participate in health work. Such mass participation not only promotes the popularization of health awareness and the development of healthy habits, but also accelerates the development of health undertakings, especially in the establishment of primary medical and health institutions and the training of health personnel.

These guidelines fully reflected the nature and characteristics of the socialist health service with Chinese characteristics, fitting China's basic conditions, the health needs of Chinese people, and the laws of the development of China's health undertakings. Under the guidance of these guidelines, China's health work achieved significant accomplishments.

2.1.1.2 The Health Work Guideline in the New Period (1978-2015)

(1) Formation of the Health Work Guideline in the New Period

The Third Plenary Session of the 11th Central Committee of the Communist Party of China held in 1978 marked the beginning of China's reform and opening-up period. With the steady establishment of the socialist market economy system and the deepening reforms and developments in social, economic, cultural, and scientific and technological fields, the health work guidelines established in the early years of the People's Republic of China faced the challenge of misalignment with the development trends of health work in the new period. To address this challenge, the "Decision of the Central Committee of the Communist Party of China and the State Council on Health Reform and Development" issued in 1997 clearly proposed the health work guideline that meets the requirements of the new period.

(2) Basic Content of the Health Work Guideline in the New Period

The health work guideline in the new period is "making rural areas the focus of our work, putting disease prevention first, supporting both TCM and Western medicine, relying on science, technology and education, mobilizing the whole society to join the efforts, improving the people's health and serving socialist modernization." This guideline reflects China's special attention to rural health work, emphasizes the central role of prevention in health work, and stresses the development philosophy of supporting both TCM and Western medicine. It also highlights the critical role of science and education in enhancing the professionalism of health services and calls for broad societal participation to achieve broader health service goals, thereby providing a solid health guarantee for socialist modernization. The strategic focus of this guideline includes making rural areas the focus of our work, putting disease prevention first, and supporting both TCM and Western medicine; the basic strategies are to rely on science, technology and education, and mobilize the whole society to join the efforts; the fundamental purpose is to improve the people's health and serve socialist modernization.

Making rural areas the focus of our work. Rural health work has always been a key area of high concern in China. Although China's rural health work has made great progress since the reform and opening-up—with the construction of medical and preventive health care network at the county, township, and village levels further strengthened, and the rural health teams gradually adjusted and enriched—it still faces many difficulties and problems. Therefore, it is imperative to significantly strengthen rural health work to curb the constraints on rural economic and social development caused by poverty due to illness and poverty returning due to illness.

Putting disease prevention first. The health work guideline in the new period continues to prioritize disease prevention. Medical, preventive, and health care institutions at all levels should implement the approach of putting disease prevention first and effectively carry out three-level prevention work.

Supporting both TCM and Western medicine. Supporting both TCM and Western medicine in the new period is an inheritance and development of the guideline of uniting TCM and Western medicine. It is also a policy guarantee for revitalizing TCM and promoting it globally. It requires TCM and Western medicine to strengthen their unity, learn from each other, jointly improve themselves, and actively explore ways and methods for the integrated development of them.

Relying on science, technology and education. Relying on science, technology and education reflects the implementation of the idea that science and technology are the primary productive forces and the strategy for invigorating China through science and education. It also summarizes the basic experience of significant development in health work since the founding of the People's Republic of China.

Mobilizing the whole society to join the efforts. Mobilizing the whole society to join the efforts is the further development and improvement of the guideline of integrating health work with mass movements. It involves the attention of party and government leaders at all levels, the collaboration of various social departments, and the active participation of the broad masses.

Improving the people's health and serving socialist modernization. The health undertakings is a public enterprise that benefits all members of society. Its development must always adhere to two core directions: one is to ensure and enhance the health level of the broad masses, and the other is to actively support and promote the process of socialist modernization. Improving the people's health means continuously meeting the growing health needs of the people and ensuring their right to health by providing comprehensive and high-quality medical services. Meanwhile, serving socialist modernization requires that the development of the health undertakings be coordinated with China's overall development strategy. By improving the people's health level, it contributes to China's economic development, social progress, and cultural prosperity.

The health work guideline in the new period effectively addressed many difficulties and problems in China's health undertakings, guiding the correct path for health development under the socialist market economy system. By clarifying strategic priorities, basic strategies, and fundamental purposes, health work can better serve the people, promote socialist modernization, improve public health, and foster social harmony and stability.

2.1.1.3 The Health and Wellness Work Guideline in the New Era (2016 to Present)

(1) Formation of the Health and Wellness Work Guideline in the New Era

Since the 18th National Congress of the Communist Party of China, the Central

Committee of the Communist Party of China has identified universal health as a fundamental foundation for a moderately prosperous society and has emphasized prioritizing health in strategic development. The focus of China's health work has gradually shifted to managing and promoting health, as well as formulating and implementing the Healthy China Initiative. From August 19 to 20,2016,the National Health and Wellness Conference was held in Beijing, where General Secretary Xi Jinping profoundly elucidated the significant importance of building a Healthy China. He also clarified the health and wellness work guideline in the new era, stating "focusing on the grassroots, taking reform and innovation as the driving force,putting disease prevention first,supporting both TCM and Western medicine,incorporating health into all policies,and promoting co-construction and sharing by the people." Subsequently,on October 25,2016,the Central Committee of the Communist Party of China and the State Council issued the "Outline of the Healthy China 2030 Plan," calling for the construction of a Healthy China and outlining the major policies and action plans.

(2) Basic Content of the Health and Wellness Work Guideline in the New Era

Focusing on the grassroots. Focusing on the grassroots is a significant reflection of the health and wellness work guideline in the new Era adapting to the new socio-economic development landscape in China. As urbanization progresses, traditional rural areas are gradually transitioning to urban settings,and farmers' identities are shifting to residents. In this context,shifting the focus of health work from "rural" to "grassroots" more accurately reflects the current social structure and population distribution and better meets the new demands of the public for medical and health services. Focusing on the grassroots means that the allocation of health resources, the provision of medical and health services,and health promotion activities should all pay more attention to the grassroots. This requires strengthening the service capabilities of grassroots medical and health institutions, improving the professional skills of grassroots health personnel, and enhancing the grassroots medical service network to ensure that grassroots people can enjoy convenient, efficient,and high-quality medical services. Simultaneously,focusing on the grassroots also emphasizes integrating health work with grassroots social governance, mobilizing and relying on grassroots people to participate in health work,and forming a beneficial situation where the government leads,society participates,and the public benefits.

Taking reform and innovation as the driving force. Taking reform and innovation as the driving force marks an important evolution of health and wellness work guideline in the new era. It transcends the traditional scope of "relying on science,technology and education,"incorporating cultural and institutional innovation as core driving forces for health work. This reflects the comprehensive implementation of the five major development concepts:innovation,coordination, green development,openness, and sharing, and it is the only way to promote the sustained development of China's health undertakings.

Putting disease prevention first and supporting both TCM and Western Medicine.

Putting disease prevention first and supporting both TCM and Western medicine are crucial principles of China's health work. Currently, the situation of infectious disease prevention and treatment remains severe, and the mortality rate of non-communicable chronic diseases is rising. Cardiovascular diseases, malignant tumors, and other chronic diseases have become the main causes of death among urban and rural residents. In health work, comprehensive prevention strategies must be implemented to effectively reduce the incidence and mortality rate of chronic diseases. The implementation of these strategies aims to build a more comprehensive medical and health system, improve the health level of the public, and lay a solid foundation for achieving the goals of Healthy China. China will leverage the advantages of TCM in prevention and treatment, accelerate the modernization and industrialization of TCM, promote the complementary and coordinated development of TCM and Western medicine, advance the high-quality development of the TCM industry, and promote TCM globally.

Incorporating health into all policies. Incorporating health into all policies is a concrete action to realize China's comprehensive health concept, reflecting a comprehensive understanding of and response to health impact factors. Globally, there is a consensus that health status is closely linked to multiple social factors such as poverty, education, environment, and employment. To ensure the sustainability of health outcomes, China must integrate the comprehensive health concept into all government policies, establishing the idea that maintaining health is a shared responsibility of all government departments and implementing comprehensive health management.

Promoting co-construction and sharing by the people. Promoting co-construction and sharing by the people further improves the guidelines of integrating health work with mass movements and mobilizing the whole society to join the efforts, reinforcing the concept of "sharing." Health and wellness involves all aspects of society, relates to every household, and is a systematic project. Only with active cooperation from various social sectors and widespread participation from the public can the goals of universal participation, shared responsibility, and universal benefit be achieved. Party committees and governments at all levels bear significant responsibilities. Only by adhering to co-construction and sharing by the people can the sustainability of health outcomes be ensured.

2.1.2 Basic Principles for Formulating Health Work Guidelines

In China, the formulation of health work guidelines adheres to the following fundamental principles:

Adhering to the comprehensive leadership of the Communist Party of China in health work. This principle reflects China's firm commitment to the development of its health undertakings and the fundamental purpose of the Communist Party of China to serve the people wholeheartedly. Only by adhering to the comprehensive leadership of the Communist Party of China in health work can effectively progress and implementation of health work be ensured.

Maintaining the welfare and public nature of health undertakings. China's health undertakings is characterized by its welfare and public nature. The welfare nature emphasizes the government's responsibility for the development of health undertakings and the health of the people, particularly the protection of vulnerable groups. The public nature stresses the shared responsibility of the government, society, and individuals in developing health undertakings and safeguarding public health. Under different economic systems, the nature of China's health undertakings varies. During the planned economy period, the health undertakings was a welfare one. However, with the establishment of the socialist market economy system, the health undertakings has evolved into a public welfare one with a certain welfare nature that does not aimed at profit.

Ensuring the fundamental position of health undertakings in economic and social development. Health departments protect people's lives and physical and mental health through the provision of medical, preventive, health care, and rehabilitation services. They participate in the enhancement of productivity and the restoration of labor force, thereby promoting economic and social development. This function cannot be replaced by any other department. Health, education, culture, science, and sports hold equally important positions as they are different aspects of the superstructure. The fundamental position of the health undertakings in economic and social development must be guaranteed, and sufficient support and attention should be given to it.

Adhering to a plan-led health reform orientation. This principle reflects the Chinese government's responsibility and commitment to health undertakings, emphasizing China's macro-control and management of the health field. Health reforms led by the plans ensure balanced development of basic health services and prevent neglect of underserved regions and vulnerable populations, while market-driven health reforms might overlook these aspects, leading to disparities in access to basic health services. In the health field, market forces cannot entirely replace the government's duties and functions. The government should ensure and improve the quality of public health services and expand service coverage, as well as guide the rational allocation and flow of health resources through the implementation of the plans to meet the basic health service needs of the people.

Prioritizing the protection of people's health in strategic development. This principle is very important. It underscores the importance of safeguarding people's health, placing it at the forefront of economic, social, and national defense development to ensure the comprehensive attention and protection of people's health rights. This principle promotes the steady development of health undertakings, helps improve overall health levels and national quality, and contributes to the sustained development of society and the economy. Therefore, it is crucial to understand the significant importance of "prosperity for all is impossible without health for all" and "striving to ensure people's health throughout the life cycle."

2.2 The Healthy China Initiative

2.2.1 The Health Development Strategy

The health development strategy is a long-term plan designed to meet the health needs of the population. It is a crucial area of economic and social development strategy, which must be coordinated with the overall economic and social development strategy. The core focus of China's health development strategy is to improve the health level of the population by strengthening the construction of basic medical and health services and achieving a combination of both qualitative and quantitative development. The guiding principle of this strategy is to maintain a balance between equity and efficiency, ensuring that all people have access to basic health services.

2.2.1.1 The Significance of the Health Development Strategy

Promoting economic development and social progress. One of the primary objectives of the health development strategy is to promote economic development and social progress. By improving the health level of the population and strengthening the construction of basic medical and health services, health work can restore workforce and enhance labor productivity, thus providing strong support for economic development. Additionally, health work can reduce the negative impacts of diseases and health issues on society, improve the quality of life for the population, and enhance social stability and sustainability of social development.

Guiding the scientific development of health undertakings. The formulation and implementation of a scientific health development strategy ensures that the health undertakings progresses in the right direction, and enhances the scientific, targeted, and effective aspects of health work, thus better serving the population and improving overall health levels. A scientific health development strategy also stimulates more innovative researches in the health field, and elevates the development level and international competitiveness of health undertakings, laying a solid foundation for its long-term development.

Facilitating the achievement of health goals. The formulation of the health development strategy allows managers to align with objective laws and circumstances, seize opportunities presented by the environment, shift from reactive response to proactive action, and facilitate the achievement of health goals.

Highlighting the development priorities of health undertakings. The formulation of the health development strategy can make the development of health undertakings more targeted and efficient. It focuses on the most pressing current and future health issues, prioritizing the development and improvement of health service quality and levels to meet the health needs of the population. By clarifying the development priorities of health undertakings, the health development strategy can guide the rational allocation and use of resources and promote substantial progress in health undertakings.

Improving national health quality. China faces both traditional health problems common to developing countries and health issues typical of developed countries, along with significant health disparities between urban and rural areas, regions, and populations. The health development strategy focuses on addressing major health problems affecting urban and rural residents and strengthens effective interventions for long-term health issues by formulating practical national health action plans to maintain and enhance national health.

2.2.1.2　Characteristics of the Health Development Strategy

The health development strategy has the characteristics of comprehensiveness, long-term perspective, leadership, programmatic nature, adaptability, and foresight. These characteristics collectively form the theoretical foundation and practical guide for the scientific development of China's health undertakings.

Comprehensiveness. The health development strategy needs to adopt a macro perspective, comprehensively considering key elements such as the formulation of health policies, resource input, and talent cultivation. It should cover various aspects of the health field, including medical services, health education, and disease prevention and control, with a focus on the future to lay a solid foundation for the sustainable development of health undertakings.

Long-term perspective. The health development strategy should be a medium- to long-term plan, focusing on the overall survival and development of health undertakings. It requires the establishment of long-term goals, continuous strengthening of infrastructure construction and talent cultivation, and the promotion of sustained progress in health undertakings through scientific development concept.

Leadership. The health administrative departments play a leading role in the development of health undertakings. They are responsible for defining the development direction, setting strategic goals, formulating relevant policies and plans, and organizing and supervising the implementation of various tasks to ensure coordinated and stable development of health undertakings.

Programmatic nature. As a programmatic document guiding the development of health undertakings, the health development strategy provides comprehensive guidance for setting health development goals and policies, as well as resource allocation, management and service planning.

Adaptability. The health development strategy should possess flexibility and adaptability to meet the changing and diverse health needs of society. Health departments need to timely adjust health service models, improve health service levels, continuously innovate and promote highly adaptable health technologies and policies, expand health service coverage, and improve health service quality.

Foresight. The formulators of the health development strategy should have foresight, anticipating potential new problems, situations, and challenges that may arise in the future and formulating corresponding coping strategies. This helps guide health undertakings towards a more targeted and sustainable development path, avoid blind following, and ensure smoother and healthier development of health undertakings.

2.2.1.3　Basic Principles for Formulating the Health Development Strategy

The core of China's health development strategy is to uphold the purpose of serving the people's health and comprehensively improve the health level of the population. The formulation of the health development strategy should adhere to the following fundamental principles:

People-centered principle. The goal of enhancing the health level of the population should be a core objective of national development and should be fully integrated into economic and social development planning. Health is not only the foundation for individual and family happiness but also a crucial cornerstone for the development of the nation and its different ethnic groups. By prioritizing the development of health undertakings and comprehensively safeguarding the health of the people, society's emphasis on health can be elevated, and the achievement of strategic goals of economic and social development can be ensured.

Equity first, balancing efficiency. It should be ensured that different groups have equitable access to basic health services while emphasizing the efficient use of health resources to achieve the greatest health outcomes with the least resource input. Additionally, there should be a focus on combining government responsibilities with market mechanisms, mobilizing the participation of the entire society, forming an orderly competition mechanism, and meeting the diverse health needs of the population.

Overall planning, focusing on key areas. When formulating the health development strategy, it is essential to consider all aspects comprehensively, balance various interests, focus on key areas, strengthen collaborative efforts, and enhance the overall coordination and coherence of the development of health undertakings. By creating comprehensive and systematic plans, the rational allocation and utilization of health resources can be achieved, thereby addressing fundamental contradictions in the health field.

Prevention-oriented, combining prevention with treatment. It is essential to emphasize the prevention and control of diseases at the source to reduce the waste of medical resources. Simultaneously, it is essential to focus on the combination of prevention and treatment, emphasize early diagnosis and treatment of diseases, and promote the shift of medical models from "disease-centered" to "people-centered," from "treatment-oriented" to "prevention-oriented," and from "patient-centered" to "health-centered."

Ensuring basic services, strengthening primary care, and building mechanisms. The provision of basic public health and medical services should be ensured to meet the basic medical needs of the population. It is essential to strengthen the capacity of primary health services, promote the establishment of a tiered diagnosis and treatment system, and focus services and resources on primary care. It is also essential to establish and improve the development mechanisms of health undertakings, strengthen the formulation and implementation of health policies and regulations, and promote the scientific, standardized, and institutionalized development of health undertakings.

2.2.2　The Content and Evolution of the Healthy China Initiative

Since the founding of the People's Republic of China, the health policy guidelines formulated at different periods have collectively contributed to the formation of China's health development strategy. The Healthy China Initiative is the core content of China's health development strategy and is currently the main health development strategy in China. The Healthy China Initiative is an essential part of building a moderately prosperous society in all respects. Health is both the goal and the source of development; it is a necessary requirement for promoting comprehensive human development, an essential condition for economic and social development, a crucial indicator of national prosperity and strength, and a common pursuit of the broad masses.

2.2.2.1　The Development Process of the Healthy China Initiative

In the 1970s, the World Health Organization proposed the strategic goal of "Health for All by the Year 2000," which the Chinese government subsequently committed to achieving. In 1988, this goal was incorporated into China's overall economic and social development objectives for the year 2000. The "Decision of the Central Committee of the Communist Party of China and the State Council on Health Reform and Development" issued in 1997 identified rural health, preventive care, and the equal importance of TCM and Western medicine as strategic priorities for the development of the health work. The Fifth Plenary Session of the 18th Central Committee of the Communist Party of China and the report of the 19th National Congress of the Communist Party of China further established the crucial status of public health.

2.2.2.2　Main Characteristics of the Healthy China Initiative

The Healthy China Initiative adheres to both goal-oriented and problem-oriented approaches, highlighting its strategic, systemic, guiding, and operational nature. It has the following distinctive characteristics:

Emphasizing the comprehensive health development concept. Currently, the main health indicators of Chinese residents are generally better than the average levels in middle- and high-income countries. However, with the advancement of industrialization, urbanization, population aging, and changes in ecological environment and lifestyles, maintaining public health faces a series of new challenges. According to the World Health Organization's research, behavioral and environmental factors have an increasingly prominent impact on health. The treatment-centered approach is inadequate and unsustainable for addressing health issues. Therefore, the Healthy China Initiative establishes the concept of "comprehensive health" and "comprehensive hygiene" with "health promotion as the center."It emphasizes integrating this concept into the entire process of public policy formulation and implementation, coordinating responses to a wide range of health impact factors, and maintaining the health of the population throughout all aspects and across the entire life-cycle.

Combining long-term and current focus. The Healthy China Initiative is aligned with the national strategies of building a moderately prosperous society in all respects and achieving the "Two Centennial Goals." It fully considers the alignment with the objectives at various stages of economic and social development and the requirements of the United Nations' 2030 Agenda for Sustainable Development. At the same time, it addresses current prominent issues by innovating systems and mechanisms, and coordinating policies and measures across health and family planning, sports and fitness, environmental protection, food and drug safety, public safety, and health education from a holistic perspective to form a concerted effort to promote health.

Having clear and operational goals. The Healthy China Initiative sets several key quantitative indicators across various aspects such as overall health levels, health impact factors, health services and guarantees, the health industry, and the health promotion system. This concretizes the goals and tasks, making the work process operational, measurable, and assessable. Accordingly, the Healthy China Initiative proposes a "three-step" goal, which includes "by 2020, main health indicators will rank among the top in middle- and high-income countries," "by 2030, main health indicators will enter the ranks of high-income countries," and "by 2050, a health nation compatible with a modern socialist country will be built."

2.2.2.3 Goals of the Healthy China Initiative

First, by 2020, a system of basic medical and health services with Chinese characteristics covering urban and rural residents will be established, the health literacy level has continued to improve, the health service system will be complete and efficient, everyone will have access to basic medical and health services and basic physical fitness services, and a health industry system with rich connotations and a reasonable structure will be basically formed, with main health indicators ranking among the top in middle- and high-income countries.

Second, by 2030, the following specific goals should be achieved:

The health level of the population has continued to improve. The physical fitness of the population has improved significantly, with the average life expectancy reaching 79 years and a marked increase in average healthy life expectancy.

Major health risk factors have been effectively controlled. The health literacy of the population has been greatly improved, a healthy lifestyle has been popularized, a healthy working and living environment has basically taken shape, food and drug safety has been effectively guaranteed, and a number of major diseases have been eliminated.

The capacity of health services has been greatly improved. A high-quality and efficient integrated medical and health service system and a well-functioning public service system for physical fitness have been fully established, the health security system has been further improved, the overall strength of health science and technology innovation ranks among the top in the world, and the quality and level of health services have been significantly improved.

The scale of the health industry has expanded significantly. A comprehensive and well-structured health industry system has been established, and a number of large enterprises with strong innovation ability and international competitiveness have been formed, becoming pillar industries of the national economy.

The institutional system for promoting health has been further improved. The system of policies, laws and regulations conducive to health has been further improved, and the system and capacity for health governance have been basically modernized.

Third, by 2050, a health nation compatible with a socialist modern country will be built.

2.2.2.4　The Content of the Healthy China Initiative

The overarching strategy of the Healthy China Initiative is to center on human health, addressing health influencing factors such as individuals' lifestyles and behaviors, medical and health services and security, and production and living environment in a sequence from internal to external, and from individual behavior to environmental conditions. The strategy encompasses five main tasks: promoting healthy lifestyles, optimizing health services, enhancing health protection, building a healthy environment, and developing the health industry.

Promoting healthy lifestyles. Starting from the source of health promotion, it emphasizes individual health responsibility. This includes strengthening health education, improving the health literacy of the entire population, extensively conducting national fitness activities, fostering self-disciplined health behaviors, and guiding the public to adopt healthy lifestyles characterized by balanced diets, adequate exercise, smoking cessation, alcohol moderation, and mental well-being.

Optimizing health services. Focusing on women and children, the elderly, impoverished populations, and people with disabilities, it implements measures from both prevention and treatment perspectives. This includes strengthening public health services that cover the entire population, increasing efforts to prevent and control chronic and major infectious diseases, implementing health poverty alleviation projects, innovating the model for medical and health service delivery, leveraging the unique advantages of TCM in preventive care, and providing higher quality health services to the public.

Enhancing health protection. By improving the universal medical insurance system, and deepening reforms in the public hospital, pharmaceutical, and medical device distribution systems to reduce inflated prices, it aims to significantly ease the financial burden of medical expenses for the public, and improve patients' medical experience. This involves strengthening the integration and alignment of various medical insurance systems, refining insurance management service systems, and ensuring the long-term sustainability of the health protection capacity.

Building a healthy environment. Addressing environmental issues that impact health, it involves initiatives such as carrying out air, water, and soil pollution prevention and treatment, strengthening food and drug safety supervision, enhancing work safety and occupational disease prevention and treatment, promoting road traffic safety, deeply engaging in patriotic health campaigns, building healthy cities and villages, and improving emergency response capabilities to minimize the impact of external factors on health.

Developing the health industry. Differentiating between basic and non-basic health industries, it aims to optimize a diversified health service delivery structure, and promote the development of non-public medical institutions toward higher standards and larger scale. This involves advancing supply-side structural reforms, supporting the development of new health service models such as health tourism, actively developing fitness and leisure industries, enhancing the development of the pharmaceutical industry, and continually meeting the increasing and diverse health needs of the population.

Case Study　The "Healthy China Initiative (2019-2030)"

To effectively advance the implementation of the "Outline of the Healthy China 2030 Plan" and the achievement of its goals, the National Health Commission formulated the "Healthy China Initiative (2019-2030)" in June 2019. In July 2019, the State Council established the Healthy China Initiative Promotion Committee, which is responsible for coordinating the implementation, monitoring, and evaluation of the "Healthy China Initiative (2019-2030)." Focusing on two core areas of disease prevention and health promotion, the "Health China Initiative(2019-2030)" proposes 15 major special actions to promote the transformation from a disease-centered approach to a health-centered approach, and strive to minimize illness and improve health outcomes among the population. These 15 special actions include: health knowledge dissemination, balanced diet promotion, national fitness campaigns, smoking control, mental health promotion, health environment promotion, maternal and child health promotion, primary and secondary school health promotion, occupational health protection, elderly health promotion, cardiovascular disease prevention and treatment, cancer prevention and treatment, chronic respiratory disease prevention and treatment, diabetes prevention and treatment, and infectious and endemic disease prevention and control.

3　China's Medical Service System

China's medical and health institutions mainly include hospitals and primary medical and health institutions. Since the reform and opening-up, the number of hospitals in China has maintained a continuous growth trend. By the end of 2021, there were 36 570 hospitals in China, 3.9 times that of 1978, of which 67.7% were private. Correspondingly, the number of hospital beds in China has also experienced continuous growth. In 2021, the number of beds in medical and health institutions per 1 000 population reached 6.7. Although large-scale medical equipment is mainly concentrated in second-level and above hospitals, the equipment allocation of primary medical and health institutions is also improving year by year. In terms of informatization construction, the hospital management information system, clinical information system and regional health information system have all achieved rapid development. Government investment in the health field is concentrated in primary medical and health institutions and basic medical security.

China's health human resources are growing rapidly, with the number of health technicians per 1 000 population reaching 7.97 in 2021, but there is a relative shortage of nursing staff. Health technicians in China's public medical and health institutions have clear career development plans, and their career development prospects are relatively broad. However, there is a certain gap between urban and rural areas in the allocation of health technicians. In 2021, the number of health technicians per 1 000 population in urban areas was 9.87, while in rural areas it was 6.27. Other challenges to the development of China's health human resources include the lack of adequate health personnel at the grassroots level and the low level of education of health technicians. Although China has initially established a continuous and unified medical education system including medical school education, post-graduation medical education and continuing medical education, this system still needs to be improved and the quality of medical education still needs to be strengthened.

3.1　Overview of China's Medical Service System

3.1.1　Medical and Health Institutions and Their Types

China's medical and health institutions can be divided into four categories: hospitals, primary medical and health institutions, professional public health institutions, and other medical and health institutions. Here is an overview of the hospitals.

Hospitals in China offer both inpatient and outpatient services. According to the objects or types of diseases they serve, hospitals can be divided into general hospitals, specialized hospitals, and others. General hospitals provide comprehensive medical services for various groups of people and diseases, while specialized hospitals such as children's hospitals, ear, nose and throat hospitals, obstetrics and gynecology hospitals, and dental hospitals provide specialized medical services. Hospitals in China include Western medicine hospitals and TCM hospitals. Most hospitals can offer Western medicine services. In China, almost every county has a TCM hospital, which provides TCM services. In some ethnic minority areas, there are also ethnic hospitals, such as Tibetan medicine hospitals and Mongolian medicine hospitals. According to different ownership systems, hospitals in China can be divided into public hospitals and private hospitals. At present, public hospitals are the main body of China's medical service system. Private hospitals have also made some progress in recent years. Most private hospitals are for-profit hospitals, while some are non-profit hospitals.

In 1989, China began to implement a hierarchical hospital management system. According to the comprehensive level of the hospitals, such as their size and function, hospitals in China are divided into three levels.

A first-level hospital is a primary hospital that directly provides prevention, medical treatment, health care and rehabilitation services to a community with a certain population. Its responsibilities mainly include providing preventive health care (such as community health and epidemic prevention, maternal and child health care, family planning surgery and technical guidance, and health education), medical services (such as outpatient and inpatient diagnosis and treatment of common and frequent diseases in the community, and community rehabilitation medicine) and other services.

A second-level hospital is a regional hospital that provides comprehensive medical services to multiple communities and undertakes certain teaching and scientific research tasks. Its responsibilities mainly include providing medical services (providing comprehensive and continuous medical care, nursing, preventive health care and rehabilitation services to the community), carrying out teaching and scientific research in combination with medical care, and guiding the primary medical and health institutions in the region to do a good job in community treatment, preventive health care, rehabilitation and mental health.

A third-level hospital is a hospital above the regional level that provides high-level specialized medical services to several regions and undertakes higher teaching and scientific research tasks. Its responsibilities mainly include providing specialized medical services, solving critical and difficult diseases, accepting second-level referrals, providing business and technical guidance and personnel training to lower-level hospitals, completing the teaching tasks of cultivating various senior medical professionals, undertaking scientific research projects at or above the provincial level, and participating in and guiding the primary and secondary prevention work.

Since the reform and opening-up, the number of hospitals in China has maintained a continuous growth trend. In 1978, there were only 9 293 hospitals in China. By 2021, the total number of hospitals reached 36 570, 3. 9 times that of 1978. Among them, the number of general hospitals, TCM hospitals and specialized hospitals has increased significantly. In 2021, 32. 3% of all hospitals in China were public hospitals and 67. 7% were private.

3.1.2 Capital Investment in Medical and Health Institutions

Most of China's medical and health institutions are public, and the government should be responsible for the construction and purchase of equipment for these public medical and health institutions. But from the 1980s to the 1990s, China's medical and health institutions gradually began to try to introduce market-oriented operation mechanisms, the government's fiscal investment in public medical and health institutions gradually decreased, and the fiscal autonomy of public medical and health institutions gradually expanded. Many hospitals and primary medical and health institutions can use their business income to build infrastructure or purchase medical equipment. Some medical and health institutions have even borrowed money to build houses and buy equipment.

Since the implementation of the new medical reform in 2009, the Chinese government has increased investment in basic medical security and primary medical and health institutions. From 2016 to 2021, China's fiscal expenditure on health care increased from 1 315. 9 billion yuan to 1 914. 27 billion yuan, including 22. 35 billion yuan from the central government. From 2016 to 2020, the central government issued a total of 1 448. 4 billion yuan in medical insurance subsidies for urban and rural residents, and the fiscal subsidy standard for urban and rural residents' medical insurance was raised from 420 yuan per person per year in 2016 to 550 yuan per person per year in 2020. From 2016 to 2020, the central government allocated a total of 50. 8 billion yuan in subsidies for the comprehensive reform of public hospitals to support local governments in consolidating the achievements of eliminating the practice of "using drug sales to supplement medical income." In 2018 and 2019, half of the annual increase in per capita government subsidies for urban and rural residents' medical insurance was used to improve the protection capacity of serious illness insurance in China. In 2017, China comprehensively implemented a comprehensive reform of public hospitals, and all public hospitals in the country abolished drug markups. In 2019, the markup for medical consumables in public hospitals was cancelled. Government investment at all levels plays different roles in the construction of hardware facilities of medical and health institutions. The central government and provincial governments play a major role in the construction of hardware facilities such as houses and equipment in primary medical and health institutions. Due to their weak fiscal capacity, county-level governments have invested less in the construction of hardware facilities apart from being responsible for paying the salaries of health technicians, especially in the underdeveloped areas of the western regions.

In addition, although China's government has increased investment in second-level and above public hospitals, the investment is not as strong as that of primary medical and health institutions. Therefore, second-level and above public hospitals still need to use business income or other financing channels to strengthen the construction of hardware facilities. China encourages private capital to run medical and health institutions, and the private medical and health institutions, whose number has been gradually increasing, mainly rely on private capital to invest in the construction of hardware facilities such as houses and equipment.

3.1.3　Status Quo of the Scale of Medical and Health Institutions

The number of beds reflects the scale of a hospital's operations. According to the official data of China health statistics, the number of hospital beds is usually counted according to the following categories: 0-49, 50-99, 100-199, 200-299, 300-399, 400-499, 500-799, and 800 and above. At the end of 2021, there were 9.45 million beds in medical and health institutions nationwide, including 7.41 million (78.5%) in hospitals, 1.71 million (18.1%) in primary medical and health institutions, and 0.30 million (3.2%) in professional public health institutions. The number of beds in urban and rural medical and health institutions remained almost the same, accounting for 52.6% and 47.4% respectively. Among hospitals, 70.2% were in public hospitals and 29.8% were in private hospitals.

In line with the trend in the number of hospitals, the number of hospital beds in China has also experienced continuous growth, and the growth rate has outpaced that of the number of hospitals. In 1978, there were only 1.10 million hospital beds in China, but by 2021, this number had increased to 7.41 million, 6.7 times that of 1978. There has also been a significant increase in the number of beds in primary medical and health institutions, but at a slower rate than in hospitals. Taking into account the growth of the population, we look at the trend of the number of beds in medical and health institutions by examining the number of beds per 1 000 population. In 2007, the number of hospital beds per 1 000 population was 2.83, and by 2021, it had reached 6.70, representing an increase of 136.7% in 14 years.

There is little difference in the number of beds between urban and rural medical and health institutions in China. In recent years, the difference in bed allocation between urban and rural medical and health institutions has gradually narrowed. In 2010, the number of beds in medical and health institutions per 1 000 population in urban areas was about 5.94, 2.28 times that of rural areas, and in 2020 this number was 1.78 times. In 2021, the number of beds in medical and health institutions per 1 000 population in urban and rural areas was 7.47 and 6.01, respectively. In addition, there are certain differences in bed allocation and services provided between different medical and health institutions due to different regions and levels.

The bed occupancy rate and average length of stay for discharged patients reflect the use of hospital beds. The bed occupancy rate is the ratio of the total number of bed days actually occupied to the total number of bed days actually opened. The average length of stay for discharged patients is the ratio of the total number of bed days occupied by discharged patients to the number of discharged patients. In 2021, the occupancy rate of hospital beds in China was 74.6%, and the average length of stay for hospital dischargers was 9.2 days.

There are significant differences in bed occupancy rates among different levels of hospitals in China. Data for 2021 shows that the bed occupancy rate in third-level hospitals in China was 85.3%, compared with 71.1% in second-level hospitals and 52.1% in first-level hospitals, respectively. The average length of stay for hospital dischargers in China peaked at 16.2 days around 1992 and has been on a downward trend since then, falling to 9.2 days in 2021.

3.1.4 Current Status of Health Human Resources

By the end of 2021, the total number of health personnel in China was 13.98 million, of which 11.24 million were health technicians. In the same year, there were 3.04 practitioners and assistant practitioners and 3.56 registered nurses per 1 000 population, and 3.08 general practitioners and 6.79 professional public health institution personnel per 10 000 population, respectively.

Since 1949, the total number of health personnel in China has generally maintained an upward trend. In the 1950s, the number of health personnel increased rapidly, by about 0.11 million per year. In the 1960s, the number of health personnel stagnated, fluctuating around 1.80 million. In the 1970s and 1980s, the number of health personnel increased rapidly again, by about 0.15 million per year, and the rate of increase slowed down after the 1990s. From 2001 to 2003, there was a negative growth in the number of health personnel. Since 2005, the number of health personnel has grown rapidly again, by more than 0.20 million per year. The number of health personnel in 2021 was 0.51 million more in 2021 (an increase of 3.8%) than in 2020.

3.1.4.1 The Structure and Distribution of Health Human Resources

In the early days of the People's Republic of China, the doctor-to-nurse ratio was about 10:1. But the number of nurses was growing significantly faster than that of doctors. By 2021, the doctor-to-nurse ratio in China reached 1:1.17. Health technicians in China are usually predominantly female. In 2018, 71.8% of China's health technicians were women, with the proportion of registered nurses being as high as 97.7%. In recent years, the age structure of China's health technicians has been dominated by young and middle-aged people. In 2018, 83.3% of China's health technicians were aged 25-54; 11% were aged 55 and over, up from 9.2% in 2017. The educational qualifications of health technicians in China are usually divided into graduate, undergraduate, junior college, technical secondary school, and others. In recent years, the educational qualifications of health technicians in China have been improving, with 42% of health technicians having a bachelor's degree or above in 2020, compared with 17.1% in 2005.

3.1.4.2   Education of Health Personnel

Since 1949, China has gradually established a continuous and unified medical education system, including medical school education, post-graduation medical education and continuing medical education. Since the 1990s, medical education in China has developed rapidly. In particular, with the encouragement of the policy of expanding the enrollment of higher education introduced in 1999, the scale of medical colleges in China has expanded rapidly. The number of students enrolled in higher medical education in 2019 was 6.7 times that of 2000. The number of medical colleges and universities had grown from 44 in the early days of the founding of the People's Republic of China to 192 in 2020. From the early days of the founding of the People's Republic of China to 2019, the number of students enrolled in medical colleges and universities increased from 15 200 to 3.32 million. In addition, 1.16 million students were enrolled in secondary medical education in 2019.

3.1.4.3   Careers of Health Personnel

There are three levels of health technician titles in China: junior, intermediate and senior. Taking doctors as an example, after graduating from technical secondary school and junior college, medical students can obtain medical assistant qualifications through examinations, and undergraduate graduates can obtain physician (or resident) qualifications. Medical assistant and physicians are both junior titles, and after working for a certain number of years (such as 5 years), they can be promoted to attending physicians (intermediate titles) through certain procedures. Senior titles include associate chief physician and chief physician. Other health personnel also have a corresponding career development system. Since the health personnel of the hospital affiliated to the medical school have the tasks of teaching, research and supervising graduate students, they also have the titles of associate professor and professor. If the medical institution has a corresponding promotion position (or title promotion quota), the health personnel who meet the promotion conditions can submit an application to the institution. After the medical institution has passed the review, it shall be reported to the health administrative department and the personnel department at the higher level for approval. Promotion to intermediate titles (such as attending physician) requires passing a provincial examination, which includes professional knowledge, foreign languages, and computer science. For promotion to senior titles (such as associate chief physician and chief physician), a defense is required. The provincial health administrative department and the personnel department invite experts in relevant fields to form a professional committee to review the applicant's qualifications and abilities. Based on the results of the defense, the provincial personnel department will make the final decision on whether to approve the applicant's promotion.

3.2 The Current Situation and Development Direction of China's Medical Services at All Levels

3.2.1 Residents' Healthcare-Seeking Pathways

In China, both urban and rural residents have their own choice to seek medical treatment in various medical and health institutions, as shown in Figures 3-1 and 3-2. However, with the improvement of the level of medical and health institutions, the proportion of medical expenses and out-of-pocket medical expenses of residents has also increased. In addition, primary medical and health institutions are mostly located in residential areas and residents generally do not need to wait for treatment, so they often choose to seek treatment in primary medical and health institutions when they judge their condition is relatively mild.

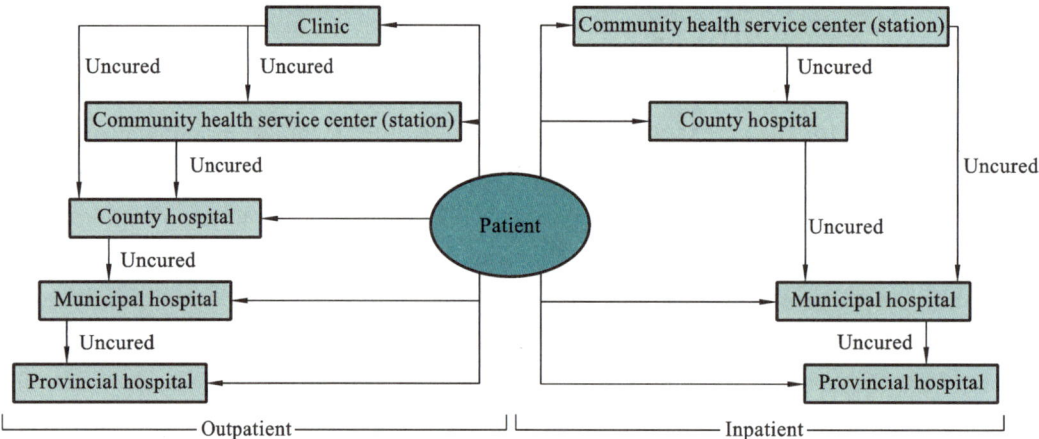

Figure 3-1 Healthcare-seeking pathways for urban residents

3.2.2 Primary Medical Services

Primary medical services in China are mainly provided by community health service centers (stations), township health centers, village clinics and other primary medical and health institutions. Community health service centers implement integrated management of their subordinate community health service stations, and other community health service stations are subject to the operational management of community health service centers. The village clinics accept the operational management and technical guidance of the township health centers, and in some areas where the integration of rural health services has been realized, the township health centers shall implement unified management of the

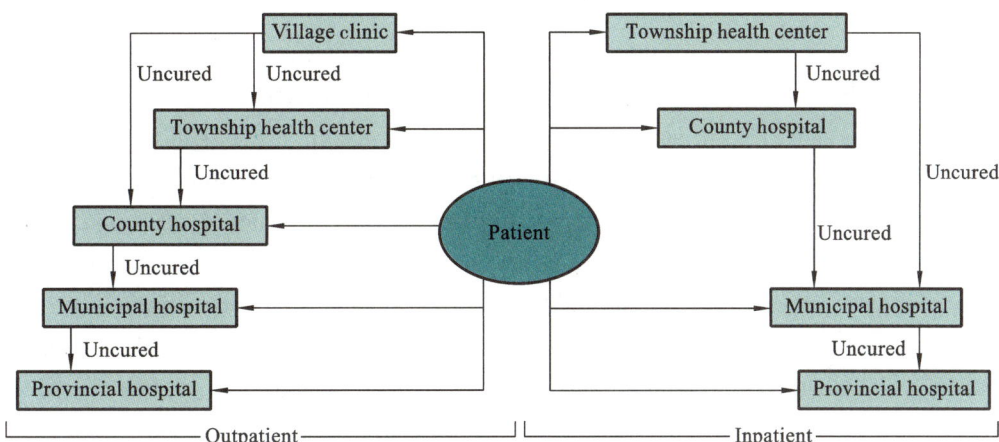

Figure 3-2　Healthcare-seeking pathways for rural residents

village clinics.

Community health service centers(stations) and township health centers are mainly responsible for providing local residents with health education, prevention, health care, rehabilitation services, as well as diagnosis and treatment services for common and frequently occurring diseases. Village clinics provide basic medical services to rural residents. The administrative departments of health are responsible for the daily supervision and management of primary medical and health institutions, and the centers for disease control and prevention, maternal and child health care hospitals (institutes, stations), specialized disease prevention and treatment centers (institutes) and other preventive health care institutions are responsible for conducting operational evaluation and guidance on the public health service work undertaken by primary medical and health institutions.

By the end of 2021, there were 36 160 community health service centers (stations), including 10 122 community health service centers and 26 038 community health service stations, 34 943 township health centers, 271 056 clinics and infirmaries, and 599 292 village clinics. Among the health personnel, there are 0.59 million health technicians in community health service centers (stations), 1.29 million health technicians in township health centers, and 1.36 million personnel in village clinics.

The number of diagnosis and treatment volume in primary medical and health institutions in China has generally shown an increasing trend. In 2021, it reached 4.25 billion (50.2% of the national total), an increase of 130 million compared with 2020, and the number of hospitalizations in primary medical and health institutions was 35.92 million (14.5% of the national total), a decrease of 1.15 million compared with 2020.

At present, China's primary medical services still have a long way to go in terms of talent team building, and the problems such as the insufficient number, low quality, and job instability of health technicians are still the bottleneck problems that restrict the further improvement of medical services and medical levels of primary medical and health institutions. In order to strengthen the capacity of primary medical services, various regions in China are actively promoting on-the-job training of rural health personnel, and implementing training programs for rural health personnel and free education programs for medical students with rural service commitments. In urban areas, China is vigorously carrying out on-the-job training for community health personnel, and implementing training programs for community health personnel and plans for the construction of primary medical and health teams focusing on general practitioners. In terms of system construction, China is improving the urban medical and health service system based on community health services, and gradually promoting the implementation of the community first diagnosis, hierarchical diagnosis and treatment, and two-way referral system.

3.2.3 Medical Services Provided by Second-Level and Third-Level Hospitals

China's second-level hospitals include general city and county hospitals, district-level hospitals in municipalities directly under the central government, as well as staff hospitals of industrial, mining, enterprises and institutions with a certain scale. Third-level hospitals include large municipal hospitals directly under the national, provincial and municipal governments, as well as affiliated hospitals of medical colleges and universities. As of the end of 2021, there were 3 275 third-level hospitals and 10 848 second-level hospitals in China. China's second-level and third-level hospitals are divided into general hospitals, TCM hospitals, hospitals of integrated traditional Chinese and Western medicine, hospitals of traditional ethic medicine, specialized hospitals and nursing homes according to the different types of services provided. General hospitals generally have specialties such as internal medicine, surgery, obstetrics and gynecology, pediatrics, otolaryngology, ophthalmology, dermatology, and TCM, as well as medical and technical departments such as laboratory and imaging. TCM hospitals, hospitals of integrated traditional Chinese and Western medicine, and hospitals of traditional ethic medicine mainly provide medical services related to TCM and ethnic medicine. Specialized hospitals are hospitals set up for the diagnosis and treatment of various specialized diseases, such as obstetrics and gynecology hospitals, infectious disease hospitals, cancer hospitals, dental hospitals, occupational disease hospitals, etc. And nursing homes are medical institutions that provide long-term medical care, rehabilitation promotion, hospice care, and other services to patients.

In 2009, China launched a new medical reform, according to which the government encourages and guides private capital to run medical institutions, and encourages the free movement of medical and health technicians between public and private hospitals. In recent years, the number of private hospitals in China has been steadily increasing. In 2021, public hospitals accounted for 32.3% of the total number of hospitals in China, while private hospitals accounted for 67.7%.

In 2021, hospitals accounted for 3.88 billion (45.8%) of the total diagnosis and treatment volume in China, primary medical and health institutions accounted for 4.25 billion (50.2%), and other medical and health institutions accounted for 340 million (4%). In 2021, the occupancy rate of hospital beds in China was 74.6% (80.3% in public hospitals). In 2021, the average length of stay for hospital dischargers in China was 9.2 days (9.0 days in public hospitals), decreased by 0.3 days (0.3 days in public hospitals) compared with the previous year. Since 2005, a number of large general hospitals have started to open day wards to provide patients with emergency day surgery and day beds that do not require hospitalization. At present, day care services in China are still in the development stage.

For a period of time, issues such as high medical costs and inconsistent service quality were prominent in some second-level and third-level hospitals in China. To address this situation, China has launched a pilot project for the comprehensive reform of urban public hospitals since 2010, striving to achieve breakthroughs in improving the service system, innovating systems and mechanisms, strengthening internal management, and accelerating the formation of a diversified medical operation pattern. Since 2012, China has launched a pilot project for the comprehensive reform of county-level public hospitals, and has explored reform methods in aspects such as the compensation mechanisms of public hospitals.

3.2.4 The Relationship between the Medical Services Provided by Second-Level and Third-Level Hospitals and Primary Medical Services

In order to guide general medical services at the primary level and promote the rational allocation of medical resources, China introduced a two-way referral system in 2016 to encourage patients to prefer primary medical and health institutions for treatment, and when necessary, primary medical and health institutions are responsible for transferring patients to second-level and third-level hospitals for treatment, and then these hospitals will transfer patients to primary medical and health institutions for rehabilitation and other follow-up treatment after the patient's condition is stable. Since the launch of the new medical reform in 2009, China has begun to explore the establishment of a division of labor and cooperation mechanism between second-level and third-level hospitals and urban and rural primary medical and health institutions, and these hospitals are responsible for driving the development of primary medical and health institutions in terms of technology, personnel and management. In order to achieve this goal, China has begun to explore the construction of medical consortiums to promote the formation of a hierarchical diagnosis and treatment pattern.

3.2.5 TCM Services and Ethnic Medical Services

Most of China's comprehensive medical institutions and primary medical and health institutions have TCM departments, which provide TCM services mostly based on traditional therapies such as herbal medicine therapy, acupuncture therapy and massage therapy. To varying degrees, these services are included in the scope of compensation for the basic medical insurance for urban employees, the basic medical insurance for non-working urban residents, and the new rural cooperative medical care. As of 2021, the total number of TCM medical and health institutions in China was 77 336, including 5 715 hospitals specialized in TCM, 71 583 outpatient departments and clinics specialized in TCM, and 38 institutions specialized in TCM research. In addition, there are a large number of private traditional medicine clinics and individual practitioners who provide TCM services. The total number of TCM health personnel reached 884 000, including 732 000 practitioners and assistant practitioners of TCM and 136 000 TCM pharmacists. The total number of consultations and treatments in TCM medical and health institutions nationwide was 1. 2 billion, and the number of discharges from TCM medical and health institutions was 38 million.

The "Regulations of the People's Republic of China on Traditional Chinese Medicine" stipulates that the establishment of TCM medical institutions shall comply with the standards for the establishment of TCM medical institutions formulated by the health administrative department of the State Council and the local regional health plan, and go through the examination and approval procedures in accordance with the provisions of the "Regulations on the Administration of Medical Institutions" to obtain the practice license. TCM practitioners shall pass the qualification examination in accordance with the provisions of the laws, administrative regulations and departmental rules on health management, and obtain a practice certificate through registration before engaging in TCM service activities.

By the end of 2015, there were 3 966 hospitals specialized in TCM in China, including 253 hospitals of traditional ethnic medicine and 446 hospitals of integrated traditional Chinese and Western medicine. There are 452 000 practitioners and assistant practitioners of TCM (including practitioners of ethnic medicine and integrated traditional Chinese and Western medicine). There are 42 528 outpatient departments and clinics of TCM, including 550 outpatient departments and clinics of ethnic medicine and 7 706 outpatient departments and clinics of integrated traditional Chinese and Western medicine. In 2015, the total number of consultations and treatments in TCM medical and health institutions in China reached 910 million, and the number of discharges from TCM medical and health institutions nationwide reached 26. 92 million.

According to the "14th Five-Year Plan for the Development of Traditional Chinese Medicine," China will build a high-quality and efficient TCM service system, improve the capacity of TCM health services, build a high-quality TCM talent team, establish a high-level TCM inheritance and protection, and scientific and technological innovation system, promote the high-quality development of the TCM industry, develop the TCM health service industry, promote the prosperity and development of TCM culture, accelerate the opening-up and development of TCM, deepen the reform of the field of TCM, and strengthen the support and guarantee for the development of TCM.

In addition to TCM therapies, there are also a large number of traditional therapies from ethnic minorities in China, and the discipline that studies this field is called "ethnic medicine." Some therapies in ethnic medicine are similar to those in TCM, such as herbal medicine therapy, cupping therapy, and acupuncture therapy. In addition, both ethnic medicine and TCM have their own unique therapies. There are dozens of categories of ethnic medicine in China, such as Tibetan medicine, Mongolian medicine, and Miao medicine. As of 2019, there were 699 integrated traditional Chinese and Western medicine hospitals and 312 hospitals of traditional ethic medicine in China. In addition to being carried out in hospitals of traditional ethic medicine, ethnic medical services are more often carried out in monasteries (for example, the educational and medical practice institutions set up in Tibetan Buddhist monasteries are called Manba Raseng), clinics and other places, or in the form of individual medical practice. Ethnic medicine is often taught in a more conservative way, such as oral transmission or even ancestral tradition, and retains more unique traditional healing methods and skills that are self-contained, but the extent of its application is not the same as that of TCM. In general, the management of ethnic physicians is carried out with reference to the management of TCM physicians.

3.3　High-Quality Development of China's Medical Service System

3.3.1　Medical Consortiums

The construction of medical consortiums is a major measure to promote the hierarchical diagnosis and treatment system in China. In 2017, the "Guiding Opinions of the General Office of the State Council on Promoting the Construction and Development of Medical Consortiums" was issued, which clarified that medical communities should be established at the county level, strengthen the combination of medical and health and elderly care services, and provide patients with integrated and convenient disease diagnosis and treatment, rehabilitation and long-term care continuity services.

On the one hand, by adjusting and optimizing the layout of medical resources, the medical consortiums can effectively sink high-quality resources and technical services to the grassroots level step by step, and improve the ability of primary medical services through various forms and means such as expert deployment to lower-level medical institutions, counterpart assistance, and telemedicine. On the other hand, as an important channel for the integration of medical resources and two-way referral, the medical consortiums can gradually break down the barriers and obstacles in administrative division, financial investment, medical insurance payment, personnel management, etc., and promote the integration of high-quality medical resources.

In terms of the organizational model of medical consortiums, China has proposed four mature models. First, in urban areas, medical groups are mainly formed, with third-level hospitals as the core and various medical institutions such as community health service institutions, nursing homes, and rehabilitation centers providing various types of services to meet the health, medical and rehabilitation needs of patients at different stages. Second, in county areas, medical communities are primarily established, focusing on exploring the integrated management of counties and townships with county hospitals as the leader, township health centers as the hub, and village clinics as the basis. A high degree of overall management and close division of labor and cooperation on personnel, finance, materials, prevention, security, and health is carried out, and a three-level linkage county-level medical service system is built. Third, for various specialized diseases, medical institutions with superior specialized medical resources are encouraged to take the lead and carry out cross-regional medical alliances. At the same time, China proposes to give full play to the resource advantages in national specialized medical care, and use specialist cooperation as a link to improve the treatment level of specialized diseases at the grassroots level and smoothen the channel of two-way referral. Fourth, China proposes to develop a telemedicine cooperation network in remote and impoverished areas, make full use of modern high-tech means such as telemedicine, distance teaching, and distance training, extend the medical technology and service capabilities of higher-level medical institutions, expand the service radius, and meet the medical needs of some grassroots areas, especially remote and impoverished areas.

At present, the construction of China's medical consortiums has been fully launched, all third-level public hospitals have participated in the construction of medical consortiums, the results of the two-way referral have initially appeared, regional medical resources have been shared, and the medical service capacity has been significantly improved. As of 2019, 607 urban medical consortium grids have been planned and constructed in 118 cities across China, and the state has promoted the pilot construction of county-level medical communities in 567 counties(cities, districts). By the end of 2020, there had been 25.08 million two-way referral patients from medical and health institutions across China. During the 13th Five-Year Plan period, the number of down-referred patients increased year by year, with an average annual growth rate of 38.4%. In 2020, the number of up-referred patients decreased for the first time, and the problem of "easy to transfer up and difficult to transfer down" gradually eased. According to the data of the Sixth National Health Service Statistical Survey, 46.9% of the two-way referral patients were referred within medical consortiums, which was higher than other referral methods.

3.3.2 Reform of Primary Medical and Health Institutions

The development of primary medical and health institutions in China faces many challenges. Over-reliance on drug revenues has hampered the provision of reasonable health services. The establishment of a reasonable compensation mechanism and the increase of government investment are the focus of the reform of primary medical and health institutions in China. In addition, primary medical and health institutions need to strengthen the construction of human resources and other conditions.

Construction of the primary medical and health system. From 2009 to 2011, the main goals of the reform was to improve the three-tiered medical and health service network at the county, township and village levels. It focused on supporting the construction of urban and rural primary medical and health institutions, including county and rural health institutions and urban community health institutions, and supported the construction of village clinics in remote areas and urban community health service centers in difficult areas. After 2012, China continued to strengthen the construction of township health centers and the capacity building of TCM services in primary medical and health institutions.

Construction of primary medical and health teams. From 2009 to 2011, China began a program to train health personnel for rural primary medical and health institutions free of charge. In 2011, the "Guiding Opinions of the State Council on the Establishment of a General Practitioner System" was promulgated, which clarified the policy measures such as gradually establishing a unified and standardized general practitioner training system and reforming the practice methods of general practitioners. In 2012, the medical reform proposed to strengthen the construction of grassroots talent teams focusing on general practitioners and continue to train medical students free of charge for township health centers and grassroots troops in the central and western regions. On-the-job training for personnel in primary medical and health institutions is an important part of improving the capacity of health personnel. Since the new medical reform, China's governments at all levels invested funds to organize various forms of on-the-job training. In addition, China has also implemented a policy of counterpart support for rural hospitals in urban hospitals, that is, each urban third-level hospital is required to establish a long-term technical assistance relationship with about three county-level hospitals to improve the service capacity of county-level hospitals.

Establishment of compensation mechanisms for primary medical and health institutions. China clarifies that government subsidies and service charges (including medical insurance fees and public health service compensation) are the main compensation methods for primary medical and health institutions. Most importantly, drug markups are no longer the main compensation channel for primary medical and health institutions. The capital construction, equipment purchase, personnel expenses, and the operating expenses for public health services approved by township health centers and urban community health service centers(stations) in accordance with state regulations shall be compensated through project subsidies or purchase of services. For the public health services provided by non-government-run primary medical and health institutions, compensation shall be made in the form of government or basic medical insurance purchasing services, and the fiscal compensation for the implementation of the basic drug system in the village clinic is clarified.

Establishment of operational mechanisms for primary medical and health institutions. The reform measures implemented include the establishment of a two-way referral system, a primary care first diagnosis system, a performance appraisal mechanism for primary medical and health institutions and personnel, and an income distribution mechanism for primary medical and health institutions. In 2012, it was clearly proposed that the income distribution of personnel in primary medical and health institutions should be based on the quantity and quality of services and be tilted in favor of the core and backbone health technicians in China.

3.3.3 Future Development

Since the implementation of the new medical reform in 2009, China has made remarkable progress in improving the service capacity of primary medical and health institutions and reforming public medical and health institutions. At the same time, due to the complexity and systemic nature of health reform, it also faces many challenges and requires long-term persistence. In view of the new problems that have arisen, it is necessary to continuously improve the content of reform and effectively promote the implementation of reform policies and measures.

The reform of China's public hospitals needs to be continuously deepened, with a focus on addressing issues within the medical service system and driving the reform from the perspective of system construction and development. At the same time, the development of the health industry and the realization of a diversified medical pattern are also important development directions in the future. In the face of ongoing challenges of health and demographic transitions, China needs a more effective medical service system to address the challenges of chronic diseases and meet growing health needs. The focus of China's medical service system reform mainly includes the following four aspects:

First, deepen the reform of the medical and health system, including deepening the comprehensive reform of primary medical and health institutions and improving the operation mechanism of networked urban and rural primary medical and health services, perfecting the reasonable hierarchical diagnosis and treatment model and establishing a contractual service relationship between community doctors and residents, making full use of information technology to promote the vertical flow of high-quality medical resources, and strengthening the integration of regional public health service resources, etc. The main task is to establish a medical and health service system with clear functions, accurate positioning, and mutual cooperation, and give full play to the role of medical and health institutions with varying functions and at different levels. This requires the integration of medical and health service systems, including the integration of medical and public health service institutions, as well as institutional cohesion and vertical integration of medical and health institutions within the region, to improve the capacity of the system as a whole and address major health challenges.

Second, accelerate the reform of public hospitals, including innovating systems and mechanisms, and mobilizing the enthusiasm of medical staff. Among them, rationalizing the price of medicine and establishing a scientific compensation mechanism are the key points. The reform of county-level public hospitals is the key work in the next few years, and the content of this reform mainly includes adhering to public welfare and fulfilling the responsibilities of the government, deepening the reform of the distribution system and fully mobilizing the enthusiasm of medical staff, establishing a modern hospital management system and strengthening internal management, promoting the reform of the payment system, optimizing the allocation of resources and strengthening industry supervision, etc.

Third, strengthen the construction of medical and health talent team and the construction of medical and health informatization. The quality, structure and distribution of the medical and health talent team has always been one of the most important factors restricting the improvement of medical and health service capacity in China. China has established a standardized training system for residents and a training system for general practitioners, and has promoted the policy of stabilizing the ranks of rural doctors. In terms of medical and health informatization, China is studying the establishment of a unified national information standard system for electronic health records, electronic medical records, drugs and devices, medical services, medical insurance and other areas, and promoting the standardization of medical and health information technology.

Fourth, encourage the community to run medical and health institutions, and give priority to supporting social forces to set up non-profit medical and health institutions, including leaving a reasonable space for the development of social medical institutions and establishing a social medical system with non-profit medical and health institutions as the main body and for-profit medical and health institutions as the supplement in the regional health planning and planning for the establishment of medical and health institutions, improving preferential policies and measures in areas such as taxation for social medical services, promoting the improvement of multi-site practice policies for physicians, and ensuring the quality of medical services provided by non-public medical and health institutions, etc.

4 China's Public Health Management System and Public Health Service System

China has established a relatively comprehensive public health management system and public health service system. In terms of public health management, health commissions at all levels, the National Disease Control and Prevention Administration, and centers for disease control and prevention at all levels are responsible for formulating and implementing public health development plans and policies. In terms of public health services, the content of services is continuously enriched and improved, the public health service network is continuously strengthened, and institutions ranging from centers for disease control and prevention at all levels to community health service centers (stations), township health centers, and village clinics are responsible for providing public health services such as infectious disease control and prevention, chronic disease prevention and treatment, health education, food safety surveillance and supervision, occupational health surveillance, handling of public health emergencies, and maternal and child health care for urban and rural residents.

Since the outbreak of SARS in 2003, the Chinese government has increased fiscal support for public health institutions and public health service programs. In recent years, the government has further adjusted the public health management system and institutional functions, which has greatly promoted the improvement of China's public health service system.

4.1 China's Public Health Management System

China's public health management system is primarily composed of national health management institutions such as the National Health Commission, the National Disease Control and Prevention Administration, and the Chinese Center for Disease Control and Prevention (China CDC), as well as these institutions at the provincial, prefectural, and county levels, each undertaking different management responsibilities. Health commissions at all levels are overall responsible for public health administrative management, disease control and prevention administrations at all levels are responsible for implementing disease control and prevention policies and decisions, and centers for disease control and prevention at all levels are responsible for technical support and work execution. From the national level to the provincial, prefectural, and county levels, the functions of planning and policy-making institutions at all levels are gradually detailed, and various decision deployments are gradually operationalized. Local public health policies sometimes serve as strong supplements to national policies.

4. 1. 1　National Health Commission

The National Health Commission is mainly responsible for organizing the formulation of national health policies, drafting laws and regulations, policies, and plans for health undertakings, formulating departmental regulations and standards, and organizing their implementation. It is also responsible for coordinating and promoting the deepening of the medical and health system reform, and researching and proposing recommendations for major guidelines, policies, and measures to deepen the medical and health system reform. In 2022, the General Office of the Central Committee of the Communist Party of China and the General Office of the State Council transferred some of the responsibilities of the National Health Commission, such as formulating and organizing the implementation of infectious disease control and prevention plans, national immunization plans, and intervention measures for major public health issues, to the National Disease Control and Prevention Administration.

Currently, the Department of Medical Emergency Response, the Department of Primary Health, the Department of Food Safety Standards, Risk Surveillance and Assessment, the Department of Maternal and Child Health, and the Department of Occupational Health under the National Health Commission are mainly responsible for the administrative management of public health-related services. Specifically, the Department of Medical Emergency Response is responsible for organizing and coordinating the response to infectious disease outbreaks, undertaking the construction of the medical emergency response system, organizing and guiding medical rescue for various public emergencies, drafting and implementing industry management policies and standards for medical safety, medical supervision, blood collection and supply institutions management and improvement of ethical conduct, drafting and supervising the implementation of major disease and chronic disease control and prevention management policies and norms, and so on. The Basic Public Health Division under the Department of Primary Health is responsible for the corresponding administrative management of grassroots public health. The Department of Food Safety Standards, Risk Surveillance and Assessment is responsible for organizing the formulation of national food safety standards, carrying out food safety risk surveillance and assessment, etc. The Department of Maternal and Child Health is responsible for drafting policies, standards, and norms for maternal and child health, promoting the construction of the maternal and child health service system, etc. The Department of Occupational Health is responsible for drafting and implementing policies and standards related to occupational health and radiation health, among others.

4.1.2　National Disease Control and Prevention Administration

In January 2022, according to the adjustment plan for the functional configuration of the National Health Commission, China abolished the National Health Commission's Bureau of Disease Control and Prevention and established the National Disease Control and Prevention Administration. The newly established National Disease Control and Prevention Administration is managed by the National Health Commission and has the status of a vice-ministerial-level national bureau.

The main responsibilities of the National Disease Control and Prevention Administration include organizing the drafting of laws, regulations, policies, plans, and standards for infectious disease control and prevention and public health supervision, leading the business work of disease control and prevention institutions at various local levels, formulating and organizing the implementation of the national immunization plans and intervention measures for major public health issues that seriously endanger people's health, coordinating and supervising the disease control and prevention work of infectious disease medical institutions and other medical institutions, planning and guiding the construction of infectious disease epidemic surveillance and early warning systems, responding to infectious disease epidemics, jointly guiding the construction of the disease control and prevention scientific research system, implementing the supervision and management of infectious disease prevention and treatment, environmental health, school health, public place health, and drinking water hygiene, and so on. Currently, provinces of China are also actively establishing provincial disease control and prevention bureaus.

4.1.3　China CDC

In China, centers for disease control and prevention are divided into four levels: national, provincial, municipal, and county levels, with different work focuses at each level. The China CDC is at the national level and is a public institution directly under the National Disease Control and Prevention Administration. The main responsibilities of the China CDC include carrying out work related to disease control and prevention, public health emergency response, environmental and occupational health, nutrition and health, aging health, maternal and child health, radiation health, and school health; organizing the formulation of national public health technical schemes and guidelines, and undertaking the comprehensive management of health standards related to public health; conducting surveillance of infectious diseases, chronic diseases, occupational diseases, endemic diseases, public health emergencies, suspected adverse reactions to vaccinations, and surveillance and assessment of the health status of the population; conducting investigations and risk assessments of major public health issues; conducting key scientific research and technological development in disease control and prevention, public health emergency response, and public health; guiding local implementation of national disease control and prevention plans and projects, providing business guidance to local disease control and prevention institutions, and participating in professional technical assessments and evaluations, and so on.

4.1.4 Other Public Health Management and Business Guidance Institutions

4.1.4.1 Mental Health Center of the China CDC

The Mental Health Center of the China CDC is the national technical center for mental health. Under the business leadership of the China CDC and entrusted by the China CDC, it mainly undertakes responsibilities include providing scientific basis and decision-making consultation for the formulation of laws, regulations, rules, policies, standards, technical specifications, and plans related to the control and prevention of mental disorders; guiding the establishment of a national mental disorder surveillance system, conducting epidemiological surveillance of the occurrence, distribution, and development patterns of common mental disorders, establishing a database, and regularly analyzing surveillance results; organizing the formulation of prevention and treatment plans for common mental disorders, and conducting quality control and effectiveness evaluation of the implementation of these plans; reporting, managing, predicting, and forecasting the information of mental disorders control and prevention; providing business guidance and technical training for mental health workers, and undertaking technical guidance in health work related to the control and prevention of mental disorders; conducting applied scientific research related to mental health, introducing, developing, and promoting new technologies and methods, and so on.

4.1.4.2 National Center for Women and Children's Health of the China CDC

The National Center for Women and Children's Health of the China CDC is the national technical guidance center for maternal and child health services. Its main responsibilities include carrying out maternal and child health work, providing technical support and consultation for the formulation of laws, regulations, policies, plans, and projects related to maternal and child health; organizing the formulation of technical schemes, guidelines, and standards for maternal and child health; conducting scientific research in the field of maternal and child health, and monitoring, evaluating, and assessing the health status of women and children and their influencing factors; undertaking the construction of maternal and child health information systems, and taking charge of technical support for the collection, management, and application service of related data; providing business guidance for local maternal and child health work, organizing business training, promoting new technologies and methods, and participating in professional technical assessments and evaluations related to maternal and child health services; conducting maternal and child health education, health science popularization, and health promotion activities; conducting graduate education and continuing education in the field of maternal and child health; conducting international exchanges and cooperation in related fields, and so on.

4.1.4.3　China Health Education Center

The China Health Education Center is a directly affiliated institution under the National Health Commission, responsible for providing technical guidance on national health education and public health communication, conducting research on related theories and practices, organizing and implementing large-scale activities related to health education and public health communication nationwide, and undertaking information management, media relations, business training, and other technical and service-related tasks. Specifically, its responsibilities include organizing research on theories, methods, and strategies in the fields of health education, health promotion, and public health communication, and providing technical consultation and policy recommendations for the government to formulate relevant laws, regulations, departmental rules, and technical standards; assisting in the organization, implementation, business training, and technical guidance of health education, health promotion, public health communication, and population education activities; assisting in the organization and coordination of news releases and major publicity activities of the National Health Commission, and conducting related policy publicity; organizing and carrying out research and promotion of practical technologies for health education policy advocacy and health science popularization, developing health science popularization information, conducting health education activities and research on tobacco control policy compliance and related publicity work, and assisting in the work related to the construction and content maintenance of the national health science popularization resource library and expert database, and so on.

4.1.4.4　Blood Collection and Supply Institutions

China's blood collection and supply institutions are divided into blood stations and single-donor plasma stations. Blood stations include general blood stations and special blood stations. They are non-profit health institutions that collect and provide blood for clinical use. General blood stations are divided into blood centers, central blood stations, and central blood banks. Special blood stations include umbilical cord blood hematopoietic stem cell banks and other blood banks. The planning and establishment of blood collection and supply institutions should be adapted to the status of local economic development, population, medical resources, and the planning and establishment of regional medical institutions. According to the *China Health Statistical Yearbook* (2022), there were a total of 628 blood collection and supply institutions in China in 2021, including 365 in urban areas and 263 in rural areas. Blood centers, central blood stations, and central blood banks are established by local people's governments, and special blood stations are set up within the administrative regions of provinces according to national planning.

Blood centers are planned and established in cities and municipalities directly under the central government where provincial and autonomous regional people's governments are located. Central blood stations are planned and established in cities where municipal-level people's governments are located. Central blood banks are set up in county-level comprehensive hospitals where central blood stations do not cover. The main responsibilities of these three institutions include recruiting voluntary blood donors, collecting and preparing blood, supplying blood for clinical use, and providing guidance on medical blood use within the designated scope in accordance with the requirements of the health administrative departments of the provincial people's governments.

4. 1. 4. 5　Specialized Disease Prevention and Treatment Institutions

Specialized diseases include various infectious diseases, occupational diseases, mental illnesses, dermatological diseases, and sexually transmitted diseases, among others. From the perspective of institutional level, specialized disease prevention and treatment institutions in China include specialized disease prevention and treatment institutes, specialized disease prevention and treatment centers, and specialized disease prevention and treatment stations. From the perspective of disease prevention and treatment types, specialized disease prevention and treatment institutions in China include institutions for the prevention and treatment of infectious diseases, tuberculosis, occupational diseases, oral diseases, mental illnesses, dermatological diseases and sexually transmitted diseases, as well as institutions for the prevention and treatment of endemic diseases and drug rehabilitation centers.

4. 2　China's Public Health Service System

China's public health service system consists of specialized public health service network and public health services provided by medical and health institutions (Figure 4-1). The specialized public health service network includes professional public health services such as disease control and prevention, health education, maternal and child health care, mental health, emergency treatment, blood collection and supply, health supervision, and specialized prevention and treatment. Specific content of specialized prevention and treatment services include the infectious disease prevention and treatment, oral disease prevention and treatment, dermatological disease and sexually transmitted disease prevention and treatment, tuberculosis prevention and treatment, occupational disease prevention and treatment, endemic disease prevention and treatment, and schistosomiasis prevention and treatment, among others. Within the medical service system, primary medical and health institutions with integrated medical and preventive functions (such as community health service institutions in urban areas and township health centers or village clinics in rural areas) not only provide basic medical services to residents in their jurisdiction but also offer basic public health services. Additionally, hospitals also provide public health services, such as specialized hospitals for infectious diseases and mental health, and public health-related departments in general hospitals (such as infectious disease departments and fever clinics).

In China, the specific content of public health services include the infectious disease prevention and treatment, epidemic surveillance and the construction of the health

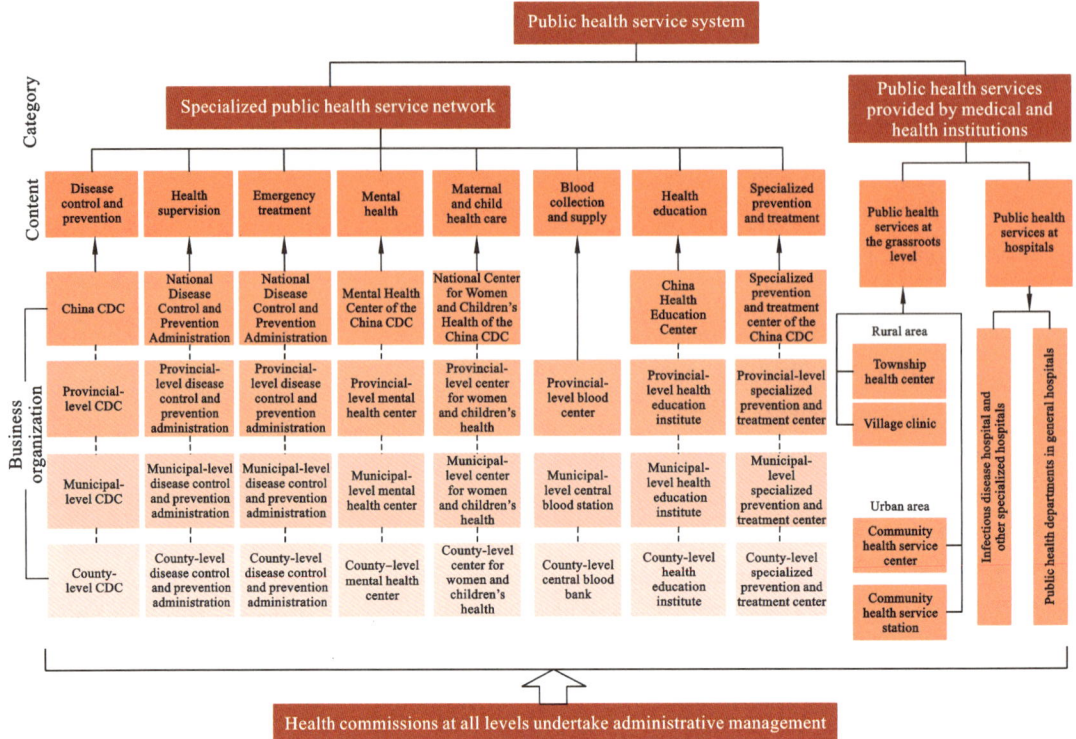

Figure 4-1 China's public health service system

Note: CDC stands for Center for Disease Control and Prevention

Source: Refer to *Health Systems in Transition* （Meng Qingyue et al.，2015），

with updates on institutional changes after 2015

emergency response network，maternal and child health surveillance and intervention，chronic disease prevention and treatment，endemic disease prevention and treatment，occupational disease prevention and treatment，environmental and health surveillance，as well as health education and health promotion. Below is an introduction to the specific content of public health services.

4.2.1 Basic Public Health Services

Since the initiation of the basic public health service equalization reform in 2009，China has been providing free basic public health services to all residents and continuously promoting the coverage of basic public health services for all residents. Basic public health services are defined as a shared fiscal responsibility between the central and local governments，with the central and local governments jointly bearing the expenditure. In 2022，the per capita fiscal subsidy standard for basic public health services in China reached 84 yuan. China's basic public health services are community-oriented，with specific public health service projects provided by a community service network covering both urban and rural areas. In 2021，a total of 119.41 million elderly people aged 65 and above，109.38 million hypertension patients，and 35.71 million type 2 diabetes patients received health management services in primary medical and health institutions. As of the end of 2021, the vaccination coverage rate at the township and street level has been kept above 95%, and basic public health service programs have achieved full population coverage.

Currently, China's national basic public health service programs include 28 items, with some changes in recent years as shown in Table 4-1. Basic public health services are mainly provided free of charge to all residents through community health service centers (stations), township health centers, village clinics and other urban and rural primary medical and health institutions. The content of China's national basic public health service programs is adjusted annually by the National Health Commission, in collaboration with the National Administration of Traditional Chinese Medicine, the National Disease Control and Prevention Administration, the Ministry of Finance and other departments, based on the economic and social development situation, public health service needs, and fiscal capacity.

Table 4-1　Changes in China's national basic public health service programs from 2009 to 2022

Year	Item number or changes	Item name
2009	1	Management of urban and rural residents' health records
	2	Health education
	3	Health management for children aged 0 to 36 months
	4	Maternal health management
	5	Elderly health management
	6	Vaccination
	7	Infectious disease reporting and management
	8	Health management for hypertension patients
	9	Health management for type 2 diabetes patients
	10	Management of severe mental illness patients
2011	New item	Health supervision and co-management
	Item renaming	Renaming of "infectious disease reporting and management" to "reporting and management of infectious diseases and public health emergencies"
	Item renaming	Renaming of "health management for children aged 0 to 36 months" to "health management for children aged 0 to 6 years"
2013	Item merging	Merging of item 8 and item 9 into "health management for chronic disease patients"
	New item	TCM health management
	Item renaming	Renaming of "management of urban and rural residents' health records" to "establishment of residents' health records"

Continued

Year	Item number or changes	Item name
2013	Item renaming	Renaming of "health management for children aged 0 to 6 years" to "child health management"
2015	New item	Health management for tuberculosis patients
2017	New item	Free provision of contraceptive devices
	New item	Healthy manners promotion campaign
2018	Item cancellation	Free provision of contraceptive devices
	Item cancellation	Healthy manners promotion campaign
2019	In addition to the above-mentioned 12 items, there are 19 new items implemented not limited to primary medical and health institutions（originally part of major public health and family planning program）	Endemic disease prevention and treatment, occupational disease prevention and treatment, surveillance of major diseases and health hazard factors, human avian influenza and SARS control and prevention program, plague prevention and treatment program, maintenance and support of national health emergency response teams, "two cancers" screening program for rural women, basic contraceptive services program, nutrition improvement program for children in poor areas, newborn disease screening program in poor areas, folic acid supplementation program for neural tube defect prevention, free pre-pregnancy health checkup program, thalassemia control and prevention program, food safety standards tracking and evaluation program, healthy manners promotion campaign program, national random supervision and inspection program, elderly health and medical care integration services, population surveillance program, supervision and management of health program
2022	Cancellation of 3 out of the 19 newly added service items in 2019	According to the joint issuance of the Ministry of Finance of the People's Republic of China and four other ministries on the "Notice on the Revision of the Management Measures for Five Subsidies including Basic Public Health Services," surveillance of major diseases and health hazard factors, national random supervision and inspection program, and population surveillance program are no longer included in basic public health services

Source: National Health Commission

4. 2. 2　Infectious Disease Prevention and Treatment

The Law of the People's Republic of China on the Prevention and Treatment of Infectious Diseases stipulates a classified management system for infectious diseases. Legally defined infectious diseases are categorized into three classes (A,B,and C),totaling 40 diseases:2 in Class A (plague and cholera),27 in Class B,and 11 in Class C. China adheres to a prevention-first policy under unified government leadership for the prevention and treatment of infectious diseases. Disease control and prevention institutions at various levels are responsible for specific tasks such as epidemic surveillance, epidemiological investigation,and epidemic reporting. Public and private medical and health institutions are responsible for reporting and clinical treatment of infectious diseases within their scope.

Currently,the major infectious diseases threatening the health of Chinese residents include tuberculosis, AIDS, and viral hepatitis. In 2021,there were 6.23 million reported cases of legally defined infectious diseases nationwide,with 22 198 deaths. The reported incidence rate was 442.16 per 100 000,and the reported mortality rate was 1.57 per 100 000. The top five diseases by death toll were AIDS,tuberculosis,viral hepatitis,rabies, and epidemic hemorrhagic fever,accounting for 99.7% of deaths from Class A and B infectious diseases. Since China expanded its national immunization program in 2007,the number of vaccines has increased from 6 to 14,preventing 15 infectious diseases. China has eradicated smallpox,achieved the goal of being polio-free,and eliminated neonatal tetanus.

4. 2. 3　Epidemic Surveillance and the Construction of the Health Emergency Response Network

Following the SARS outbreak in 2003,China gradually established the world's largest direct reporting system for infectious disease epidemics and public health emergencies. This system enables medical and health institutions of all levels, including township health centers,to report infectious disease epidemics and public health emergencies directly to the national level,and has reduced the average reporting time from five days to within four hours. It covers 168 000 medical and health institutions nationwide,with 350 000 users,and achieves a timely reporting rate of over 99% for legally defined infectious diseases. Over the years,the effective operation of this system has reduced underreporting of infectious diseases and significantly improved the timeliness of the reporting of infectious diseases. Currently,100% of disease control and prevention institutions above the county level,98% of medical and health institutions above the county level,and 94% of primary medical and health institutions in China have achieved real-time online reporting of legally defined infectious diseases. Recently, this system has further enhanced the efficiency of China's health statistics work,providing robust data support for close contact tracing of infected individuals, epidemiological investigation, epidemic assessment, and big data comparative analysis.

4.2.4　Maternal and Child Health Surveillance and Intervention

China has established a relatively comprehensive maternal and child health care network. By the end of 2021, there were 3 032 maternal and child health care institutions in China, including 26 at the provincial level, 377 at the prefectural (municipal) level, and 2 554 at the county (district, county-level city) level, with 454 000 health technicians in these institutions. In terms of maternal and child health informatization construction, China has successively established the Maternal and Child Health Annual Report Information System, the Maternal and Child Health Surveillance Information System, and the Maternal and Child Health Care Institutions Surveillance Information System. China actively promotes hospital deliveries to ensure maternal and infant safety. In 2021, the prenatal examination rate for pregnant women reached 97.6%, the postpartum visit rate reached 96%, and the hospital delivery rate was 99.9% (100% in cities and 99.9% in counties), basically achieving full hospital deliveries; the systematic management rate for children under three years old reached 92.8%. China conducts screening work to prevent and treat common diseases among women. By 2020, the "two cancers" screening work has covered nearly 2 600 counties (cities, districts) nationwide, and nearly 200 million people have been screened for the "two cancers" free of charge, including 130 million for cervical cancer and 64 million for breast cancer. In 2023, China released the "Action Plan for Accelerating the Elimination of Cervical Cancer (2023-2030)" to actively respond to the "Global Strategy to Accelerate the Elimination of Cervical Cancer" proposed by the World Health Organization, accelerating the process of cervical cancer elimination in China to protect and promote women's health. The action plan proposes the following goals: by 2025, promote pilot human papilloma virus (HPV) vaccination services for girls of appropriate age, achieve a 50% cervical cancer screening rate for women of appropriate age, and reach a 90% treatment rate for cervical cancer and precancerous lesions; by 2030, continue to promote HPV vaccination pilot work for girls of appropriate age, achieve a 70% cervical cancer screening rate for women of appropriate age, and reach a 90% treatment rate for cervical cancer and precancerous lesions.

In recent years, China has further strengthened comprehensive prevention and treatment of reproductive health and birth defects. China actively promotes premarital health care services; in 2018, 10.2 million newlyweds received premarital medical examinations, with a premarital examination rate of 61.1%. China has carried out the national pre-pregnancy health checkup program; from 2010 to 2018, free checkups were provided for 83.49 million couples planning to conceive. China has implemented a program of folic acid supplementation to prevent neural tube defects, providing free folic acid supplements to nearly 102 million women of childbearing age from 2009 to 2018. Prenatal screening and prenatal diagnosis coverage has gradually expanded, with a 61.1% serum screening rate for Down syndrome in 2018. Efforts to control and prevent thalassemia have been strengthened, with free screening for 1. 65 million couples in 10 southern provinces by 2018,effectively reducing the birth of children with severe thalassemia. The coverage of neonatal disease screening has steadily expanded, with a 97. 5% screening rate for neonatal genetic metabolic diseases nationwide in 2017. In 2018,neonatal congenital heart disease screening was initiated.

4.2.5 Chronic Disease Prevention and Treatment

The most common chronic diseases in China include cardiovascular diseases,diabetes, malignant tumors, and chronic respiratory diseases. To effectively control and prevent chronic diseases and curb the rapid rise in premature mortality caused by them,China began formulating a national chronic disease prevention and treatment plan in 2012. The "China's Medium- to Long-Term Plan for Prevention and Treatment of Chronic Diseases (2017-2025)"formulated by the Chinese government proposed the goals that by 2020, the environment for chronic disease control and prevention should be significantly improved, and the premature mortality rate from chronic diseases should be reduced,aiming to lower the premature mortality rate from cardiovascular diseases, cancer, chronic respiratory diseases,and diabetes among people aged 30-70 by 10% compared with 2015; by 2025,the risk factors for chronic diseases should be effectively controlled,the health management for the entire population across the life span should be achieved,and the goal is to lower the premature mortality rate from cardiovascular diseases,cancer,chronic respiratory diseases, and diabetes among people aged 30-70 by 20% compared with 2015; gradually increase residents' health life expectancy and effectively control the burden of chronic diseases.

To achieve these goals,China proposes to establish a division of labor and hierarchical management mechanism among disease control and prevention institutions, hospitals, specialized disease prevention and treatment institutions,and primary medical and health institutions in chronic disease prevention and treatment, with clear responsibilities and tasks. Disease control and prevention institutions and specialized disease prevention and treatment institutions should assist health administrative departments in formulating and implementing chronic disease control and prevention plans and programs, and provide business guidance and technical management. Hospitals are responsible for chronic disease-related information registration and reporting, providing diagnosis, treatment, and rehabilitation services for patients with severe and critical chronic diseases, offering technical guidance for primary medical and health institutions in chronic disease diagnosis, treatment, and rehabilitation, and establishing a two-way referral mechanism between themselves and primary medical and health institutions. Primary medical and health institutions are responsible for implementing chronic disease control and prevention measures. Moreover, China has made it clear that health education institutions are responsible for researching chronic disease health education strategies and methods, disseminating core information on chronic disease prevention and treatment, and guiding other institutions in conducting chronic disease health education activities. Maternal and child health care institutions provide consultation and guidance on chronic disease prevention related to women and children.

Currently, an important task in China's chronic disease prevention and treatment is to ensure the successful construction and innovative development of chronic disease comprehensive control and prevention demonstration areas. Since 2010, China has been creating chronic disease comprehensive control and prevention demonstration areas. In these demonstration areas, community surveys and diagnoses are conducted to identify major local health problems and risk factors, and appropriate technologies are applied to develop suitable chronic disease control and prevention strategies, measures, and long-term management models. Regarding the promotion of innovative development of chronic disease comprehensive control and prevention demonstration areas, the following measures are proposed in the "China's Medium- to Long-Term Plan for Prevention and Treatment of Chronic Diseases (2017-2025)": using the construction of national chronic disease comprehensive control and prevention demonstration areas as a starting point to cultivate chronic disease comprehensive control and prevention models suitable for different regions; the construction of demonstration areas should closely align with the requirements of creating healthy cities and towns, integrate with hierarchical diagnosis and treatment and family doctor contract services, comprehensively enhance the construction quality of demonstration areas, as well as play a leading role in strengthening the main responsibilities of the government, implementing the responsibilities of various departments, and providing comprehensive chronic disease prevention and treatment management services for the entire population throughout the life cycle, so as to drive the overall improvement of regional chronic disease prevention and treatment management levels.

4.2.6 Endemic Disease Prevention and Treatment

Endemic diseases are caused by geochemical and biological factors, as well as production and lifestyle habits, leading to region-specific occurrences. These diseases often occur in impoverished and rural areas, contributing significantly to poverty due to illness and poverty returning due to illness. Endemic disease prevention and treatment is a complex social system project and a significant livelihood project. In China, disease control and prevention institutions at various levels and specialized institutions for endemic disease prevention and treatment are responsible for the surveillance and health education of endemic diseases. They are also responsible for formulating endemic disease control and prevention measures and evaluating their effectiveness, as well as coordinating with relevant departments to implement control and prevention measures such as universal iodized salt use and improvement of water quality. China was once severely affected by endemic diseases, with iodine deficiency disorders, water-borne high iodine goiter, endemic fluorosis, endemic arsenic poisoning, Kashin-Beck disease, and Keshan disease being the main concerns. However, after years of efforts, most regions have effectively controlled or eliminated these hazards. The "three-year campaign on the prevention and treatment of endemic diseases" launched in 2018 has achieved sustained elimination of iodine deficiency disorder, basically eliminated coal-burning type fluorosis and arsenic poisoning, Kashin-Beck disease, and Keshan disease, and effectively controlled drinking water type fluorosis and arsenic poisoning, tea-drinking type fluorosis, and water-borne high iodine hazards. The prevention and treatment goals were achieved alongside poverty alleviation tasks, marking historic achievements in endemic disease prevention and treatment. Nevertheless, as endemic diseases are biogeochemical in nature, long-term consolidation and maintenance of prevention measures are required to prevent recurrence. Therefore, in the future, China will, on the basis of the "three-year campaign on the prevention and treatment of endemic diseases," further enhance nationwide comprehensive endemic disease prevention and treatment capabilities, establish long-term prevention and treatment management mechanisms, address key and difficult issues in current endemic disease prevention and treatment, and continuously consolidate and improve prevention and treatment outcomes to protect the health of the population.

4.2.7 Occupational Disease Prevention and Treatment

Occupational health is a fundamental and integral part of building a Healthy China, concerning the health and well-being of the vast workforce as well as economic development and social stability. China currently faces new challenges and requirements in safeguarding workers' health: the intertwining of new and old occupational disease hazards, and increasing difficulty in controlling and preventing occupational diseases and work-related illnesses; expanding scope of occupational health management and services, and prominent contradictions between the growing demand for occupational health services and the unbalanced and inadequate development of occupational health work. Additionally, the capacity for supporting services and guarantees for occupational disease prevention and treatment needs urgent strengthening, with lagging occupational health information system development. The foundation of occupational health needs to be further consolidated, and the regulatory responsibilities of some local governments and the main responsibilities of employers are not fully implemented.

China implements an occupational health supervision system. The work safety supervision and administration departments, health administrative departments, and labor security administrative departments under the State Council are responsible for supervising and managing occupational disease prevention and treatment nationwide according to the law. The diagnosis of occupational diseases and occupational health examinations are conducted by medical and health institutions approved by the provincial health administrative departments. In the event of an acute occupational disease hazard accident, employers must immediately take emergency rescue and control measures and report to the local health administrative departments and related departments. The health administrative departments are responsible for organizing medical treatment. The diagnosis, treatment, and rehabilitation costs for occupational disease patients, as well as social security for those who are disabled or have lost labor capacity due to occupational diseases, are covered by the national work-related injury insurance in which employers participate. If an employer does not participate in the national work-related injury insurance, the medical care and living security of the patient shall be borne by the employer.

In 2021, China issued the "National Occupational Disease Prevention and Treatment Plan (2021-2025)," setting the following goals: by 2025, establish a more complete occupational health governance system, significantly improve conditions regarding occupational disease hazards, notably improve working conditions in the workplace, further standardize the management of labor employment and working hours, effectively control key occupational diseases such as pneumoconiosis, realize the continuous enhancement of occupational health service capacity and guarantee level, significantly increase awareness of occupational health across society, and further improve the health of workers.

4.2.8　Environmental and Health Surveillance

In 2007, China issued the "National Action Plan on Environment and Health (2007-2015)," the first programmatic document in the field of environment and health in China. In 2022, the "14th Five-Year Plan for Environmental Health Work" formulated by the Chinese government proposed the goals that by 2025, the distribution characteristics of high environmental health risk sources in key areas nationwide will be basically understood, the layout of environmental health risk surveillance will be initially formed, the environmental health standard system will be further improved, and a batch of environmental health risk assessment technical specifications and model calculation software will be developed. Additionally, pilot projects for environmental health management will be carried out in 10-15 regions, achieving multi-level, diversified, and characteristic development of environmental health management. A professional team will be built, with cumulative business training for 50 000 people. A good social atmosphere supporting and participating in environmental health work will be fostered, with the national residents' environmental health literacy level reaching more than 20%.

4.2.9　Health Education and Health Promotion

China has initially established a health education system led by professional health education institutions, based on primary medical and health institutions in urban and rural areas, and including other medical and health institutions and key places such as schools, enterprises, government agencies, and public institutions. Professional health education institutions include health education centers, health education institutes, and health education stations. The China Health Education Center is responsible for providing technical guidance on health education and health news publicity nationwide, conducting related theoretical and practical research, organizing and implementing large-scale health education and health news publicity activities, and undertaking information management, media contacts, business training, and other technical and service work. At the local level, health education institutes or health education stations are set up to handle specific health education work. To promote the health of urban and rural residents, the Chinese government departments, social groups, and enterprises have jointly or independently carried out various health education and health promotion activities, covering areas such as tobacco control, maternal and child health, children's nutrition, and hepatitis prevention and treatment.

China has established a combined approach to population health surveillance, integrating routine surveillance and health checkups. Routine surveillance refers to the regular health surveillance work carried out by primary medical and health institutions as part of basic public health services. These surveillance efforts are mainly organized and implemented by township health centers and community health service centers, with village clinics and community health service stations conducting specific health surveillance under the management of them respectively. In recent years, health checkups have developed rapidly in China, primarily provided by health checkup institutions affiliated with hospitals, with some independent professional health checkup institutions also offering services.

Moreover, China has conducted special health surveillance programs, such as the Chinese Residents' Nutrition and Health Status Surveillance, which started in 1959. In recent years, other programs, including cause of death surveillance, tumor follow-up registration, chronic disease and nutrition surveillance, have also been carried out, with the coverage of surveillance sites expanding annually. All work has become increasingly standardized, and a chronic disease surveillance and information management platform covering morbidity, prevalence, mortality, and risk factors is gradually taking shape.

Case Study Ⅰ　Schistosomiasis Prevention and Treatment in China

According to the World Health Organization, as of 2021, schistosomiasis transmission has been reported from 78 countries. However, preventive chemotherapy for schistosomiasis, where people and communities are targeted for large-scale treatment, is only required in 51 endemic countries with moderate-to-high transmission. In 2021, at least 251.4 million people worldwide needed preventive treatment for schistosomiasis. Schistosomiasis is a chronic parasitic disease caused by schistosomes. The Schistosomiasis prevention and treatment program is one of China's major infectious disease prevention and treatment programs. Statistics indicate that in the early days of the People's Republic of China, there were 11. 6 million schistosomiasis patients, and over 100 million people were at risk. After more than half a century of efforts, by the end of 2004, the number of schistosomiasis patients in China had dropped to 843 000 (including 28 000 with advanced schistosomiasis), and the area infested with the host Oncomelania snails had reduced to a quarter of its original size. The number of infections and people at risk had significantly decreased, showcasing the tremendous achievements in China's schistosomiasis prevention and treatment efforts. These achievements are inseparable from China's emphasis on adopting a science-based approach and the participation of the entire population. The key experience from China's efforts is summarized as follows:

Adhering to the party's centralized and unified leadership and form synergy. In the early days of the People's Republic of China, Chairman Mao Zedong called for "mobilizing the whole party and the entire population to eliminate schistosomiasis." Under the unified leadership of the Communist Party of China, a leadership group for schistosomiasis prevention and treatment was established, rather than just health departments working alone. This group fully integrated resources from various departments, including health, agriculture, water conservancy, chemical industry, commerce, education, and civil affairs, as well as organizations like the military, Communist Youth League, and Women's Federation. The entire population was widely mobilized, including not only the residents of schistosomiasis-endemic areas but also a large number of farmers, students, and the People's Liberation Army from non-endemic regions.

Adopting a science-based approach and integrating traditional Chinese and Western medicine. China adhered to adopting a science-based approach. The Central Committee of the Communist Party of China carefully listened to the opinions of scientists and professionals, such as adopting fire-burning instead of soil-burying methods for captured Oncomelania snails. Scientific research was supported and promoted, and a combination of traditional Chinese and Western medicine was used, with comprehensive surveillance targeting humans, livestock, and host Oncomelania snails.

Mobilizing the entire population, adapting to local conditions, and doing the right thing at the right time. Taking the elimination of schistosomiasis as a political task, China has closely relied on the masses and mobilized the entire population to participate in various aspects such as Oncomelania snail elimination, patient treatment, fecal management, safe water use, and personal protection. For example, during the winter when farmers were less busy and water levels were low, most Oncomelania snails were exposed on the ground. The prevention and treatment focus was on mass treatment for able-bodied labor force, combined with water conservancy projects to bury soil and reclaim land to eliminate Oncomelania snails, along with fecal management.

During the summer and autumn, when farmers frequently engaged in activities like cutting grass, collecting fertilizer, transplanting rice seedlings, and fertilizing, the risk of schistosomiasis infection was high. The prevention and treatment focus was on fecal management and personal protection, combined with treating semi-able-bodied labor force and children patients.

China is currently conducting planned, continuous, and systematic schistosomiasis surveillance, which is crucial for continuing effective control and prevention efforts. This includes the following aspects:

Establishing a nationwide surveillance network. China has been establishing and improving the epidemic surveillance system at county, township, village, and urban community levels to closely monitor the epidemic situation, socioeconomic conditions, and changes in the human and natural environment. The patient surveillance and new case reporting mechanisms are being improved, and comprehensive surveillance sites are being established to monitor not only the human population but also livestock, Oncomelania snails, and suspicious environments.

Carrying out timely epidemic reporting and case investigation. Various medical institutions, disease control and prevention institutions (schistosomiasis control institutions), health quarantine institutions, and their medical staff are required to report schistosomiasis cases within 24 hours of diagnosis using an infectious disease report card through the network direct reporting system after distinguishing between acute and chronic cases. County-level disease control and prevention institutions are responsible for individual case investigations of reported acute schistosomiasis cases within one week, filling out case investigation forms, and promptly entering the data into the database, and then reporting through the schistosomiasis information reporting system network.

Conducting Oncomelania snail inspections and environmental surveillance. The significant success of China's schistosomiasis prevention and treatment efforts lies in the nationwide mobilization and Oncomelania snail elimination campaigns, which cut off the host transmission route. Despite the achievements, the Chinese government continues to conduct annual spring Oncomelania snail inspections. The inspection scope includes existing Oncomelania snail environments (including susceptible environments and other Oncomelania snail habitats) and suspicious environments. Systematic sampling and environmental sampling methods are used to check Oncomelania snail infection status.

Case Study Ⅱ　Malaria Prevention and Treatment in China

According to the World Health Organization, globally in 2022, there were an estimated

249 million malaria cases and 608 000 malaria deaths in 85 countries. Malaria is a life-threatening disease transmitted to humans through the bites of certain types of mosquitoes. However, malaria is preventable and treatable. On June 30, 2021, the World Health Organization announced that China had been certified malaria-free, recognizing China's remarkable achievement of eliminating malaria after reporting around 30 million malaria cases annually in the 1940s and eradicating the disease entirely after 70 years of relentless effort. This accomplishment marks another significant eradication of a major infectious disease in China, following smallpox, poliomyelitis, filariasis, and neonatal tetanus, and represents a crucial milestone in both China's public health history and the global campaign to eliminate malaria.

Malaria was once one of China's most historically pervasive, widespread, and deadly infectious diseases. Before the founding of the People's Republic of China, approximately 30 million people contracted malaria annually, of which 300 000 died, with a fatality rate as high as 1‰. Following the founding of the People's Republic of China, the Central Committee of the Communist Party of China and the State Council led the Chinese people in combating malaria through five arduous phases: carrying out key investigations and prevention and treatment measures (1949-1959), controlling severe epidemics (1960-1979), reducing the incidence rate (1980-1999), consolidating prevention and treatment achievements (2000-2009), and eliminating malaria (2010-2020).

In 2010, the Chinese government actively responded to the United Nations' global malaria eradication initiative by setting the goal of eliminating malaria by 2020. Through persistent efforts, China reduced the annual number of indigenous malaria cases from 30 million to zero, safeguarding the health and lives of its people. China established scientifically precise malaria control and prevention strategies, along with a sensitive and efficient system for reporting, detecting, treating, monitoring, and emergency response, thereby gaining the capacity to prevent the reintroduction and spread of malaria. China also developed artemisinin and other effective antimalarial drugs and treatment regimens and innovated the "1-3-7" malaria elimination protocol, which includes completing malaria case report within 1 day, case review and epidemiological investigation within 3 days, and focus investigation and response within 7 days. Additionally, China implemented multi-departmental and regional joint control and prevention measures and cooperated on malaria control and prevention in border areas, contributing Chinese expertise to global malaria control and elimination efforts. China reported its last local primary case of malaria in April 2016, has not detected any local primary case for four consecutive years since 2017, and submitted an application for malaria elimination certification to the World Health Organization in November 2020. After an on-site assessment by the World Health Organization, China passed the national malaria elimination certification on June 30, 2021.

5 China's Medical Security System

The medical security system is an essential component of the social security system, encompassing common medical issues in most areas of social security system, such as illness, injury, childbirth, and elderly care. The establishment of a medical security system is a social responsibility that plays an increasingly important role in national affairs and social development. Countries around the world are attempting to improve their entire social security system by establishing a relatively comprehensive medical security system, so as to promote social harmonious development, and progress. China has already established a basic medical security system that covers all urban and rural residents. China's medical security system plays a significant role in safeguarding citizens' health and survival rights, improving population health levels, promoting the development of medical and health services, improving social fairness, and maintaining social stability.

China's medical security system includes multiple layers such as basic medical insurance, medical assistance, supplementary medical insurance, and commercial medical insurance (Figure 5-1). Basic medical insurance, medical assistance, and supplementary medical insurance fall within the scope of social medical security, with funding and benefit policies formulated by the government and security services mainly provided by

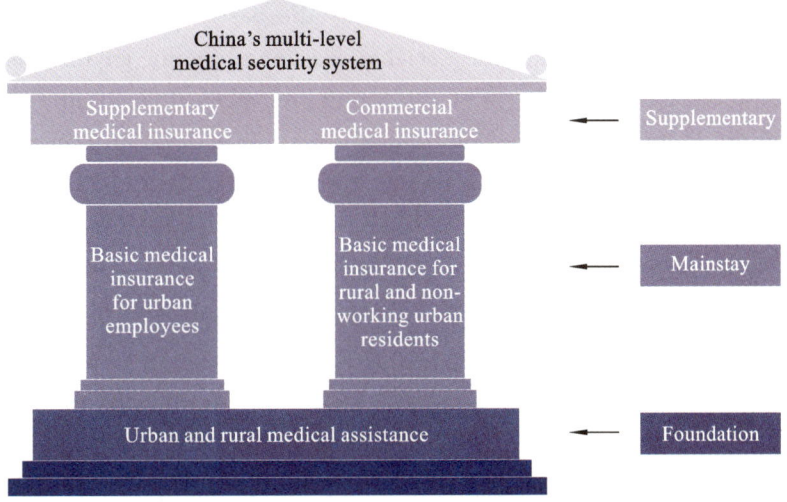

Figure 5-1 China's multi-level medical security system

government-affiliated institutions, while commercial medical insurance is offered by insurance companies through market-oriented mechanisms. Basic medical insurance includes basic medical insurance for urban employees and basic medical insurance for rural and non-working urban residents. Urban employees are required to participate in basic medical insurance for urban employees, while non-working urban residents and rural residents voluntarily participate in basic medical insurance for rural and non-working urban residents on a household basis. The urban and rural medical assistance serves as the foundation of China's multi-level medical security system, encompassing urban medical assistance and rural medical assistance. The urban and rural medical assistance system raises funds through multiple channels such as government allocations and social donations, primarily providing financial assistance to urban and rural low-income households, households enjoying five guarantees, and other economically disadvantaged families to ensure that impoverished populations enjoy basic medical services.

The following text will first provide a detailed introduction to basic medical insurance for urban employees and basic medical insurance for rural and non-working urban residents, and then introduce the urban and rural medical assistance, commercial medical insurance, and supplementary medical insurance.

5.1　Basic Medical Insurance for Urban Employees

5.1.1　Institutional Background

To safeguard the medical rights and interests of urban employees, China has successively established the socialized medicine and the labor insurance medical system (during the planned economy period), as well as the basic medical insurance for urban employees (which emerged under the socialist market economy environment). Starting from the comprehensive reform pilot of employee medical insurance conducted in Zhenjiang, Jiangsu Province, and Jiujiang, Jiangxi Province in 1994, to the promulgation of the "Decision of the State Council on Establishing the Basic Medical Insurance for Urban Employees" (hereinafter referred to as the "Decision") in December 1998, the framework of the basic medical insurance for urban employees was basically established in China. Currently, China's basic medical insurance for urban employees has been universally established nationwide.

The "Decision" proposes that the main task of the medical insurance system reform is to adapt to the socialist market economy system and establish a social medical insurance system that guarantees the basic medical needs of employees based on the fiscal, enterprise, and individual affordability. The "Decision" also proposes that the principles for establishing the basic medical insurance system for urban employees are as follows: the level of basic medical insurance should be commensurate with the level of productive forces in the primary stage of socialism; all urban employers and their employees must participate in basic medical insurance and this shall be subject to territorial administration; basic medical insurance premiums are jointly borne by both employers and employees; and the basic medical insurance funds implement a combination of social pooling funds with individual accounts.

5.1.2　Main Content

5.1.2.1　Coverage Range

According to the "Decision," the basic medical insurance system for urban employees should cover all urban employers, including enterprises (state-owned enterprises, collective enterprises, foreign-invested enterprises, private enterprises, etc.), government agencies, public institutions, social organizations, private non-enterprise units, and their employees. In other words, all formally employed individuals must participate in basic medical insurance to achieve "wide coverage."

With the further deepening of China's economic system reform and the adjustment of its industrial structure, the number of employees in flexible forms of employment such as part-time, temporary, and flexible work has gradually increased. To address the medical insurance issues of flexible employment personnel, in 2003, the Ministry of Labor and Social Security of the People's Republic of China issued the "Guiding Opinions on Urban Flexible Employment Personnel Participating in Basic Medical Insurance," which explicitly includes flexible employment personnel within the scope of the basic medical insurance system and encourages them to achieve overall participation through labor security agencies or community labor security service agencies.

Since entering the 21st century, the migration of rural labor to cities in China has accelerated, and the tide of migrant workers has further expanded. Although these individuals work and live in cities, they cannot enjoy the security and benefits of the cities they reside in. To improve the medical security for migrant workers, the Ministry of Labor and Social Security of the People's Republic of China launched a special campaign in 2006 to expand the coverage of medical insurance for migrant workers. As a result, all urban laborers are now covered by the basic medical insurance system for urban employees. By the end of 2022, the number of participants in China's basic medical insurance for urban employees reached 362 million.

5.1.2.2　Fund Collection

According to the "Decision," the basic medical insurance premiums for employees are jointly paid by employers and employees. The employers' contribution rate should be controlled at around 6% of the total wages of employees, while the employees' contribution rate is generally 2% of their personal income. With the development of the economy, the contribution rates of employers and employees can be adjusted accordingly. This funding level was formulated based on the actual situation of China's relatively low productivity level and limited fiscal and corporate affordability at that time. This document also stipulates that retirees participating in basic medical insurance do not pay basic medical insurance premiums personally. Currently, the average employer contribution rate in China is approximately 7.5%, and the average employee contribution rate is 2%. To address the medical insurance issues of retirees from closed and bankrupt state-owned enterprises, in May 2009, the Ministry of Human Resources and Social Security and three other ministries jointly issued the "Notice on Appropriately Addressing Issues Related to Medical Insurance for Retirees from Closed and Bankrupt State-Owned Enterprises." The notice clarifies that when an enterprise is closed or bankrupted, the required costs for retirees to participate in medical insurance should be paid through the enterprise's bankruptcy assets according to relevant provisions of the Enterprise Bankruptcy Law of the People's Republic of China. If the enterprise's bankruptcy assets are insufficient, they can be raised through various channels such as the proceeds from land sales that are not included in the bankruptcy assets, fiscal subsidies, and adjustments to the balance of medical insurance funds. Provincial governments should provide assistance and support to struggling cities and counties. For retirees from locally bankrupt state-owned enterprises participating in the basic medical insurance system for urban employees, the central government will provide a one-time subsidy based on the principle of "combining rewards and subsidies."

5.1.2.3 Fund Operation and Management

China's basic medical insurance funds consist of social pooling funds and individual accounts. According to the "Decision," all the basic medical insurance premiums paid by employees are credited to their individual accounts. The basic medical insurance premiums paid by employers are divided into two parts, one for establishing the social pooling funds and the other for crediting to individual accounts. The proportion credited to individual accounts is generally around 30% of the employers' contribution. The social pooling funds and individual accounts are accounted for separately according to their respective payment scopes and must not be misappropriated. In 2021, to further improve the basic medical insurance system for employees with mutual assistance and shared responsibility, the General Office of the State Council issued the "Guiding Opinions of the General Office of the State Council on Establishing and Improving the Outpatient Co-Insurance Mechanism for Employee Basic Medical Insurance," which modified the method of calculating individual accounts credits. In principle, the individual accounts credit standard is controlled at 2% of the individual's insured contribution base, and the basic medical insurance premiums paid by the employer are all credited to the social pooling funds. After adjusting the structure of the social pooling funds and individual accounts, the increased social pooling funds are mainly used for outpatient co-insurance and improving the outpatient benefits for insured individuals.

China's basic medical insurance funds are managed through special fiscal accounts.

Fund collection is the responsibility of the medical insurance administrative institutions in the pooling area. The medical insurance funds first enter the fund income account of the administrative institutions, and then are handed over to the special fiscal account managed by the local financial department for unified management. Based on the payment plan of the medical insurance administrative institutions, the local financial department will allocate funds from the special fiscal account to the fund expenditure account of the medical insurance administrative institutions. Finally, the funds flow from the fund expenditure account of the medical insurance administrative institutions to medical institutions.

5.1.2.4　Scope of Coverage and Benefit Payment

China's basic medical insurance payment system implements a catalog management approach, primarily to ensure that insured individuals enjoy basic medical services legally, regulate reasonable prescriptions from medical institutions, and reasonably control medical expenses. The payment catalog includes the drug catalog, the diagnosis and treatment item catalog, and the medical service facility catalog. Among them, the drug catalog adopts an "admission method" for management, meaning that the listed drugs fall within the scope approved for payment by basic medical insurance; the diagnosis and treatment item catalog currently mainly adopts an "exclusion method" for management, but some regions adopt an "admission method" for management; the medical service facility catalog adopts an "exclusion method" for management.

The benefit payment of the basic medical insurance for urban employees covers three aspects: general outpatient services, outpatient services for major illnesses, and inpatient services. The basic medical insurance funds for urban employees implement a combination of social pooling funds and individual accounts (unified accounting). Specifically, the individual accounts cover outpatient services for minor illnesses, while the social pooling funds cover inpatient services and outpatient services for major illnesses. The basic medical insurance for urban employees sets a deductible threshold, coinsurance ratio, and ceiling limit. According to the requirements of the "Decision," the deductible threshold is controlled in principle at around 10% of the local employees' annual average salary, and the maximum payment limit is controlled in principle at around four times the local employees' annual average salary. Medical expenses below the deductible threshold are paid from the individual accounts or borne by the individual. Medical expenses above the deductible threshold and below the maximum payment limit are primarily paid from the social pooling funds, with individuals also bearing a certain proportion.

5.1.2.5　Medical Service Management

The purpose of medical service management conducted by China's medical insurance institutions is to reasonably control medical expenses and ensure the quality of medical services. The content of medical service management can be summarized as "designated medical treatment and three catalogs." Designated medical treatment refers to the practice that the medical insurance administrative institutions and medical institutions sign the designated medical treatment agreements, the medical institutions accepts the assessment and supervision of the medical insurance administrative institutions, and only when insured individuals seek medical treatment at designated medical institutions can they obtain reimbursement from medical insurance. Designated medical institutions include general hospitals, specialized hospitals, and community health service institutions within the jurisdiction. With the expansion of medical insurance coverage, the number of designated medical institutions has also increased significantly. Generally, public medical institutions and private medical institutions with a certain scale within the jurisdiction are included in the scope of designated medical institutions.

The "three catalogs" refer to the drug catalog, the diagnosis and treatment item catalog, and the medical service facility catalog mentioned above. All three catalogs are formulated based on the principles of clinical necessity, safety, effectiveness, and appropriate pricing. Among them, the drug catalog is formulated by the Ministry of Human Resources and Social Security, while the diagnosis and treatment item catalog and the medical service facility catalog are formulated by the human resources and social security departments of various provinces. The drug catalog is divided into Class A and Class B. Class A is uniformly formulated by the state, and cannot be adjusted by local authorities. Class B is formulated by the state, but provinces, autonomous regions, and municipalities directly under the central government can make appropriate adjustments based on local conditions. The sum of the number of drugs added and reduced must not exceed 15% of the total number of drugs in the national Class B catalog. The human resources and social security departments of prefectural and county-level overall planning areas have no authority to adjust the drug catalog, but they can adjust the reimbursement ratio appropriately. Generally, about 20% of the self-paid expenses for drugs in Class B catalog are deducted, and the remaining amount can be reimbursed.

5.1.2.6 Medical Insurance Payment

Since 2011, China's medical and health system reform has taken the reform of medical insurance payment methods as an important task. An increasing number of regions have been transitioning from fee-for-service payment to mixed payment models.

Total budget control. It stipulates that the growth rate of medical institutions' business income must not exceed an agreed-upon value. For example, Shanghai and other places have adopted this approach.

Average cost per hospitalization. It stipulates that the average cost per hospitalization in medical institutions must not exceed an agreed-upon value. For instance, Nanjing, Zhenjiang, Guangzhou, Shenzhen, and other regions have implemented this method.

Diagnosis related groups (DRGs). For several specific diagnoses, fixed payment methods are implemented. For example, Beijing implemented DRGs in six pilot hospitals in 2011, covering 108 different diagnoses. Throughout the city, this payment method has been implemented for a small number of diseases such as appendicitis, goiter, cataract, benign ovarian tumor, uterine fibroid, hallux valgus, and gallstone. In Mudanjiang, Heilongjiang Province, however, single-diagnosis payment is implemented for the vast majority of diseases, with a total of 830 diagnoses in 2010.

Capitation. This method is primarily implemented in the management of chronic outpatient diseases (such as mental illnesses). Patients sign a contract with a designated medical institution, committing to seeking initial consultation at that institution for the entire year. The medical insurance institution then pays the designated medical institution a capitation fee for the outpatient services provided to chronic patients for one year. However, patients still need to pay a certain proportion of out-of-pocket expenses when seeking medical treatment.

Diagnosis-intervention packet (DIP). This is a payment method originally created in China. It relies on big data and groups cases based on the "diagnosis + operation" classification rule after collecting a large number of real-world cases. Medical insurance payments are then made according to certain settlement rules.

In China's practice, the prepaid system is combined with a risk-sharing mechanism. If the actual expenses of a medical institution exceed the pre-determined budget, the medical insurance institution will share a portion of the overrun expenses. The specific sharing method is negotiated between the medical insurance institution and the medical institution and is reflected in the designated medical treatment agreement.

5.1.2.7　Medical Service Regulation

In China, medical service regulation primarily includes aspects such as designated access, real-time monitoring, annual assessment, and reward and punishment mechanisms.

5.2　Basic Medical Insurance for Rural and Non-Working Urban Residents

Case Study　China's Rural Cooperative Medical Care System Being Hailed as the "Chinese Model"

In the 1980s, the World Health Organization and the World Bank pointed out in their investigation report on China that the rural cooperative medical care system implemented in China was the only model for developing countries to solve health funding issues. Dr. Mahler, the then Director-General of the World Health Organization, actively recommended China's rural health work experience to developing countries.

China's rural cooperative medical care system has been praised by the World Health

Organization and the World Bank as the "Chinese Model" that achieved the greatest health benefits with the least investment. It can be traced back to the earliest health pharmacies and health cooperatives in the 1930s, having undergone the embryonic stage in the 1930s to 1940s, the initial stage in the 1950s, the development and peak stage in the 1960s to 1970s, the disintegration stage in the 1980s, and the recovery and development stage since the 1990s (when the new rural cooperative medical care system was established). The development and improvement of China's rural cooperative medical care system laid the foundation for China to address the basic health issues of 800 million farmers with relatively low health expenditure in the 1960s to 1970s. In 1978, the coverage of China's rural cooperative medical care system reached over 90%. This system has improved the rural medical situation in China and enhanced the health level of the broad masses of the people. After implementing the rural cooperative medical care system, by 2003, China's infant mortality rate had dropped from 200‰ in the early days of the founding of the People's Republic of China to 25.5‰, the maternal mortality rate had decreased from 1 500 per 100 000 to 51.3 per 100 000, the population mortality rate had declined from 17‰ to 6.4‰, and the average life expectancy had increased from 35 years to 72.4 years.

The early rural cooperative medical care system in China had the following characteristics: First, it was an important manifestation of promoting the development of the cooperative economy and improving its social service functions at that time. China's rural cooperative medical care system emerged in the form of health pharmacies and adhered to the principle of putting disease prevention first. Second, medical personnel played a significant role. These medical personnel did not receive salaries. They were busy with farm work most of the time, and served as doctors when needed, known as "barefoot doctors." They were trained by "mobile medical teams," which were a crucial pillar for consolidating and developing China's rural cooperative medical care system. Third, China's rural cooperative medical care system was primarily funded by farmers' voluntary contributions. Daily expenses of health pharmacies were secured through three sources: "health care fees" paid by farmers, 15% to 20% of the public welfare funds extracted from agricultural cooperatives, and medical income. Fourth, China's rural cooperative medical care system was a low-cost, widely covered rural health insurance system, enabling rural residents to enjoy basic primary health services nearby and ensuring fairness and accessibility of medical and health services for sick farmers.

Issues with the early rural cooperative medical care system in China include: First, there was a lack of relevant legal and organizational guarantees. Without formal legal documents, there was no legal basis, and management lacked scientific rigor. Second, during the "cultural revolution," there was an eagerness for quick success and immediate benefit. Under the influence of extreme left-wing ideologies, there was an overemphasis on catering to political needs, disregarding objective and subjective conditions as well as medical and health characteristics in health policy-making and management, which damaged the healthy development of the medical and health system and hindered the healthy development of rural medicine. Third, the technical level of health personnel was relatively low, resulting in an overall low performance of the rural cooperative medical care system. Fourth, the funding level was limited, and the ability to resist risks was poor. After the disintegration of the rural collective economy, the rural cooperative medical care system lost its primary source of funding, which was one of the fundamental reasons why it was difficult for the system to exist for a long time. Fifth, the rural cooperative medical care system adopted an approach that focused on outpatient clinics and minor illnesses. This increased the benefit coverage, but the level of protection was low, making it difficult to meet the multi-level needs of the rural population.

The basic medical insurance system for rural and non-working urban residents was established in 2016 by integrating the basic medical insurance system for non-working urban residents and the new rural cooperative medical care system. This section will first introduce the relevant content of basic medical insurance for non-working urban residents and new rural cooperative medical care separately, and then describe the integration of the basic medical insurance system for non-working urban residents and the new rural cooperative medical care system.

5.2.1 Basic Medical Insurance for Non-Working Urban Residents

5.2.1.1 Institutional Background

In 2007, the pilot project for basic medical insurance for non-working urban residents was officially launched in China. 88 cities were selected across the country as pilot cities. In March 2008, the State Council issued the "Guiding Opinions of the State Council on Carrying Out the Pilot Project for Basic Medical Insurance for Non-Working Urban Residents" (hereinafter referred to as the "Guiding Opinions"). In 2010, the pilot project for basic medical insurance for non-working urban residents was fully implemented nationwide. The most distinctive feature of basic medical insurance for non-working urban residents is the government's universal subsidy for every insured resident.

Different from the main goal of basic medical insurance for urban employees, which is to guarantee the basic medical needs of the employed population in urban areas and establish a social insurance system combining individual accounts with social pooling funds, the goal of the basic medical insurance system for non-working urban residents is to establish a social security system that covers all non-working urban residents, with a reasonable funding mechanism, sound management system, and standardized operational mechanism, focusing primarily on comprehensive insurance for major illnesses.

The principles of the pilot project for basic medical insurance system for non-working urban residents are as follows: starting at a low level, determining the funding level and security standards reasonably based on the level of economic development and the affordability of all parties, focusing on guaranteeing the medical needs for major illnesses of non-working urban residents, and gradually improving the level of security; adhering to the principle of voluntariness and fully respecting the wishes of the people; clarifying the responsibilities of the central and local governments, with the central government determining the basic principles and major policies, and the local governments formulating specific measures to implement territorial management for insured residents; adhering to overall planning and coordination, ensuring the connection between the basic policies, standards, and management measures of various medical security systems.

5.2.1.2 Main Content

Similar to the basic medical insurance for urban employees, the basic medical insurance for non-working urban residents is also mostly formulated by the social security management departments of various localities, and managed by medical insurance administrative institutions. The basic medical insurance for non-working urban residents implements a catalog and management policy similar to that of the basic medical insurance for urban employees. Here, only the provisions that are inconsistent with the basic medical insurance for urban employees will be elaborated.

(1) Coverage Range

According to the "Guiding Opinions," the coverage range of the basic medical insurance system for non-working urban residents includes "students in primary and secondary schools (including vocational high schools, technical secondary schools, and technical schools), children, and other non-working urban residents who are not covered by the basic medical insurance system for urban employees." Together with the basic medical insurance system for urban employees that covers all employed populations, it has achieved full coverage of urban residents' medical insurance.

(2) Fund Collection

The basic medical insurance funds for non-working urban residents mainly come from two aspects: fiscal subsidies and individual contributions. When the pilot project was launched in 2007, the government provided subsidies at a standard of no less than 40 yuan per capita annually. For disadvantaged residents such as those receiving low-income assistance and severely disabled persons who have lost their ability to work, the government provided additional subsidies. The fiscal subsidy funds were included in the fiscal budgets of governments at all levels. With the introduction of the "Opinions of the Central Committee of the Communist Party of China and the State Council on Deepening the Reform of the Medical and Health System" in March 2009, the support of governments at all levels for the basic medical insurance system for non-working urban residents has gradually been strengthened, and the per capita fiscal subsidy standard for basic medical insurance for non-working urban residents has also been gradually increased, from 80 yuan per capita in 2009 to 450 yuan per capita in 2017, greatly improving the level of residents' medical and health security.

Regarding personal contributions, China currently does not have a unified standard. Local governments determine the appropriate level based on the local economic development level, basic medical consumption needs of different groups, and the affordability of local residents' families and the fiscal budget. In 2017, the per capita individual contribution standard for basic medical insurance for non-working urban residents reached 180 yuan.

(3) Scope of Coverage and Benefit Payment

The basic medical insurance funds for non-working urban residents implement social pooling funds without setting up individual accounts. The funds are mainly used for the medical expenditures of inpatient services and outpatient services for major illnesses of insured residents. When the pilot project was launched in 2007, the basic medical insurance for non-working urban residents only covered inpatient services and outpatient services for major illnesses, and general outpatient services were not reimbursed. In 2009, the "Guiding Opinions of the Ministry of Human Resources and Social Security, the Ministry of Finance, and the Ministry of Health on Implementing the Risk Pooling of Outpatient Services for the Basic Medical Insurance for Non-working Urban Residents" was issued, requiring all localities to gradually include medical expenses for outpatient services for minor illnesses into the fund payment scope while focusing on ensuring the medical expenditures of inpatient services and outpatient services for major illnesses of insured residents.

When covering inpatient services and outpatient services for major illnesses, the basic medical insurance for non-working urban residents implements the same reimbursement catalog as the basic medical insurance for urban employees, but the level of benefits enjoyed by insured residents is generally lower than that of the basic medical insurance for urban employees. The specific thresholds for initiating medical insurance payments, payment ratios, and maximum limits for the basic medical insurance for non-working urban residents are determined by local authorities. During the 12th Five-Year Plan period, the reimbursement ratio for inpatient expenses covered by the basic medical insurance for non-working urban residents reached 75%. Currently, China has implemented the risk pooling of outpatient services for the basic medical insurance for non-working urban residents, which includes the outpatient expenses of insured residents into the reimbursement scope of the pooling funds, effectively addressing the burden of general outpatient medical expenses for non-working urban residents. The risk pooling of outpatient services generally requires insured residents to seek medical treatment at primary medical and health institutions, and the maximum limit is usually only a few hundred yuan.

5.2.2　New Rural Cooperative Medical Care

5.2.2.1　Establishment of the New Rural Cooperative Medical Care System

To address the issue of farmers lacking medical security and the increasingly serious problem of poverty due to illness and poverty returning due to illness among rural residents, in October 2002, the Central Committee of the Communist Party of China and the State Council issued the "Decision of the Central Committee of the Communist Party of China and the State Council on Further Strengthening Rural Health Work," proposing the gradual establishment of the new rural cooperative medical care system. In 2003, the General Office of the State Council forwarded the "Opinions on Establishing a New Rural Cooperative Medical Care System" issued by the Ministry of Health and other departments, marking the official commencement of the establishment of the new rural cooperative medical care system. Since then, a new medical security system has gradually been implemented nationwide.

The new rural cooperative medical care system is a mutual medical assistance system for farmers that is organized, guided, and supported by the government. Farmers voluntarily participate in the system, with funding coming from individuals, collectives, and the government. The system focuses on providing comprehensive protection for major illnesses.

5.2.2.2　Objectives and Principles of the New Rural Cooperative Medical Care System

(1) Objectives of the New Rural Cooperative Medical Care System

The new rural cooperative medical care system differs from any previous medical security system and has distinct Chinese characteristics. Its objectives are to establish a basic medical security system that meets the health service needs of the vast majority of farmers, address the issues of poverty due to illness and poverty returning due to illness among farmers, reduce farmers' economic burden of medical treatment, increase the utilization rate of health services, promote the construction of rural health service systems, and improve the health level of the population.

(2) Principles of the New Rural Cooperative Medical Care System

The new rural cooperative medical care system follows unique principles that differ from previous cooperative medical care systems and align with China's rural development philosophy and the characteristics of farmers.

First, the principle of voluntary participation on a household basis. The most significant feature of the new rural cooperative medical care system is that it upholds the basic principle of "voluntary participation by farmers." The purpose is to allow farmers to recognize this beneficial system on their own and voluntarily participate in it, leveraging the situation to ultimately achieve full coverage of the new rural cooperative medical care system.

Second, the principle of government fiscal funding as the main source. In previous cooperative medical care systems, individual farmers or collective economies were the main funding sources. However, practice has shown that the amount of funding raised was relatively limited, the ability to resist risks was poor, and the systems were not sustainable. Since its inception, the new rural cooperative medical care system has clearly defined the principle of "government fiscal funding as the main source," specifying that central and local governments should provide certain subsidies to participating farmers.

Third, the principle of focusing on comprehensive protection for major illnesses while also considering outpatient services. The new rural cooperative medical care system primarily subsidizes hospitalization expenses while also compensating for outpatient expenses.

Fourth, the principle of using the county level as the unit of overall planning. In previous cooperative medical care systems, overall planning was conducted at the township level, which resulted in weaker management and lower risk resistance capabilities. Therefore, the new rural cooperative medical care system adopts the county level as the unit of overall planning and implementation, thus enhances the risk resistance capabilities and regulatory oversight.

Fifth, the principle of "operating through the health system with coordinated cooperation from various departments." China stipulates that people's governments at the county level and above are responsible for the unified coordination and guidance of the new rural cooperative medical care system within their respective administrative areas. The new rural cooperative medical care management committees shall be established, composed of relevant departments such as finance, health, and civil affairs, to clarify the responsibilities and tasks of the regulatory bodies and operating agencies.

5.2.2.3 Main Content

(1) Fund Collection

The new rural cooperative medical care funds mainly come from fiscal subsidies and individual contributions. At the beginning of its launch in 2003, the per capita fund collection level for the new rural cooperative medical care system was only 30 yuan, with the central government and local governments each providing subsidy funds at a standard of 10 yuan per capita, and farmers paying 10 yuan out of their own pockets. In recent years, the per capita funding standard for the new rural cooperative medical care system has gradually increased, and the government finances have taken on the role of the main funding source for the new rural cooperative medical care system.

(2) Compensation Mode

The new rural cooperative medical care funds primarily subsidize the inpatient medical expenses and outpatient expenses for major illnesses of participating farmers (some areas have already implemented risk pooling of outpatient services). Each region determines the scope, standards, and amount of fund payments based on the total funding amount, combined with local conditions. The competent departments of the new rural cooperative medical care system formulate a reimbursement drug catalog (generally at the provincial level) to constrain the scope of drug compensation. The reimbursement drug catalog is designed in a tiered manner, including the village level, township level, and county level and above. The higher the level of the designated medical institutions, the more types of drugs are allowed for use and reimbursement. The reimbursement drug catalog at the township level is primarily based on the National Essential Medicine List (primary level), with appropriate additions based on local outstanding health needs and the payment capacity of the new rural cooperative medical care funds. The reimbursement drug catalog at the county level adopts the National Essential Medicine List (primary level), and if there is a genuine need to add traditional ethnic medicines or drugs for special local diseases based on local conditions, appropriate additions can be made. The reimbursement rate for drugs within the National Essential Medicine List under the new rural cooperative medical care system is significantly higher than that for drugs outside the national essential medicine list.

(3) Payment Method

The new rural cooperative medical care system implements total outpatient payment for designated medical institutions. Based on the handling method for the total outpatient budget surplus, it is divided into three types: outpatient total prepayment, outpatient total budget + flexible settlement, and outpatient total limit. The main inpatient payment methods under the new rural cooperative medical care system include single-diagnosis payment, per diem payment, total payment, and mixed payment.

5.2.3　Integration of the Basic Medical Insurance System for Non-Working Urban Residents and the New Rural Cooperative Medical Care System

In January 2016, the State Council issued the "Opinions of the State Council on Integrating the Basic Medical Insurance System for Rural and Non-Working Urban Residents," merging the basic medical insurance system for non-working urban residents and the new rural cooperative medical care system into a unified basic medical insurance system for rural and non-working urban residents. This integration is a significant measure to promote the reform of the medical and health system, ensure that rural and non-working urban residents enjoy equal rights to basic medical insurance, promote social fairness and justice, and enhance people's well-being. It is of great significance for promoting the coordinated economic and social development of urban and rural areas and building a moderately prosperous society in all respects.

5.2.3.1　Integration of Basic Policies

The basic medical insurance for rural and non-working urban residents has achieved "six unifications." First, a unified coverage scope. The coverage scope of the basic medical insurance system for rural and non-working residents includes all individuals eligible for participation in the existing basic medical insurance system for non-working urban residents and the new rural cooperative medical care system, covering all urban and rural residents except those who should be covered by the basic medical insurance system for urban employees. Second, a unified fund collection policy. The basic medical insurance for rural and non-working urban residents continues to adopt a fund collection method that combines individual contributions with government subsidies, encouraging support or funding from collectives, units, or other social and economic organizations. Third, a unified benefit protection. Following the principles of moderate security and balanced revenue and expenditure, it ensures balanced urban and rural benefit protection, gradually unifying the scope of coverage and payment standards. The basic medical insurance funds for rural and non-working residents are mainly used to cover the inpatient and outpatient medical expenses of participants, with the inpatient reimbursement rate within the policy range maintained at around 75%. Fourth, a unified medical insurance catalog, including the drug catalog, diagnosis and treatment item catalog, and medical service facility catalog for basic medical insurance for rural and non-working urban residents. Fifth, a unified designated management. The management measures for designated medical institutions of basic medical insurance for rural and non-working urban residents have been unified, and a comprehensive evaluation and assessment mechanism as well as a dynamic entry and exit mechanism have been established and improved. Sixth, a unified fund management. The basic medical insurance for rural and non-working urban residents implements a unified national fund financial system, accounting system, and fund budget and final account management system. The basic medical insurance funds for rural and non-working urban residents are included in the special fiscal account and managed under the "two-line management" system of revenue and expenditure. The funds are independently accounted for and managed in a special account.

5.2.3.2　Integration of Management Systems

First, regions with suitable conditions are encouraged to streamline the management system of medical insurance and unify the administrative management functions of basic medical insurance. This includes integrating the medical insurance administrative institutions, personnel, and information systems of basic medical insurance for rural and non-working urban residents, standardizing operational procedures, and providing integrated service delivery. On the basis of integrating these institutions, it is further recommended to improve the management and operational mechanisms, and optimize the operational procedures. Second, regions with suitable conditions are encouraged to innovate in service delivery models, promote the separation of management from operations and introduce competitive mechanisms. Under the premise of ensuring the safety of the insurance funds and effective supervision, governments can purchase services and entrust qualified commercial insurance institutions and other social entities to participate in the operation of basic medical insurance, thereby invigorating the operational vitality.

5.3 Urban and Rural Medical Assistance, Commercial Medical Insurance, and Supplementary Medical Insurance

5.3.1 Urban and Rural Medical Assistance

The medical assistance system is able to provide medical security for the vast impoverished population, improve their health levels, and help them escape from the plight of poverty and illness as soon as possible. For China, the medical assistance system plays an important role and is of great significance in safeguarding people's rights and interests, fulfilling government responsibilities, embodying social fairness, and promoting higher-quality, more efficient, and fairer national economic development. Therefore, building a medical assistance system for impoverished people plays a crucial role in the harmonious development of China's economy and society. The medical assistance system is an essential component of the medical security system, and its construction occupies an important position in the construction of the medical security system.

5.3.1.1 Collection and Management of Urban and Rural Medical Assistance Funds

Currently, the urban and rural medical assistance funds in China are raised through multiple channels, including fiscal allocations from the government, lottery welfare funds, social donations, and income from fund interest. Improving the health status of the impoverished population is an unshirkable responsibility of the government, and medical assistance for the impoverished requires a certain level of fiscal support from the government. In China, the central government allocates special funds to subsidize urban and rural medical assistance in disadvantaged areas, while local governments, especially provincial governments, effectively adjust the fiscal expenditure structure, increase investment, and further expand the scale of medical assistance funds. As China is still in the primary stage of socialism, with varying levels of economic development across regions, government fiscal allocations for medical assistance are heavily constrained by local economic development levels. In addition to government fiscal allocations, social donations are also an important component of the sources for urban and rural medical assistance funds.

Most of China's medical assistance funds are deposited in special fiscal accounts and managed in dedicated ledgers, ensuring that the funds are used specifically for their intended purposes (in this regard, China still lacks experience in maintaining and increasing the value of these funds through certain financial operations). For instance, establishing foundations to entrust specialized agencies with the operation of both fiscal funds and non-fiscal funds (funds obtained through social donations and other channels). These foundations are responsible for settling medical assistance expenses with medical institutions, strictly enforcing fund usage procedures, and assisting recipients in restoring their health.

To achieve legal and standardized management of medical assistance funds, the following points must be adhered to. First, implement specialized account storage and dedicated management. Civil affairs departments are the main entities responsible for managing medical assistance funds, while financial departments exercise oversight powers over the funds and assume corresponding responsibilities. It is necessary to establish a special fiscal account and implement budget-based management of medical assistance funds. Departments such as civil affairs, finance, and auditing at the county (city, district) level must conduct supervision and inspection of the use of medical assistance funds, promptly correct any issues found, and report them to the local people's government. Second, implement closed-loop operation. Closed-loop operation can be simply summarized as the separation of money and accounts, meaning that those in charge of money do not handle accounts, and those handling accounts do not manage money. Funds should always flow between the government's special fiscal accounts and the bank accounts of medical institutions. Third, the use of funds must be open and transparent. Information such as the collection, management, and use of medical assistance funds, as well as the recipients and the amount of assistance provided, should be regularly disclosed to the public through methods such as public notices. Fourth, continuously improve management efficiency and minimize management costs. All relevant departments involved in the management of medical assistance funds should coordinate with each other to continuously improve fund management efficiency and reduce management costs.

5.3.1.2　Target Recipients of Urban and Rural Medical Assistance

In China, urban and rural medical assistance serves as a supplementary form to the basic medical insurance for urban employees, basic medical insurance for rural and non-working urban residents, and commercial medical insurance. The target recipients of it are low-income groups.

Rural medical assistance is aimed at rural families receiving the "five guarantees," rural poverty-stricken household members, and other eligible rural poor farmers as stipulated by local governments. Urban medical assistance mainly targets those who are not enrolled in the basic medical insurance for urban employees among the recipients of the urban residents' minimum living security allowance, those who have participated in the basic medical insurance for urban employees but still face heavy personal financial burdens, and other specifically impoverished groups. In addition, China has also included members of low-income families with serious or critical illnesses, low-income elderly, severely disabled individuals, and other impoverished individuals who have difficulty paying for medical expenses due to serious or critical illnesses into the scope of urban and rural medical assistance.

Since the establishment of the urban and rural medical assistance system, the scope of recipients has been continuously expanded, including not only traditional disadvantaged groups but also other eligible recipients. The specific criteria for defining the recipients are formulated by local civil affairs departments, jointly with relevant departments such as finance, based on factors such as local economic conditions, the collection of medical assistance funds, the payment ability of impoverished populations, and their basic medical needs. These criteria are then submitted to the people's government of the same level for approval and implementation.

5.3.1.3   Methods and Services for Urban and Rural Medical Assistance

Medical assistance can be provided through various approaches. Different regions have adopted multiple medical assistance methods, taking into account factors such as local economic and social development levels, as well as fiscal revenue status. The primary methods are subsidizing insurance participation and reimbursing medical expenses. Subsidizing insurance participation involves assisting individuals who cannot afford to pay medical insurance premiums by funding part or all of their premiums, enabling them to obtain medical insurance coverage. Reimbursing medical expenses involves providing a certain percentage or amount of subsidy to recipients for their personal out-of-pocket medical expenses that exceed a certain threshold or for special diseases, after deducting the amounts covered by various medical insurance schemes, reimbursable portions from employers, and social assistance.

Currently, urban and rural medical assistance services primarily focus on inpatient assistance, while also taking into account outpatient assistance. Inpatient assistance is mainly used to cover the medical expenses borne by the recipients due to hospitalization for illness. Outpatient assistance is primarily used to cover the medical expenses for common illnesses, chronic diseases, long-term medication maintenance, as well as emergency and first-aid treatment, which are borne by the recipients themselves.

5.3.1.4   Management Departments for Urban and Rural Medical Assistance Work

Medical assistance involves multiple departments, and its management is jointly conducted by civil affairs departments, financial departments, human resources and social security departments, health departments, and other relevant departments.

The urban and rural medical assistance work in China is primarily managed by the civil affairs departments, which have set up specialized agencies from the central to local levels. These agencies are responsible for formulating the medical assistance system, coordinating the relationship between the various departments involved in its implementation, as well as the distribution and utilization of assistance funds. The financial departments are primarily responsible for compiling the annual budget for medical assistance funds, establishing special fiscal accounts for urban and rural medical assistance funds, managing the accounts, conducting accounting, and overseeing the use of funds. The human resources and social security departments are responsible for cooperating in the organization and implementation of medical assistance work, ensuring the integration of medical insurance and medical assistance policies. The health administrative departments are responsible for coordinating and overseeing the provision of medical services to ensure the specific implementation of medical assistance work. Other departments, such as audit departments, as well as organizations such as the Federation of Trade Unions and the Red Cross, also participate in the management of medical assistance work.

5.3.2 Commercial Medical Insurance

5.3.2.1 Market Position and Scale

With the further improvement of China's market economy system and the increase in residents' income, the demand for medical and health services among residents has been continuously increasing, and the role of commercial medical insurance in the medical security system has become increasingly significant. The new medical reform explicitly proposes to accelerate the establishment and improvement of a multi-level medical security system with basic medical security as the mainstay, supplemented by various forms of supplementary medical insurance and commercial health insurance, and covering both urban and rural residents. This clarifies the complementary role of commercial medical insurance in the medical security system. In the current commercial medical insurance market, student medical insurance, supplementary medical insurance, and comprehensive insurance that includes medical insurance, accident insurance, property insurance, and life insurance are relatively common. In 2012, the "Guiding Opinions on Carrying Out Critical Illness Insurance for Urban and Rural Residents" further clarified that commercial insurance institutions are supported to undertake critical illness insurance, leveraging market mechanisms to improve the operational efficiency, service level, and quality of critical illness insurance.

5.3.2.2 Market Structure

In China, collective participation in commercial medical insurance by enterprises or collectives is a relatively common form of group insurance. As enterprises provide benefits to their employees, they also enhance their employees' labor productivity. Such commercial medical insurance often serves as a supplement to basic medical insurance. For example, some commercial medical insurance can cover certain medications that are not included in the reimbursement catalog of basic medical insurance, and can also provide nutritional subsidies to insured individuals after illness. Collective participation by students is also common. Students can participate in the basic medical insurance for rural and non-working urban residents that covers hospitalization services, and those who have also participated in commercial medical insurance can obtain better coverage after falling ill. Participants in basic medical insurance can also obtain a higher reimbursement ratio or a wider reimbursement scope by participating in commercial medical insurance. Factors such as age, gender, economic status, education level, and geographical location have a certain influence on the choice of commercial medical insurance. At the same time, age, gender and other factors can also be limiting conditions for the purchase of commercial medical insurance.

In 2015, the "Opinions of the General Office of the State Council on the Full Implementation of Critical Illness Insurance for Urban and Rural Residents" was issued, further clarifying support for commercial insurance institutions to undertake critical illness insurance. The specific measures include the local government's departments of human resources and social security, health and family planning, finance, and insurance supervision jointly formulate basic policies for the financing, payment scope, minimum payment ratio, medical treatment, and settlement management of critical illness insurance, and solicit opinions through appropriate channels. In principle, commercial insurance institutions undertaking critical illness insurance are selected through government bidding. The bidding mainly includes specific payment ratios, profit and loss ratios, and the strengths of the undertaking and management team. Commercial insurance institutions that meet the basic entry conditions set by the insurance regulatory department voluntarily participate in the bidding. After winning the bid, they undertake critical illness insurance by signing insurance contracts, assuming operational risks, and being responsible for their own profits and losses.

5.3.2.3　Market Behavior

China encourages employers and individuals to participate in commercial medical insurance. The premiums of commercial medical insurance are generally calculated based on the positioning of the insurance, the payment capacity of the target population, combined with the operating costs of the insurance institutions. For individual insured persons, they are generally required to provide relevant health information before participating in the insurance to determine the premiums. If the participation is in the form of an enterprise or other groups, the personnel can enjoy group insurance rates.

Since the current market share of commercial medical insurance is relatively low, it is difficult to form negotiating power with medical institutions. Therefore, the coverage of commercial medical insurance is generally focused on reimbursement of medical expenses after treatment and subsidies for days off work such as hospitalization, and commercial medical insurance may have corresponding requirements for the medical institutions available for insured individuals to choose from.

The demand group for commercial medical insurance in China includes residents who already enjoy basic medical insurance. Such insured individuals have a greater demand for special examinations, treatments, and medications outside the scope specified by basic medical insurance. Commercial medical insurance can meet these non-basic medical service needs.

5.3.2.4　Public Policy

In China, commercial medical insurance is regulated by the National Financial Regulatory Administration. The "Measures on Administration of Health Insurance," which was first issued in 2006 and reissued in 2019 after revision, has unified the regulatory standards for the operation of health insurance businesses. To accelerate the development of the health service industry, the State Council has put forward the goal of "enriching commercial health insurance products, significantly increasing the number of insured individuals, significantly increasing the proportion of commercial health insurance expenditures in total health expenditures, and forming a relatively complete health insurance mechanism," laying a policy foundation for the development of commercial medical insurance. In addition, some regions have explored the operation of basic medical insurance models by commercial medical insurance institutions, which may provide more development opportunities for commercial medical insurance in the future.

5.3.3 Supplementary Medical Insurance

5.3.3.1 Overview of the Development of Supplementary Medical Insurance

China's supplementary medical insurance emerged along with the reform of the medical system. In 1993, the "Decision of the Central Committee of the Communist Party of China on Several Issues Concerning the Establishment of the Socialist Market Economic System" clearly stated that "a multi-level social security system should be established." In 1994, the "Pilot Opinions on the Reform of the Medical System for Employees" stipulated that employee medical mutual assistance funds and commercial medical insurance should be developed as a supplement to social medical insurance to meet medical needs beyond the basic medical security stipulated by the state, but the principle of individual voluntary participation and independent choice should be adhered to.

Under the guidance of the national macro policy, various regions have actively explored different forms of supplementary medical insurance. Many regions and cities have actively prepared and formulated various forms of supplementary medical insurance while establishing the basic medical insurance system for urban employees, and have formulated relevant policies and specific implementation measures.

5.3.3.2 Commercial Operation of Supplementary Medical Insurance

Currently, the management of supplementary medical insurance in China mainly falls into two categories: bundled operation and commercial operation. Bundled operation refers to the government's social security agencies operating supplementary medical insurance in the same way as basic medical insurance. Its characteristics include management difficulties, operational challenges, and heavy fiscal and corporate burdens. Commercial operation involves social security agencies utilizing commercial insurance institutions to manage and operate supplementary medical insurance. This approach can alleviate fiscal pressure, save human resources, optimize the allocation of medical resources, strengthen the management of medical institutions, and ultimately promote the standardization and scientization of basic medical insurance management. Supplementary medical insurance has received widespread attention. In China, commercial medical insurance is often operated as supplementary medical insurance, so the commercial operation of supplementary medical insurance will become an important aspect of improving the medical security system.

（1）Development Potential for the Commercial Operation of Supplementary Medical Insurance

The unique advantages of commercial insurance institutions can increase their potential to occupy the medical insurance market. If they possess advanced management methods and flexible business strategies, they can also accept specific project management delegations from social security agencies and other supplementary medical insurance institutions. Overall, medical insurance demand in China has been growing rapidly in recent years. Due to the dual functions of commercial medical insurance as a health care and investment tool, individual commercial medical insurance products offered by various medical insurance institutions have been continuously increasing.

（2）Issues to Consider in the Process of Commercial Operation of Supplementary Medical Insurance

First, it is important to reasonably define the nature of supplementary medical insurance. The government should only address basic medical issues, leaving the remaining medical issues to be resolved by the market. Additionally, the enthusiasm of medical insurance institutions should be fully mobilized.

Second, social security agencies and medical insurance institutions should strengthen the regulation of the behavior of both the supply and demand sides in medical services. It is necessary to establish a competition system among hospitals to improve the efficiency of medical services. At the same time, measures such as information management and irregular spot checks should be taken to prevent the waste of medical resources or collusion between doctors and patients for fraud.

Third, it is necessary to continuously strengthen the development of supplementary medical insurance products to meet the diverse needs of different levels of supplementary medical insurance.

Fourth, it is important to improve the professional level of institutions that offer supplementary medical insurance.

6　China's Drug Supply Guarantee System

Drugs play an irreplaceable role in disease prevention and treatment, rehabilitation, health care, disaster relief, and epidemic prevention for the public. Their significance in economic development and national security has become increasingly prominent. As a special commodity, drugs face great challenges in research and development innovation, require strong professional technical expertise in production and use, can trigger adverse reactions even under normal use, and pose significant risks to patient health and social stability when of low quality or misused. The drug supply guarantee system stands alongside the public health service system, medical service system, and medical security system as one of the four beams of China's basic medical and health system. Moreover, the guarantee of drug supply is also one of the key tasks in the construction of Healthy China.

6.1　China's Drug Supply Guarantee Organization System

China's drug supply guarantee organization system can be divided into the following components: drug administrative supervision and management organization system, drug technical supervision and management organization system, pharmaceutical education, research organizations, and associations system, drug production and distribution organization system, and pharmaceutical organization system in medical institutions.

6.1.1　The Drug Administrative Supervision and Management Organization System

China's drug supervision and management institutions are divided into four levels, namely, the National Medical Products Administration (NMPA), the medical products administrations at provincial (autonomous region, municipality directly under the central government) level, the market supervision and management institutions at municipal (prefecture, league) level, and the market supervision and management institutions at county (district) level. The basic framework is illustrated in Figure 6-1.

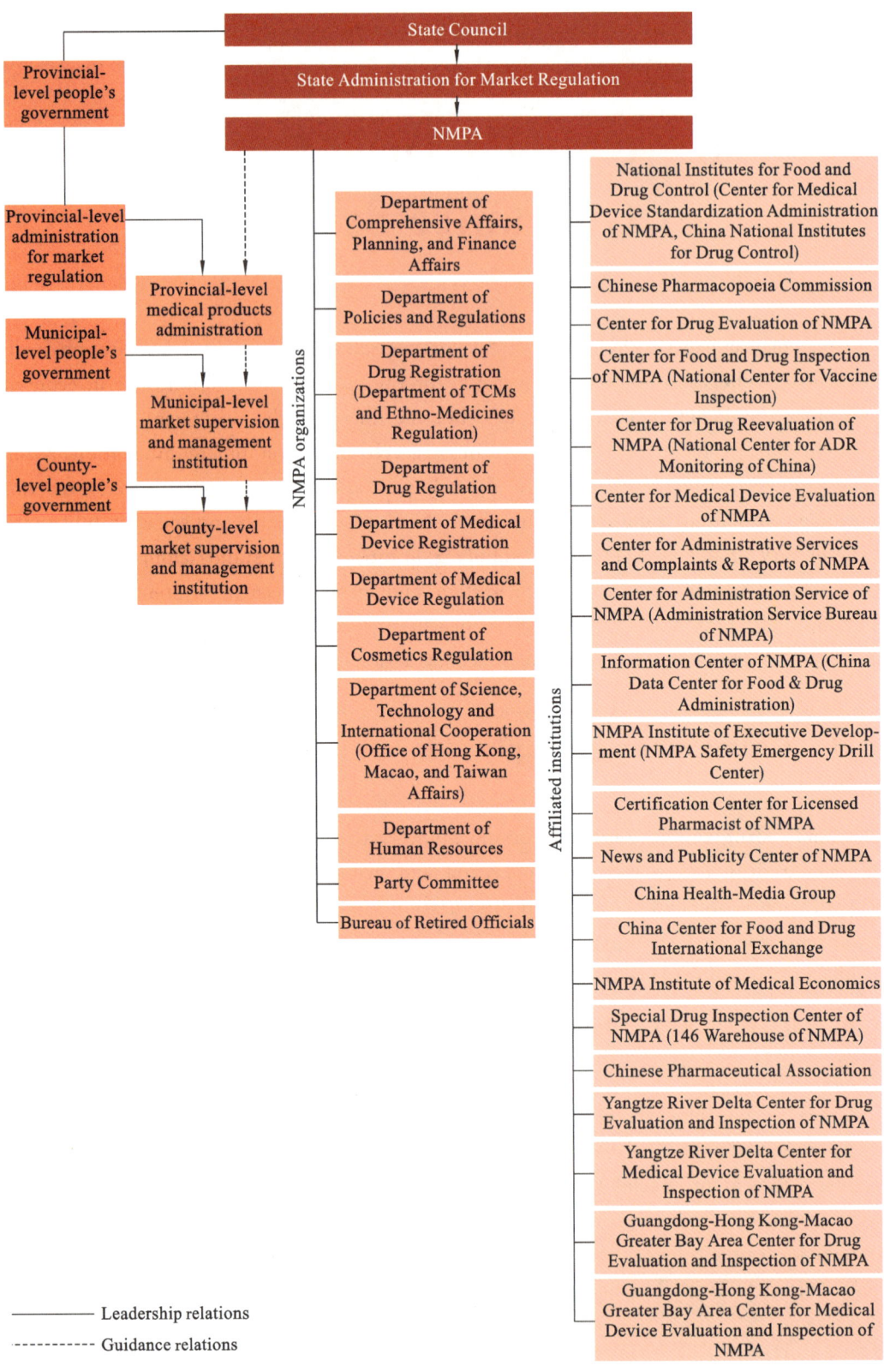

Figure 6-1　The basic framework of China's drug supervision and management institutions

6.1.1.1　The NMPA

The NMPA is a national agency under the supervision of the State Administration for Market Regulation. It holds vice-ministerial status and is primarily responsible for the safety supervision and management, standardization management, registration management, quality management, supervision inspections, and post-market risk management of drugs, medical devices, and cosmetics.

6.1.1.2　Provincial and Lower-Level Drug Supervision and Management Institutions

The provincial-level medical products administration in China functions as a working body under the provincial people's government and is responsible for statutory drug supervision and management within its jurisdiction. Its functional offices typically include Comprehensive Affairs, Planning and Finance Affairs Office, Policies and Regulations Office, Administrative Approval Office, Drug Registration Management Office, Drug Production Supervision and Management Office, Drug Circulation Supervision and Management Office, Medical Device Supervision and Management Office, and Cosmetics Supervision and Management Office. Drug supervision and management institutions below the provincial level are managed in a hierarchical manner by local governments, with their operations guided and supervised by higher-level authorities.

6.1.1.3　Other Institutions Related to Drug Supervision and Management

(1) Market Supervision and Management Institutions

The market supervision and management institutions are responsible for registering and issuing business licenses to relevant market entities, investigating and penalizing illegal activities related to market access, production, operation, and transactions. They enforce anti-monopoly laws, conduct price supervision and inspection, and address unfair competition. Additionally, they oversee the review and monitoring of advertisements for drugs, health foods, medical devices, and special medical purpose formula foods. The market supervision and management institutions also supervise drug supervision and management institutions at the corresponding level. At the city and county levels, market supervision and management institutions are responsible for issuing permits, conducting inspections, and imposing penalties related to drug retail and medical device operation, and conducting inspections and imposing penalties related to cosmetics sales, and quality for drug and medical devices used in healthcare settings.

(2) Health Administrative Institutions

Health administrative institutions are institutions responsible for medical and health administration at various governmental levels. The highest health administration body in China is the National Health Commission. The National Health Commission is tasked with refining the national essential medicine system, drafting national drug policies and the essential medicines list, and conducting drug usage monitoring, clinical comprehensive evaluations, and early warnings for drug shortages. It also proposes recommendations on drug pricing policies and supportive measures to produce drugs listed in the National

Essential Medicine List. In collaboration with the NMPA, the National Health Commission convenes the Chinese Pharmacopoeia Commission to compile, revise, and translate the *Pharmacopoeia of the People's Republic of China*. Together, they establish mechanisms for mutual notification and joint handling of serious adverse drug reactions and medical device events, ensuring a coordinated response to critical issues affecting public health and safety.

(3) TCM Management Institutions

TCM management institutions are responsible for drafting strategies, plans, policies, and relevant standards for the development of TCM and ethnic medicine. They guide the discovery, organization, summarization, and enhancement of theories, medical techniques, and drugs of ethnic medicine. These institutions also organize comprehensive surveys of medicinal resources, and promote their protection, development, and rational utilization.

(4) Medical Security Management Institutions

Medical security management institutions are responsible for drafting policies, plans, and standards for medical insurance, maternity insurance, medical assistance, and other medical security systems, and implementing them. They supervise the related medical security funds, improve medical expense settlement platforms, and organize the formulation and adjustment of prices and fee standards for drugs and medical services. These institutions also develop procurement policies for drugs and medical consumables and supervise their implementation, and oversee the service behaviors of medical institutions and medical expenses covered by medical insurance.

In addition, various departments in China such as the macroeconomic regulation and development department, the human resources and social security department, the industry and information technology management department, the Office of the Central Cyberspace Affairs Commission, the commerce management department, customs, as well as the public security department, undertake specific responsibilities within their respective scopes for drug supervision and management.

6.1.2 Drug Technical Supervision and Management Organization System

Drug supervision and management is highly technical, and technical support is necessary during the implementation of administrative supervision and management. Drug technical supervision and management institutions are integral to drug supervision and management, providing technical support and guarantees for administrative supervision. China's drug technical supervision and management institutions include drug testing institutions and other technical institutions directly under the NMPA.

6.1.2.1 Drug Testing Institutions

Drug testing institutions are statutory professional inspection institutions responsible for national drug quality supervision and inspection. They represent the state in supervising and inspecting drugs, and their results have legal effect. In China, drug testing institutions are divided into four levels: the National Institutes for Food and Drug Control, drug testing institutions at provincial (autonomous region, municipality directly under the central government), municipal (prefecture, league), and county levels.

According to the "Reply of the State Commission Office for Public Sector Reform on the Organization and Staffing of Institutions Directly Under the National Medical Products Administration," the National Institutes for Food and Drug Control is a public welfare institution of Category II under the NMPA, and it is the statutory institution and highest technical arbitration institution for national drug and biological product quality testing. The main responsibilities of the National Institutes for Food and Drug Control include testing and inspection of food, drugs, medical devices, cosmetics, and related drug excipients, packaging materials, and containers, conducting experimental research on the causes of serious adverse reactions and events of related products, organizing the planning, research, preparation, calibration, distribution, and management of national standard substances, conducting the verification of bacterial strains and cell lines for production, undertaking the collection, identification, preservation, distribution, and management of medical standard strains and cell lines, and so on.

6. 1. 2. 2 Other Technical Institutions Directly Under the NMPA

(1) Chinese Pharmacopoeia Commission

The Chinese Pharmacopoeia Commission is the earliest established standardization institution in China. It is responsible for organizing the compilation of the *Pharmacopoeia of the People's Republic of China* and formulating and revising national drug standards. The Chinese Pharmacopoeia Commission is the statutory professional management institution for national drug standards. The permanent office of the Chinese Pharmacopoeia Commission operates under the responsibility of the secretary general and includes the following departments: Business Management Department (Quality Management Department), Information Management Department (Editorial Office), TCM Department, Chemical Medicine Department, Biological Products Department, Office, Personnel and Party Affairs Department (Discipline Inspection Office), Finance Department, and General Provisions, Excipients, and Packaging Materials Department. It also has branches such as the "Drug Standards of China" magazine agency.

(2) Center for Drug Evaluation of NMPA

The Center for Drug Evaluation of NMPA is the technical review institution for drug registration, providing technical support for drug registration. It includes the following departments: Business Management Department, Personnel Department (Services and Management Department for Retired Cadres), Quality Management Department, Compliance Department, Clinical Trial Management Department, Data Management Department, Office, Finance Department, Party Committee Office, Discipline Inspection Office, TCM and Ethnic Medicine Pharmacy Department, TCM and Ethnic Medicine Clinical Department,

Chemical Medicine Pharmacy Department Ⅰ, Chemical Medicine Pharmacy Department Ⅱ, Pharmacology and Toxicology Department, Chemical Medicine Clinical Department Ⅰ, Chemical Medicine Clinical Department Ⅱ, Statistics and Clinical Pharmacology Department, Biological Products Pharmacy Department, and Biological Products Clinical Department.

(3) Center for Drug Reevaluation of NMPA

The Center for Drug Reevaluation of NMPA includes the following departments: Office, Comprehensive Business Department, Chemical Medicine Monitoring and Evaluation Department, Biological Products Monitoring and Evaluation Department, TCM Monitoring and Evaluation Department, Medical Devices Monitoring and Evaluation Department, Cosmetics Monitoring and Evaluation Department, Scientific Research and Information Management Department, and Party Discipline Office (Personnel Department).

(4) Center for Food and Drug Inspection of NMPA

The Center for Food and Drug Inspection of NMPA is a Category Ⅱ public welfare institution directly under the NMPA (retaining bureau-level status). It includes the following departments: Office, Comprehensive Business Department (Quality Management Department), Information Management Department, Inspection Department Ⅰ, Inspection Department Ⅱ, Inspection Department Ⅲ, Inspection Department Ⅳ, Inspection Department Ⅴ, Inspection Department Ⅵ, Personnel Department (Party Committee Office), and Finance Department.

(5) Certification Center for Licensed Pharmacist of NMPA

The Certification Center for Licensed Pharmacist of NMPA operates under the supervision and guidance of the Personnel Department of NMPA. It includes the following departments: Office (Personnel and Party Affairs Department), Examination Department, Registration Management Department, and Information Department.

6.1.3 Pharmaceutical Education, Research Organizations, and Associations System

Pharmaceutical education, research organizations, and associations are important components of China's pharmaceutical affairs organizations. Pharmaceutical associations include the Chinese Pharmaceutical Association and various pharmaceutical societies approved by Chinese government. Since the government institution reform, the industry management functions of pharmaceutical associations have been strengthened.

6.1.3.1 Pharmaceutical Education Organizations

Pharmaceutical education in China has developed over more than a century and consists mainly of higher pharmaceutical education, secondary pharmaceutical education, and continuing pharmaceutical education. This has resulted in a multi-type, multi-level, and multi-form educational system.

As of the end of 2016, China had 458 regular higher education institutions offering undergraduate programs related to pharmaceuticals, with 35 under the supervision of the

Ministry of Education and 407 under the supervision of provincial, autonomous region, and municipal authorities. By 2021, China had 143 institutions authorized to award academic degrees in pharmacy, 46 institutions enrolling master's degree students in professional pharmacy programs, and a total of 498 higher education institutions offering pharmacy-related programs nationwide.

Continuing pharmaceutical education is primarily provided by higher education institutions and secondary schools with pharmacy programs, as well as pharmaceutical societies.

6.1.3.2　Pharmaceutical Research Organizations

Pharmaceutical research organizations in China mainly include independent drug research institutes and those attached to higher pharmaceutical education institutions, large pharmaceutical enterprises, and major hospitals. Independent drug research institutes are affiliated with national and local academy systems such as the Chinese Academy of Sciences, the Chinese Academy of Medical Sciences, the Academy of Military Medical Sciences, as well as relevant departments of central and local governments.

6.1.3.3　Pharmaceutical Associations

Pharmaceutical associations serve as a link between pharmaceutical affairs organizations, pharmacy personnel, and government institutions, assisting the government in management functions. Their roles include industry or professional social management, with tasks such as academic research and technical management of the industry and profession. Examples of these associations include the Chinese Pharmaceutical Association, the Chinese Pharmacists Association, and the China Pharmaceutical Enterprises Association.

6.1.4　Drug Production and Distribution Organization System

Drug production and distribution organizations are economic entities, mainly including drug production enterprises, drug wholesale enterprises, and drug retail enterprises. Drug production enterprises, commonly known as drug factories, are specialized or general enterprises legally established to engage in drug production activities and provide drugs to society, possessing corporate status. Drug distribution enterprises are also specialized or general enterprises that can be divided into drug wholesale enterprises and drug retail enterprises. Drug wholesale enterprises are typically referred to as drug companies or TCM companies, while drug retail enterprises are commonly known as retail pharmacies (drugstores).

6.1.5　Pharmaceutical Organization System in Medical Institutions

Pharmaceutical organizations in medical institutions are composed of departments that provide qualified drugs and engage in patient-centered, clinical pharmacy-based pharmaceutical technical services aimed at promoting the rational use of drugs and related drug management tasks. To achieve the transformation of pharmaceutical work functions under medical and health system reform, the "Regulations on Pharmaceutical Affairs Management in Medical Institutions" in China requires that medical institutions set up corresponding departments of pharmacy based on their functions, tasks, and scale and equip these departments with professional technical personnel, equipment, and facilities suitable for their tasks. The various departments within the departments of pharmacy are generally divided by function. Basic functional departments are those directly involved in drug supply and pharmaceutical services, such as outpatient and emergency pharmacies, inpatient pharmacies, TCM pharmacies, intravenous medication preparation center, and clinical pharmacy offices. Derivative functional departments are those that guarantee drug supply and support pharmaceutical services, such as drug logistics centers, formulation rooms, drug testing rooms, and pharmaceutical research offices.

The "Regulations on Pharmaceutical Affairs Management in Medical Institutions" in China clearly stipulates that second-level or above hospitals must establish a pharmaceutical affairs management and pharmacotherapeutics committee, while other medical institutions should form a pharmaceutical affairs management and pharmacotherapeutics group. These organizations are supervisory bodies for drug management in medical institutions and professional technical organizations that make specialized decisions on important pharmaceutical affairs. They develop policies for drug use in medical institutions based on national laws and policies, unify understanding, and collaboratively solve various drug-related issues. By supervising and guiding their affiliated medical institutions in scientific drug management and rational drug use, these organizations enhance drug management and improve medication practices in medical institutions.

Pharmaceutical organizations in medical institutions hold a significant position and proportion in pharmaceutical affairs organizations, and in China, they comprise the largest number of pharmacists. Figure 6-2 depicts the possible organizational chart of the department of pharmacy in a third-level general hospital in China. Hospitals can refer to this and set up the necessary departments according to their specific circumstances.

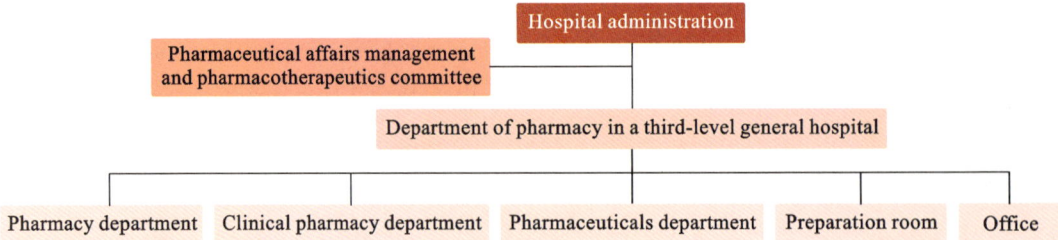

Figure 6-2　The possible organizational chart of the department of pharmacy in a third-level general hospital in China

6.2　China's Drug Supply Guarantee Management System

The Drug Administration Law of the People's Republic of China clearly states that the purpose of this law is to "strengthen drug administration, ensure drug quality, protect drug safety and legitimate rights and interests of the public, and protect and promote public health." To achieve these objectives, China's drug supply guarantee management system focuses on several core areas.

6.2.1　Quality Management of New Drug Research and Drug Registration Management

From the perspective of drug registration management, new drugs refer to drugs that have not been marketed in China or abroad, categorized into innovative drugs and modified new drugs. New drug development research must verify the safety, efficacy, and quality stability of candidate drugs, involving a complex system engineering requiring multi-disciplinary and multi-departmental collaboration. The research process of new drugs mainly includes preclinical research, clinical research, and post-marketing surveillance, as shown in Figure 6-3.

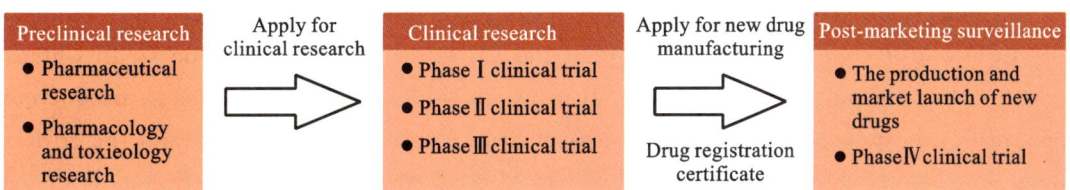

Figure 6-3　The research process of new drugs

Source: Drug Management (2nd Ed.) by Zhang Xinping and Liu Lanru, 2023

The safety evaluation of drug preclinical research must comply with the "Good Laboratory Practice for Non-Clinical Laboratory Studies." It is the guideline for conducting drug efficacy and toxicity animal studies, applicable to non-clinical studies conducted for drug registration applications. It is also a directive document guiding scientific research institutions to develop safe and effective drugs, aiming to ensure the safety of preclinical researches and the reliability of data. The current "Good Laboratory Practice for Non-Clinical Laboratory Studies" in China was reviewed and approved by the State Food and Drug Administration on June 20, 2017, and has been in effect since September 1, 2017.

The "Good Clinical Practice" is the quality standard that regulates the entire process of drug clinical trials, including protocol design, implementation, monitoring, auditing, recording, analysis, summary, and reporting. Its purpose is to ensure the standardization of the clinical trial process and the scientific, true, and reliable nature of the data and results, as well as protect the rights, interests and safety of subjects and other parties involved in the research. With the rapid development of China's drug research and development and the deepening reform of the drug evaluation and approval system, the NMPA, together with the National Health Commission, issued the newly revised "Good Clinical Practice" on April 23,2020, which took effect on July 1,2020, to meet the needs of drug regulation.

Drug registration refers to the process where drug registration applicants submit applications for clinical trials, marketing authorization, and re-registration, as well as supplementary applications according to legal procedures and related requirements. The drug regulatory department reviews the safety, efficacy, and quality controllability based on laws, regulations, and current scientific knowledge, and decides whether to approve the application. The "Provisions for Drug Registration" in China classifies drug registration management into categories such as TCM, chemical drugs, and biological products, based on the nature of the drugs and the actual clinical use in China. Each major category is further subdivided based on the level of maturity of drug research and development, that is, people's understanding of the pharmaceutical properties, pharmacological and toxicological characteristics, and clinical characteristics of the drug developed, whether this type of drugs has already been marketed domestically or abroad, as well as whether there is an existing national drug standard.

6.2.2　Supervision and Management of Drug Production Quality

"Good Manufacturing Practice" (GMP) is a universally adopted statutory technical specification for supervising and managing the entire drug production process. In China, GMP is the fundamental guideline for drug production enterprises to manage production and quality. It applies to the entire process of drug formulation production and the critical processes in active pharmaceutical ingredient (API) production that affect the quality of the final product. The current GMP in China has been in effect since March 1,2011. It has played a positive role in promoting the concentration of pharmaceutical industry resources in advantageous enterprises, eliminating outdated production capacity, adjusting the pharmaceutical economic structure, promoting industrial upgrading, fostering internationally competitive enterprises, and accelerating the entry of pharmaceutical products into the international market. Although the newly revised Drug Administration Law of the People's Republic of China in 2019 abolished the certification of the GMP, this does not mean the elimination of the GMP system. Instead, it is replaced by GMP compliance inspections conducted by provincial drug supervision and management institutions, changing the five-year certification inspection to random GMP compliance inspections, thereby imposing higher requirements on enterprises to continuously meet GMP standards.

6.2.3　Supervision and Management of Drug Distribution Quality

The newly revised Drug Administration Law of the People's Republic of China in 2019 stipulates that drug distribution enterprises must comply with the "Good Supply Practice"

(GSP) for conducting drug distribution activities. The fundamental purpose of this regulation is to ensure that drug distribution enterprises focus on quality in all their operations, guaranteeing the quality of drugs.

In 2000, the China's NMPA revised the GSP based on the "Quality Management Standards for Pharmaceutical Commodities(Trial)." In the same year, the "Implementation Rules for Good Supply Practice" and the "Trial Measures for the Certification of Good Supply Practice (GSP)" were issued. This year marked a milestone for the implementation of drug distribution quality management in China. Subsequently, due to reforms in the governance mechanisms of China's pharmaceutical industry and changes in supporting laws and regulations, the GSP underwent two revisions and one amendment in 2012, 2015, and 2016, respectively. The GSP, along with its supporting documents such as the "Implementation Rules for Good Supply Practice" and the "Guiding Principles for On-Site Inspection of Good Supply Practice," collectively forms the normative system for drug distribution quality management in China.

6.2.4　Pharmaceutical Affairs Management in Medical Institutions

Pharmaceutical affairs management in medical institutions refers to the effective organization and management of the entire clinical medication process in medical institutions, with patients as the center and clinical pharmacy as the basis. It aims to facilitate pharmaceutical technical services supporting clinical scientific and rational use of drug, as well as related drug management. Specific responsibilities include drug supply management, management of institution-prepared medications, compounding and prescription management, clinical application management of medications, clinical pharmacy services, and pharmaceutical care, etc. This section primarily discusses management aspects such as drug procurement, prescription evaluation, and rational use of drug.

Drug procurement is a critical task to ensure the supply of drugs in medical institutions, essential for meeting medical service needs. The quality of drug procurement directly impacts the quality of medical services and economic efficiency of medical institutions. The main goals of drug procurement management include lawful and timely acquisition of high-quality drugs at appropriate prices. Methods for drug procurement include centralized bidding, invitation bidding, and inquiry-based procurement. China's implementation of centralized drug procurement involves specifying quantities during centralized drug procurement bids or negotiations, where companies bid and negotiate prices based on these specified quantities, with the lowest bid winning the contract. The core concept involves "quantity in exchange for price," akin to large-scale group purchasing or bulk buying. The "Opinions of the General Office of the State Council on Promoting the Normalization and Institutionalization of the Centralized Drug Procurement" issued in January 2021 marked the normalization, institutionalization and standardization of China's centralized drug procurement efforts, serving as a guideline for these activities.

Prescription evaluation involves assessing the compliance of prescriptions as well as the appropriateness of clinical drug use (including indications, drug selection, administration routes, dosage, drug interactions, and compatibility contraindications), identifying existing or potential issues, formulating and implementing interventions and improvement measures, and promoting rational clinical drug use according to relevant regulations and technical specifications. Prescription evaluation within hospitals is conducted under the leadership of the pharmaceutical affairs management and pharmacotherapeutics committee (group) and the medical quality management committee, organized jointly by the hospital's medical management and department of pharmacy.

Rational use of drug refers to the appropriate use of drugs in terms of their proper selection, dosage, timing, route of administration, and duration for the right patients to achieve appropriate treatment outcomes. Clinical rational drug use management involves overseeing the entire process of drug use in clinical diagnosis, prevention, and treatment within medical institutions. Medical institutions are required to formulate basic drug clinical application management methods in accordance with national macro-management regulations, establish and implement a graded management system for antibiotic clinical use, and establish systems for monitoring, evaluating, and early warning of clinical drug use safety, effectiveness, and economy, conducting reviews and interventions for prescriptions and medication orders, as well as monitoring and reporting adverse drug reactions, medication errors, and drug-related incidents. Upon discovery of such incidents, clinical departments must promptly treat patients, report to the department of pharmacy, and maintain observation and records. According to relevant national regulations, medical institutions are also mandated to report adverse drug reactions to relevant departments. And medication errors and drug-related incidents should be promptly reported to county-level health administrative departments.

6.3　China's National Essential Medicine System

The concept of essential medicines (EM) was introduced by the World Health Organization in 1977. In 2019, the Law of the People's Republic of China on Basic Medical and Health Care and the Promotion of Health defined essential medicines as those that satisfy basic medical needs of disease prevention and treatment, are adapted to the current basic national conditions and security capacities, and intended to be equitably available in appropriate dosage forms, at an appropriate price, and in adequate supply.

6.3.1 Objectives and Significance of China's National Essential Medicine System Construction

As a core policy in deepening reform of the medical and health system, China's national essential medicine system aims to ensure the accessibility, affordability, high quality, and rational use of essential medicines. This system encompasses the selection, production, distribution, use, pricing, reimbursement, monitoring, and evaluation of essential medicines, integrated with public health, medical service, and medical security systems. Since the new medical reform, the establishment and implementation of China's national essential medicine system have played a crucial role in improving the drug supply guarantee system, meeting basic medical and health needs, ensuring access to essential medicines for the population, and reducing the financial burden on patients.

6.3.2 Overview of China's National Essential Medicine System Construction

In April 1979, China actively responded to and participated in the World Health Organization's Essential Medicines Programme. Under the organization of the Ministry of Health and the State Administration of Medicine, the "National Essential Medicine Selection Group" was established to initiate the formulation of the national essential medicine list. In 1982, China officially issued the first edition of the "National Essential Medicine List," comprising 278 drugs, and the number of drugs in the list increased to 307 by 2009, covering major global diseases such as malaria, AIDS, tuberculosis, reproductive health diseases, as well as chronic diseases like cancer and diabetes.

The implementation of the new medical reform in 2009 marked a new phase for China's national essential medicine system. Policy documents such as the "Implementation Opinions on Establishing the National Essential Medicine System," "Management Measures for the National Essential Medicine List (Trial)," "National Essential Medicine List (Part of Primary Care)"(2009 Edition), "National Guidelines for Clinical Application of Essential Medicines (Part of Primary Care)," "National Formulary for Essential Medicines (Part of Primary Care)," and "Guidelines on Establishing and Standardizing a Mechanism for Purchasing Essential Medicines in Government-Run Primary Medical and Health Institutions" established an implementation system led by the government, supported by the market, and grounded in legal frameworks for the production, distribution, supply, use, and regulation of essential medicines.

From 2014 onwards, efforts have focused on consolidating and improving the national essential medicine system, addressing issues such as system coherence, shortages of some medicines, inadequate service capacity, ensuring supply of essential medicines, consistency in quality assessment, and promoting rational clinical use. On October 25, 2018, the "2018

National Essential Medicine List" was formally released by the National Health Commission, expanding the variety of drugs, optimizing the structure of the list, standardizing formulations and specifications, while maintaining the principle of emphasizing both TCM and Western medicine.

6.3.3 Overall Requirements of China's National Essential Medicine System

The fundamental goal of China's national essential medicine system is centered around promoting people's health, reinforcing the functional positioning of essential medicines to emphasize their basic nature, necessity for prevention and treatment, supply assurance, priority usage, quality assurance, and financial burden reduction. This comprehensive approach spans policies from the selection, production, distribution, use, payment, and monitoring of essential medicines, aiming to enhance the drug supply guarantee system, ensure that drugs are safe and effective, reasonably priced, and adequately supplied, alleviate the issue of high medical costs, facilitate the coordination of drug use between different levels of medical institutions, and support the development of a tiered diagnosis and treatment system. It also contributes to the transformation and upgrading of the pharmaceutical industry and supply-side structural reform.

6.3.4 Main Content of China's National Essential Medicine System

China's national essential medicine system effectively manages various aspects of essential medicines, including selection, production, distribution, use, payment, and monitoring.

6.3.4.1 Selection of Essential Medicines

The principles for selecting essential medicines include necessity for prevention and treatment, safety, effectiveness, reasonably pricing, ease of use, emphasizing both TCM and Western medicine, basic guarantee, clinical preference, and suitability for primary healthcare facilities. The selection and adjustment of the National Essential Medicine List should adhere to scientific, fair, transparent, and open principles, establishing evidence-based medicine and pharmacoeconomic evaluation standards and mechanisms. Scientific and reasonable formulation of the list should involve extensive consultation with all sectors of society and accept social supervision.

6.3.4.2 Production and Supply of Essential Medicines

The system emphasizes centralized procurement and implements categorized purchasing of medicines. Efforts are made to align drug use between different levels of medical institutions, promote centralized drug procurement for public medical institutions in cities and counties to lower drug prices, and ensure supply through measures such as market-based price determination, designated production, unified distribution, or inclusion in reserves for shortage-prone essential medicines.

6.3.4.3　Procurement Management of Essential Medicines

In 2019, the General Office of the State Council issued the "Pilot Plan for National Centralized Drug Procurement and Use," outlining strategies such as national organization, alliance procurement, and platform operations, principles including volume-based procurement, price based on quantity, linking quantity and price, unified bidding and procurement, quality assurance, and payment guarantee, and organizational forms like the Pilot Office and the Joint Procurement Office. The Joint Procurement Office conducts centralized procurement on behalf of the alliance regions and is supported by a supervision group, an expert group, and a centralized procurement team.

6.3.4.4　Management of the Use of Essential Medicines

Maintaining the leading role of essential medicines, the system specifies the proportion of essential medicines used in public medical institutions. It implements clinical usage monitoring and comprehensive evaluation of drug clinical efficacy. Reforms in medical insurance payment methods are deepened, with standards set for drug insurance payments, guiding medical institutions and personnel towards rational diagnosis, treatment, and drug use.

6.3.4.5　Quality Supervision of Essential Medicines

Comprehensive random checks are conducted on all types of essential medicines, strengthening supervision over their production processes to ensure quality and safety. Consistency evaluations of the quality and efficacy of generic drugs are promoted, and those passing such evaluations are prioritized for inclusion in the essential medicine list. Gradually, the essential medicine varieties that have not passed the consistency evaluation will be transferred out of the essential medicine list.

6.3.4.6　Performance Evaluation of the National Essential Medicine System

The implementation of the national essential medicine system is integrated into the performance evaluation systems at all levels of government to enhance supervision and assessment. A robust system for supervisory evaluation of the implementation of the essential medicine system is established to leverage third-party assessments and effectively utilize evaluation results.

6.3.5　Adjustment and Optimization of China's National Essential Medicine System

The "Outline of the Healthy China 2030 Plan" explicitly calls for the consolidation and improvement of the national essential medicine system. In September 2018, the General Office of the State Council issued the "Opinions of the General Office of the State Council on Improving the National Essential Medicine System" (hereinafter referred to as the "Opinions"). The "Opinions" reinforces the functional positioning of essential medicines to emphasize their basic nature, necessity for prevention and treatment, supply assurance, priority usage, quality assurance, and financial burden reduction. The "Opinions" focuses on improving the policy from the selection, production, distribution, use, payment, and monitoring of essential medicines.

First, in terms of the selection of essential medicines, there is a stronger emphasis on highlighting the clinical value of medicines, maintaining dynamic adjustments, and balancing additions and removals. Newly approved medicines with definite efficacy, reasonable pricing, and better suitability for disease prevention and treatment may also be considered for inclusion. At the same time, considering that the national essential medicine system has achieved full coverage in government-run primary medical and health institutions, allowing local supplements to the list is a transitional measure in the early stages of the system construction. The "Opinions" stipulates that, in principle, local supplements should not be allowed. This will facilitate comparative analysis of the use of essential medicines across different medical institutions.

Second, in terms of supply assurance, there is an increased focus on optimizing the roles of both government and market forces. Drawing from effective practices in recent years such as centralized procurement and addressing drug shortages, systematic arrangements are made to encourage technological upgrades in enterprises, improve procurement and distribution mechanisms, and strengthen early warning and response to shortages. Special emphasis is placed on preemptively preventing drug shortages through monitoring, early warnings, and timely responses, ensuring continuous availability and supply stability of essential medicines through multiple channels and methods.

Third, in terms of distribution and usage, there is a heightened focus on aligning drug use between grassroots and second-level medical institutions and above to support the development of tiered diagnosis and treatment system. Emphasis is placed on comprehensive provision and prioritized usage of essential medicines at all levels of medical institutions, standardizing the variety, dosage forms, and specifications of drugs used between different levels of medical institutions to ensure seamless coordination. This provides medication assurance for primary care first diagnosis, two-way referrals, managing minor ailments at the grassroots level, and facilitating recovery back to communities. Additionally, incentives and constraints for rational diagnosis, treatment, and medication are established for medical institutions and personnel through reforms in medical insurance payment methods and fiscal subsidies.

Fourth, in terms of quality assurance, there is an increased emphasis on linkage with consistency evaluations of generic drug quality and efficacy. It is stressed that medicines passing consistency evaluations should be prioritized for inclusion in the essential medicine list according to procedures, gradually phasing out generic versions of essential medicines that fail these evaluations. This further reinforces the concept that essential medicines are safe and reliable.

Fifth, in terms of financial burden reduction, there is an increased focus on aligning with medical insurance reimbursement policies, considering needs in public health and disease prevention and treatment. The treatment medicines within the essential medicine list are clearly defined. When adjusting the medical insurance catalog, medicines meeting criteria are prioritized for inclusion or reclassification as Class A or B, gradually improving the level of actual protection and maximizing reductions in patient medication expenses to enhance public satisfaction.

7　TCM Services and Management

TCM is a gem of Chinese civilization, with its philosophy of "preventative treatment of disease" being integrated into the Healthy China Initiative. Currently, a preliminary TCM service system that encompasses both urban and rural areas, combining preventive care, disease treatment, and rehabilitation, has been established in China. The level and efficiency of TCM services are continually enhancing. Since the 21st century, China has undergone two large-scale public health campaigns against epidemics, creating a miracle in human history as a populous nation successfully emerging from major disease outbreaks. The combination of TCM and Western medicine, as well as the use of both TCM and Western medicine, has played a pivotal role in these campaigns, becoming distinctive features and highlights of China's epidemic control and prevention efforts. TCM, with its millennia-old heritage, has withstood numerous practical tests, safeguarding the health of the Chinese people, demonstrating the contemporary value of the Chinese treasure, and offering solutions to the world in combating infectious diseases and ensuring the health of all peoples.

7.1　TCM Services

7.1.1　TCM Service System

7.1.1.1　TCM Preventive Health Care Service System

The TCM preventive health care service system, primarily focusing on delivering TCM services, embodies the TCM principle of "preventative treatment of disease." Reinforcing the development of this system is a pivotal strategy in propelling medical reforms and advancing the growth of TCM undertakings in China. Presently, China has established a preliminary regional network for TCM preventive health care services, alongside a systematic and comprehensive content framework for such services that connects the entire care continuum. Distinct platforms showcasing TCM characteristics and capable of autonomously conducting preventive health care work have also been assembled. This system in China encompasses three integral parts: the provision system of TCM preventive health care services, the technology (and product) system of these services, and the support system backing them. Specifically, TCM preventive health care services are rendered by TCM preventive health care departments in various tiers of TCM hospitals, similar departments within general hospitals, as well as primary medical and health institutions like community health service centers and township health centers. The technology (and product) system encompasses methodologies and technologies for gathering, storing, integrating, and dynamically assessing and monitoring individual health status data. The construction of the support system includes establishing mechanisms for technological innovation and research and development institutions, cultivating specialized personnel, refining TCM-centric health assurance models, instituting pertinent management systems and standards, and promoting TCM health culture.

Currently, the TCM preventive health care service system in China is experiencing vigorous growth. A number of TCM medical institutions have set up preventive health care departments, effectively integrating existing resources to actively provide TCM preventive health care services, including therapies like massage and moxibustion. Privately-run TCM wellness and health preservation establishments are emerging in large numbers, akin to bamboo shoots after a spring rain, enriching the spectrum of services available and acting as a complement to the TCM preventive health care service system. Furthermore, the Ministry of Human Resources and Social Security has specifically designated occupations for those engaged in TCM preventive health care work, accompanied by the formulation of corresponding standards and regulations, which have significantly propelled the advancement of TCM preventive health care services.

7. 1. 1. 2 TCM Medical Service System

The TCM medical service system constitutes a vital part of China's medical service system. In accordance with the "Several Opinions of the State Council on Supporting and Promoting the Development of Traditional Chinese Medicine," the TCM medical service system is jointly composed of TCM medical institutions and other medical institutions' TCM health resources, forming an interconnected system in the provision of TCM medical services. This includes both urban and rural TCM medical service networks. Currently, China has essentially established a comprehensive TCM medical service system covering both urban and rural areas. In urban settings, a TCM medical service network has taken shape, primarily consisting of TCM hospitals (hospitals of traditional ethnic medicine and integrated traditional Chinese and Western medicine), outpatient departments and clinics specialized in TCM, clinical department of TCM in general hospitals, and community health service institutions. In rural areas, another TCM medical service network is primarily built around county-level TCM hospitals, clinical department of TCM in general hospitals (specialized hospitals, and maternal and child health care hospitals), TCM departments in township health centers, and village clinics, providing basic TCM medical, preventive, and healthcare services. For details, see Figure 7-1.

Most comprehensive medical institutions and primary medical and health institutions in

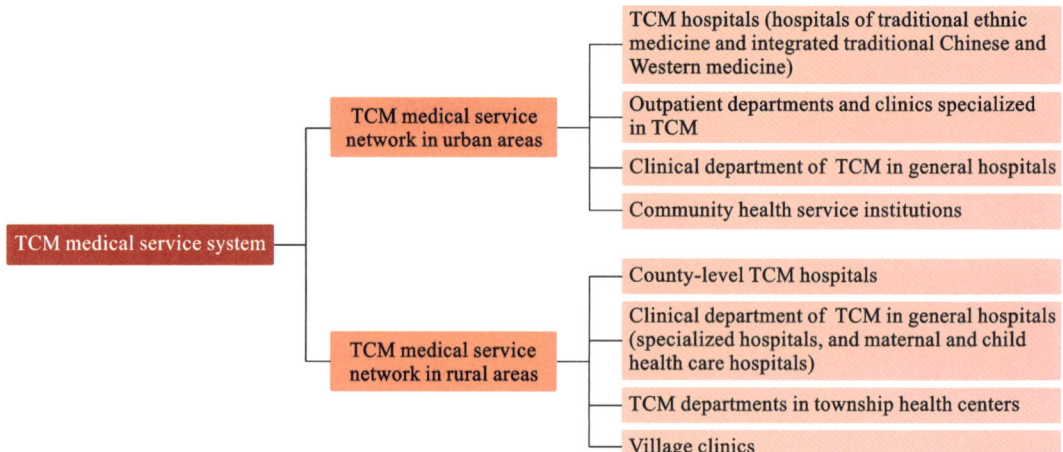

Figure 7-1　China's TCM medical service system

China have TCM departments, offering TCM services primarily based on traditional therapies such as herbal medicine, acupuncture, and massage. These services are, to varying degrees, included in the reimbursement scope of basic medical insurance for urban employees and basic medical insurance for rural and non-working urban residents.

By the end of 2020, China was home to 5 482 hospitals specialized in TCM, comprising 2 332 public TCM hospitals and 2 094 private TCM hospitals. Among these, there were 535 third-level, 1 926 second-level, and 1 155 first-level TCM hospitals. In the effort to elevate TCM service standards, 6 hospitals specialized in TCM were included in the nurturing category for national medical centers, 20 TCM hospitals were incorporated into the scope of national regional medical centers as exporting hospitals, and 8 TCM projects were identified as national regional medical center construction projects.

7. 1. 1. 3　Primary-Level TCM Service System

The primary-level TCM service network in China, featuring county-level TCM hospitals as leaders, community health service centers, community health service stations, township health centers, and village clinics as the main bodies, TCM departments in non-TCM medical institutions such as county-level general hospitals, maternal and child health care institutions as key supports, and privately-owned TCM hospitals, TCM outpatient departments and clinics as supplements, has gradually become more refined. By the end of 2020, 99. 0% of community health service centers, 90. 6% of community health service stations, 98. 0% of township health centers, and 74. 5% of village clinics were capable of providing TCM services. The enhancement of primary-level TCM service capabilities has yielded significant results, markedly improving the fairness, accessibility, and convenience for the public in seeking TCM services.

7.1.2　Types of TCM Services

7.1.2.1　TCM's "Preventive Treatment of Disease" Services

The concept of "preventive treatment of disease" in TCM originates from the *Yellow Emperor's Inner Canon*, which states that "the superior physician treats disease before it manifests, not after—it is this principle that is meant." The idea of "preventive treatment of disease," traceable to the *Yellow Emperor's Inner Canon*, emphasizes prevention over treatment, encapsulated in the principles of prevention before a disease arises, guarding against pathological changes when falling sick, and protecting recovering patients from relapse. This is also the basic idea that China's health sector has generally adhered to so far. "Preventive treatment of disease" in TCM necessitates not only treating diseases but also preventing their onset; it involves not just disease prevention but also forecasting disease trends, seeking remedies before pathology emerges, and seizing initiative during treatment.

In numerous Chinese policy documents, "preventive treatment of disease" in TCM is equated with TCM preventive health care. Promoting TCM health initiative of "preventive treatment of disease" and the construction of a TCM preventive health care service system constitute key directions for China's medical reforms and the development of TCM. Centered on individual wellness, TCM's "preventive treatment of disease" services employ unique preventive techniques to avert diseases. Over a decade has seen the development of China's TCM health initiative of "preventive treatment of disease." As China's new medical reform deepens, "preventive treatment of disease" in TCM is increasingly applied in safeguarding the health of urban and rural residents and preventing diseases. According to the *National Compilation of Traditional Chinese Medicine Statistics* by National Administration of Traditional Chinese Medicine, from 2019 to 2021, the number of health check-ups and "preventive treatment of disease" services completed in hospitals specialized in TCM in China notably increased, with an annual growth rate of 8.8%, marking a phased achievement in establishing the TCM preventive health care service system of "preventive treatment of disease."

7.1.2.2　TCM Outpatient Services

TCM outpatient services refer to the comprehensive application of fundamental TCM theories and clinical experience in diagnosing and treating patients, so as to offer them a holistic and systematic TCM health care experience. The scope of practice for TCM outpatient services in China is extensive, encompassing several key areas. First, TCM diagnosis. This involves using traditional diagnostic methods such as inspection, auscultation and olfaction, inquiry, and palpation to ascertain patients' conditions. Second, TCM treatment. Patients are treated using various TCM modalities, including herbal medicine, acupuncture, massage and cupping therapy, and others. Third, TCM preventive health care. Based on theories and methods of TCM wellness and health preservation, patients receive guidance on maintaining good health and preventing diseases. Four, integrated treatment of traditional Chinese and Western medicine. In TCM comprehensive clinics, integration of Western medical examinations and therapies with TCM practices is employed for a combined therapeutic approach. Five, TCM health counseling. Through TCM theories and methods related to health, patients can receive guidance aimed at promoting and maintaining their overall well-being.

According to the "Guidelines for Medical Institution Setup and Planning (2016-2020)," China's provinces have essentially established clear functional roles for provincial, municipal, and county-level TCM hospitals, as well as township health centers and village clinics in TCM practices. This has led to the formation of a hierarchical, structurally sound, and functionally comprehensive TCM service system. Alongside China's sustained and rapid economic and social development, improvements in living standards and a rising demand for medical services have fueled the continuous advancement of China's medical services. As a vital component of these services, TCM outpatient services have also experienced substantial growth. In 2020, hospitals specialized in TCM in China provided approximately 596.99 million patient visits, among which outpatient departments specialized in TCM accounted for about 31.14 million visits, and clinics specialized in TCM saw around 157.38 million visits. Since 2013, the proportion of patient visits to TCM medical institutions out of the total patient visits nationwide has been on a consistent rise. By 2020, patient visits to TCM medical institutions accounted for 16.8% of all patient visits in China.

7.1.2.3 TCM Inpatient Services

TCM inpatient services refer to the comprehensive medical services provided within TCM medical institutions, where TCM practitioners, adhering to the core concepts of Yin Yang and the Five Phases, zang-fu organs, meridians and collaterals, holism, and treatment based on syndrome differentiation, comprehensively utilize the four diagnostic methods (inspection, auscultation and olfaction, inquiry, and palpation) along with auxiliary instruments. Primarily employing herbal formulations as the main therapeutic modality, these services also incorporate distinctive TCM treatments such as acupuncture, massage, cupping, and seasonal therapies (like treating winter ailments in summer) to offer inpatients a holistic approach to medical care.

In April 2019, the National Administration of Traditional Chinese Medicine in China issued the "Performance Appraisal Indicators for Third-Level Public Traditional Chinese Medicine Hospitals," aiming to conduct a comprehensive and unified data collection and evaluation of all third-level public TCM hospitals nationwide. This set clear standards and requirements specifically for TCM inpatient services. In 2020, approximately 29.07 million patients were discharged from hospitals specialized in TCM across China, accounting for 83% of the total discharges from TCM medical institutions nationally. The role of hospitals specialized in TCM in providing inpatient services has thus become increasingly prominent.

7. 1. 3 The Concept, Characteristics and Advantages of TCM Services

7. 1. 3. 1 The Concept of TCM Services

The concept of TCM embodies the notion of "man is an integral part of nature," a perspective that emerged from a natural philosophical medical model over 2 000 years ago. This concept underscores a human-centered approach, respects individuals' natural and social attributes, and pays close attention to the impact of psychological, emotional, environmental, and other subjective and objective factors on physical health. Through prolonged clinical practice, TCM has developed a unique theoretical framework and therapeutic approach centered on the "holism" and "treatment based on syndrome differentiation." With the transformation of disease spectrum, TCM's individualized "treatment based on syndrome differentiation" methodology and the notable efficacy of Chinese herbs in treating common and frequently-occurring diseases are gaining increasing global attention. Based on the patient's subjective experience, TCM offers distinctive perspectives and methods in addressing both physical and mental ailments, effectively tackling suboptimal health issues in populations.

7. 1. 3. 2 The Characteristics of TCM Services

The concept of "harmony between form and spirit" in TCM aptly embodies the distinct characteristics of TCM services. TCM considers both the "spirit" (abstract thought) and the "form" (concrete expressions), recognizing that the well-being of both is essential for holistic health. In summary, the characteristics of TCM services are twofold. First, it resides in TCM's comprehensive and distinct theoretical framework, encompassing the theory of holism, treatment based on syndrome differentiation, and constant movement. Second, it is manifested in the TCM techniques employed in disease diagnosis and treatment, such as the four diagnostic methods of inspection, auscultation and olfaction, inquiry, and palpation, as well as therapies like acupuncture, massage, and cupping. In essence, TCM services are delivered under the guidance of TCM's characteristic theoretical system, utilizing TCM diagnostic and therapeutic techniques. TCM is often hailed as the "fifth great invention" alongside China's Four Great Inventions, and its resilience and continuing enhancement in service quality over 2 000 years can be attributed to its unique diagnostic and therapeutic methods, efficacious treatments, and distinct theoretical system.

7. 1. 3. 3 The Advantages of TCM Services

The TCM diagnostic and therapeutic equipment is simple and its techniques are straightforward, which helps alleviate the burden on medical institutions. TCM services boast the advantages of low investment and cost-effectiveness. The concept of "preventive treatment of disease" in TCM encompasses both prevention before a disease arises and guarding against pathological changes when falling sick, echoing the primary medical and health service's emphasis on an integrated approach that includes prevention, health protection, medical care, rehabilitation, health education, family planning, and technical guidance. Guided by this concept, shifting the focus of health upstream involves differential diagnosis and treatment tailored to different population groups, regulating body balance to prevent diseases, thereby fostering a healthy living environment and enhancing the quality of life. This approach presents a novel solution to break the vicious cycle of poverty due to illness and poverty returning due to illness.

TCM theories embody a health paradigm that starkly contrasts with the reductionism of Western medicine. Unlike modern Western medicine's focus on treating existing diseases, TCM advocates "preventive treatment of disease," aiming to achieve the goals of prevention before a disease arises, guarding against pathological changes when falling sick, and protecting recovering patients from relapse. One of China's earliest surviving medical classics, the *Yellow Emperor's Inner Canon*, clearly records this concept of "preventive treatment of disease," stating that "the superior physician treats disease before it manifests, not after—it is this principle that is meant." In recent years, a series of policy documents issued and implemented in China, such as the "13th Five-Year Plan for the Development of Traditional Chinese Medicine" and the "Guidelines for the Establishment and Management of 'Preventive Treatment of Disease' Departments in Traditional Chinese Medicine Hospitals (Revised Edition)," highlight a prominent orientation towards "preventive treatment of disease." This concept, characterized by promoting health, putting disease prevention first, and combining prevention with treatment, is gradually gaining recognition and importance among the people in China.

7.1.4 TCM Service Resources

7.1.4.1 TCM Medical and Health Institutions

According to the "Statistical Bulletin on Health Development in China," the structure of China's medical and health institutions consists of hospitals, primary medical and health institutions, professional public health institutions, and other institutions. Among these, TCM medical and health institutions encompass hospitals specialized in TCM, outpatient departments specialized in TCM, clinics specialized in TCM, institutions specialized in TCM research, as well as clinical departments of TCM within non-TCM medical institutions. These institutions serve as the main providers of TCM services. The total number of TCM medical and health institutions across China has grown from 46 541 in 2015 to 80 319 in 2022, demonstrating an average annual growth rate of 8.1%, and representing a 72.6% increase compared with 2015.

(1) Hospitals Specialized in TCM

According to the "Statistical Bulletin on Health Development in China," hospitals specialized in TCM in China encompass TCM hospitals, hospitals of integrated traditional Chinese and Western medicine, and hospitals of traditional ethnic medicine. By the end of 2022, there were a total of 5 862 hospitals specialized in TCM in China, among which 4 779 were TCM hospitals, accounting for 81.5% of the total. Hospitals of integrated traditional

Chinese and Western medicine and hospitals of traditional ethnic medicine represented 13% and 5.5% respectively.

(2) Outpatient Departments and Clinics Specialized in TCM

According to the "Statistical Bulletin on Health Development in China," outpatient departments specialized in TCM in China consist of TCM outpatient departments, outpatient departments of integrated traditional Chinese and Western medicine, and outpatient departments of traditional ethnic medicine, while clinics specialized in TCM include TCM clinics, clinics of integrated traditional Chinese and Western medicine, and clinics of traditional ethnic medicine. These outpatient departments and clinics form part of the grassroots network for TCM services, with the majority being established by social entities. From 2015 to 2020, the number of outpatient departments specialized in TCM in China experienced an average annual growth rate of 16.6%, significantly higher than that of clinics specialized in TCM. By 2022, there were 3 786 outpatient departments specialized in TCM and 70 631 clinics specialized in TCM in operation.

(3) Institutions Specialized in TCM Research

According to the "Statistical Bulletin on Health Development in China," institutions specialized in TCM research in China comprise TCM institutions, institutions of integrated traditional Chinese and Western medicine, and institutions of traditional ethnic medicine. By the end of 2020, China was home to a total of 43 institutions specialized in TCM research, including 34 TCM institutions, 2 institutions of integrated traditional Chinese and Western medicine, and 7 institutions of traditional ethnic medicine.

(4) Clinical Departments of TCM within Non-TCM Medical Institutions

According to relevant Chinese standards, the clinical departments of TCM in general hospitals should be established as primary clinical departments within the hospital. The general hospitals should provide TCM beds, with the number not less than 5% of the hospitals' standard bed capacity. Larger hospitals, based on actual needs, may establish independent TCM wards. Furthermore, independent TCM outpatient services must be set up, with third-level general hospitals offering no fewer than three TCM specialties and second-level general hospitals offering no fewer than two. By the end of 2020, among China's general hospitals, 4 071 had clinical department of TCM, constituting the highest proportion (86.7%) among similar institutions. Among community health service centers and township health centers, 4 590 and 17 414 respectively had clinical department of TCM, accounting for 63.1% and 50.1% of their respective categories.

7.1.4.2   The Number of TCM Beds

TCM beds refer to those provided by TCM medical and health institutions including hospitals specialized in TCM, outpatient departments specialized in TCM, and clinical departments of TCM within non-TCM medical institutions, with hospitals specialized in

TCM being the predominant provider. In 2020, China had approximately 9.10 million beds in medical and health institutions in total, among which around 1.43 million were in TCM medical and health institutions, accounting for 15.7%. Specifically, the beds in hospitals specialized in TCM numbered around 1.15 million (a 40.1% increase compared with 2015), representing 16.1% of all hospital beds nationwide, and indicating a steady growth trend. Among the beds in hospitals specialized in TCM, TCM hospitals provided about 0.98 million beds (accounting for 85.5%), hospitals of integrated traditional Chinese and Western medicine had roughly 0.13 million beds (accounting for 10.9%), and hospitals of traditional ethnic medicine had 42 379 beds (accounting for 3.7%).

7.1.4.3 TCM Resources

(1) Definition and Classification of TCM Resources

TCM resources are integral components of natural ecological resources and constitute a crucial material foundation for the development of TCM. These resources encompass medicinally used animals, plants, and minerals scattered within specific regions or areas, which are utilized under the guidance of TCM's fundamental theories for traditional medicinal purposes. The term does not solely refer to the narrow definition of TCM resources; it also encompasses folk herbal medicines and ethnic medicinal resources such as Zhuang and Miao medicines. With the continuous exploitation and utilization of natural resources, some have become scarce, leading to the development of artificially cultivated, bred, or manufactured medicinal resources through biochemical technologies, known as artificial TCM resources. Natural TCM resources, in contrast to artificial ones, can be broadly classified into two categories: biological resources and non-biological resources. Approximately 99.4% of these resources fall under biological resources, including medicinal animals and plants, which are renewable. Conversely, medicinal mineral resources, classified as non-biological resources, are non-renewable and account for about 0.6% of the total.

(2) The Status Quo of the Existing TCM Resources

Information regarding the types, distribution, and reserves of TCM resources is primarily obtained through conducting national surveys of them. China has carried out four such surveys since 1960. According to the data from the Fourth National Survey of TCM Resources, China boasts a total of 18 817 species of TCM resources. Among these, there are 826 species of medicinal fungi (approximately 4.39%), 15 227 species of medicinal plants (about 80.92%), 2 611 species of medicinal animals (around 13.88%), and 153 species of medicinal minerals (about 0.81%). Furthermore, to understand the regional variations in the distribution of TCM resources, China has conducted detailed classifications based on administrative regions. Specifically, Hainan province possesses nearly 2 500 species of TCM resources, while Yunnan province has 8 875, highlighting a significant difference in distribution across regions.

7.1.4.4 TCM Human Resources

TCM human resources encompass three main categories: practitioners and assistant practitioners of TCM (encompassing practitioners of TCM, integrating traditional Chinese and Western medicine, and ethnic medicine), TCM pharmacists, and intern practitioners of TCM. Personnel engaged in TCM management tasks are not included in this statistical count.

(1) Total Human Resources of TCM

As China attaches greater importance to TCM and the demand from the public for TCM services rises, the total volume of TCM human resources in the country has seen a rapid increase. By 2021, the overall number of TCM human resources in medical and health institutions nationwide reached 884 815. From 2017 to 2022, both the total number of practitioners and assistant practitioners nationwide and those specializing in TCM categories experienced continuous growth, increasing from 3.39 million to 4.44 million and from 527 000 to 764 000 respectively, with average annual growth rates of 5.5% and 7.7%. During the same period, the number of TCM pharmacists grew from 120 000 in 2017 to 139 000 in 2022, with an average annual growth rate of 3%. Evidently, within TCM human resources, the number of practitioners and assistant practitioners of TCM was expanding at a faster pace, whereas the growth in the number of TCM pharmacists was slower.

(2) The Allocation and Age Structure of TCM Human Resources

During the 13th Five-Year Plan period, the allocation of TCM human resources per 10 000 population in various regions of China steadily increased, with the maximum allocation rising from 4.43 to 5.87 personnel, and the minimum allocation of TCM pharmacists per 10 000 population growing from 0.84 to 0.93. In central regions, the overall allocation of TCM personnel, practitioners and assistant practitioners of TCM, and TCM pharmacists per 10 000 population was lower than the national average. However, the allocation of health technicians per 10 000 population in TCM hospitals in these regions, which was in the middle range during the 12th Five-Year Plan period, rose to lead the nation by the end of the 13th Five-Year Plan period. Regarding the allocation of practitioners and assistant practitioners of TCM per 10 000 population, western regions consistently held the lead. Given the relatively smaller population in these areas, the number of practitioners per 10 000 population tended to be higher. As for the allocation of TCM pharmacists per 10 000 population, eastern regions exceeded the national average. These regions enjoy relatively abundant TCM human resources, and despite having a larger population base, they maintain their leading position.

Compared with 2017, there were changes in the age structure of TCM human resources in China in 2021. Specifically, for practitioners and assistant practitioners of TCM in public

TCM hospitals, the proportion of those aged below 25 increased by 0.5%, those aged 25 to 34 rose by 7%, those aged 35 to 54 decreased by 6.3%, those aged 55 to 59 saw an increase of 1.3%, while the percentage of those aged 60 and above declined by 2.5%.

7.2　TCM Management

7.2.1　TCM Management System

Since the founding of the People's Republic of China, to ensure and promote the development of TCM, the state has established specialized organizations for TCM management and built a hierarchical TCM management system extending from the central government to local levels. Through ongoing practical exploration, central-level TCM management bodies have undergone four major transitions, evolving from the Department of Traditional Chinese Medicine, to the Bureau of Traditional Chinese Medicine, then to the State Administration of Traditional Chinese Medicine, and finally to the current National Administration of Traditional Chinese Medicine. As the central-level TCM administrative institutions have continually upgraded, local governments have also successively established corresponding TCM management agencies. Currently, China's TCM management structure encompasses four tiers: central, provincial, municipal, and county levels, with management responsibilities covering areas such as medical services, education, scientific research, and cultural dissemination.

The National Administration of Traditional Chinese Medicine of China, serving as the national governing body, is responsible for planning and guiding the development of TCM management across the country. By 2018, all 31 provincial-level administrative regions had completed institutional reforms, with basically established TCM administrations (bureaus, offices) at the provincial level. The municipal-level TCM management system was further refined, and the grassroots TCM management system witnessed a leap from nonexistence to establishment. Provinces including Hebei, Jilin, and Sichuan have set up relatively independent TCM administrations under the provincial health commission. Most provincial-level TCM administrations are at the deputy director-general level, with Jilin Province being a notable example. This province has formed a relatively complete TCM management system. The model of relatively independent TCM administrations, which grants these institutions independent staffing quotas, personnel authority, and dedicated financial budgets, facilitates autonomous operations of them. This, to a certain extent, promotes the implementation of TCM policies.

China's TCM undertakings operates under a divided departmental and hierarchical regulatory framework, involving multiple ministries and commissions, chiefly including the National Development and Reform Commission, the Ministry of Agriculture and Rural

Affairs, the National Health Commission, and the National Administration of Traditional Chinese Medicine. At the national level, the National Administration of Traditional Chinese Medicine is established to oversee TCM affairs comprehensively. Both provincial and municipal levels have set up TCM administrations, while each county-level health administrative body houses a TCM management department. Relevant departments at all levels collaborate to ensure the effective implementation of policies and regulations pertaining to TCM. This multi-department cooperative management system provides a reliable organizational guarantee for the development of TCM in China.

7.2.2　The Legal System of TCM

The development of TCM is inseparable from legal safeguards. The issuance of the "Regulations of the People's Republic of China on Traditional Chinese Medicine" in 2003 played a vital role in promoting and regulating the development of TCM. However, with the rapid economic and social development, a series of issues emerged in the development of TCM in China, including insufficient service capabilities of TCM, a decline in the TCM service market, and difficulties for the current physicians, clinics, and drug management systems to adapt to the characteristics and development needs of TCM. To further ensure and facilitate the development of TCM, in 2008, the Standing Committee of the 11th National People's Congress included the TCM law in its legislative plan. The Law of the People's Republic of China on Traditional Chinese Medicine was officially adopted at the 25th Session of the Standing Committee of the 12th National People's Congress on December 25, 2016, and came into effect on July 1, 2017. This marked a milestone event in the history of TCM development. As the first comprehensive and systematic law that fully embodies the characteristics of TCM, the Law of the People's Republic of China on Traditional Chinese Medicine codifies China's policies and guidelines for managing the development of TCM, legally affirming the significant position of TCM and embodying the expectations and demands of the people for TCM in a legal form. Based on the Constitution of the People's Republic of China, the Law of the People's Republic of China on Traditional Chinese Medicine ensures the legal status of TCM and provides fundamental guidance for its development.

7.2.3　TCM Quality Control

7.2.3.1　Whole Process Quality Control

TCM encompasses a variety of forms, such as Chinese crude drugs (derived from plants, animals, and minerals), TCM decoction pieces, and Chinese patent medicines, which constitute the primary manifestations of medicines found in a Chinese pharmacy. TCM decoction pieces and Chinese patent medicines, among other TCM preparations, are processed and prepared from Chinese crude drugs through specific stages. High-quality medicines form the material basis for effective treatment, and superior TCM decoction pieces and Chinese patent medicines ensure optimal clinical outcomes in TCM practice. Thus, the quality assurance of TCM necessitates rigorous control starting from the sourcing of raw materials. Chinese crude drugs possess multiple attributes as pharmaceuticals, commodities, and agricultural and sideline products, and their circulation process spans cultivation, harvesting, processing, packaging, storage, transportation, and sales, with potential quality issues arising at any step along this chain. This complexity inherents in these steps consequently dictates the intricacy of quality control required.

Chapter Ⅲ of the Law of the People's Republic of China on Traditional Chinese Medicine contains provisions specifically addressing the "Protection and Development of TCM." Article 21 stipulates the overarching requirements for the supervision of the entire process from the production to circulation of Chinese crude drugs, stating that "the state shall formulate technical norms and standards for the cultivation, breeding, collection, storage, and primary processing of Chinese crude drugs, and strengthen the quality supervision and management throughout the entire process of production and circulation of Chinese crude drugs to ensure their quality and safety." Article 24 sets regulations for the establishment of a quality monitoring system for Chinese crude drugs and the construction of a traceability system for their circulation. Furthermore, Article 31 provides regulations concerning the preparation of TCM preparation formulations by medical institutions.

From a legal standpoint, China's current TCM supervision system is centered around the Drug Administration Law of the People's Republic of China, complemented by administrative regulations and departmental rules including the "Regulations for the Implementation of the Drug Administration Law of the People's Republic of China," "Good Manufacturing Practice," "Good Supply Practice," and "Good Agricultural Practice for Chinese Crude Drugs." The "Regulations for the Implementation of the Drug Administration Law of the People's Republic of China" outlines the rules governing drug research and development, production, distribution, usage, and supervision, encompassing TCM. The "Good Manufacturing Practice," "Good Supply Practice," and "Good Agricultural Practice for Chinese Crude Drugs" establish detailed guidelines and operational standards for drug production and distribution practices. Additional normative documents also play a pivotal role. For instance, the national food and drug administration authorities have issued a series of notices, including "Notice on Strengthening Supervision over the Administration of TCM Decoction Pieces," "Notice of the China Food and Drug Administration on Further Strengthening the Supervision over the Production and Operation of TCM Decoction Pieces," and "Notice of the China Food and Drug Administration on Further Strengthening Quality Supervision over Special Chinese Crude Drug Markets," which lay down explicit regulations for the production and management supervision of TCM decoction pieces, Chinese crude drugs, and Chinese patent medicines. Overall, a preliminary legal and regulatory system for TCM has been established in China.

In terms of the organization and management of TCM, after the reform and opening-up, the

State Council established the State Pharmaceutical Administration to oversee drug regulation. With the emergence of dispersed drug supervision, the authority for TCM regulation was transferred to the State Administration of Traditional Chinese Medicine. During the institutional reform in 1998, the State Council integrated the relevant functions of the Pharmaceutical Administration Bureau of the Ministry of Health, the State Pharmaceutical Administration, and the State Administration of Traditional Chinese Medicine, forming the National Medical Products Administration, which reported directly to the State Council and was responsible for comprehensive supervision of drugs from research and development to sales. In 2003, with the addition of food and cosmetic supervision responsibilities, the National Medical Products Administration was renamed the State Food and Drug Administration, assuming administrative and technical oversight of drugs (including Chinese crude drugs, TCM decoction pieces, and Chinese patent medicines) throughout their lifecycle from research and development, production, distribution to usage. The management below the provincial level was organized on a vertical basis. Under the context of the large-scale institutional reform in 2008, the State Food and Drug Administration changed from being a directly affiliated agency of the State Council to being under the jurisdiction of the Ministry of Health, and the drug regulatory bodies below the provincial level shifted from vertical management to local management. In 2013, the State Food and Drug Administration was renamed the China Food and Drug Administration, and in 2018, it was again renamed the National Medical Products Administration, which is managed by the State Administration for Market Regulation, overseeing the unified regulation of drugs across different stages such as production, distribution, and consumption.

7.2.3.2　Construction of the Quality Traceability System

The International Organization for Standardization defines traceability as the ability to track and identify the history, usage, or location of goods or actions through recorded identification codes. Establishing a traceability system is a critical measure to reinforce quality and safety supervision. The concept of a quality traceability system for Chinese crude drugs was first proposed at the 3rd International Conference on the Modernization of Traditional Chinese Medicine in 2010, aiming at enforcing quality control throughout the entire process of production and usage of these materials. The TCM quality traceability system employs modern Internet of Things (IoT) technology, block chain, cloud computing, big data, and other information technologies to manage key information throughout the entire process of TCM production, from planting, processing, manufacturing, distribution to usage. This enables the realization of a system where "the source is identifiable, the destination is traceable, the quality is verifiable, and the responsibility is accountable," essentially achieving "traceability from farm to patient" or "traceability regulation from patient back to farm." The development of such a traceability system for TCM quality is a public welfare project that ensures the safety, efficacy, and controllability of TCM quality, thereby safeguarding public health.

Case Study　Chinese Pharmaceutical Chemist Tu Youyou Discovered an Anti-Malaria Medicine——Artemisinin

Since ancient times, humans have been engaged in a protracted battle against malaria, with records dating back to China's *Yellow Emperor's Inner Canon: Basic Questions*, compiled before the Common Era. Even to this day, malaria continues to wreak havoc in numerous countries, posing a threat to people's health and lives.

On October 5, 2015, the Karolinska Institute in Sweden announced the awarding of the 2015 Nobel Prize in Physiology or Medicine to pharmaceutical chemist Tu Youyou and two other scientists, in recognition of their contributions to the research on treatments for parasitic diseases such as malaria. Tu Youyou thus became the first Chinese native scientist to win a Nobel Prize in a scientific discipline.

Before artemisinin was discovered, quinine and chloroquine were the primary medicines used to combat malaria. However, the effectiveness of these medicines against malaria did not persist for long. In the 1960s, many regions of the world began to witness the emergence of malaria parasites resistant to these medicines, particularly in Southeast Asia and Africa, reaching a point where no effective medicines were available. Consequently, the development of new anti-malaria medicines became imperative. By 1972, after screening over 2 000 traditional Chinese herbal medicine recipes, Tu Youyou and her team found that an extract from the Artemisia annual plant, a member of the Compositae family, showed some inhibitory effects on mouse malaria parasites. Initially, the effectiveness was limited due to improper extraction methods resulting in low concentrations of the active ingredient. Inspired by Ge Hong, a medical scholar from China's Eastern Jin Dynasty, and adopting a low-temperature ether extraction method instead, the team successfully extracted the effective antimalarial compound, artemisinin, which achieved a 100% inhibition rate against the malaria parasites.

Compared with other anti-malaria medicines, artemisinin-based medicines exhibit high efficiency and rapid clearance of malaria parasites. However, due to the short half-life of artemisinin compounds in the human body, researchers recommend combining artemisinin and its derivatives with other anti-malaria medicines to achieve complete eradication of the parasites and mitigate the development of resistance. A 2004 publication in *The Lancet* demonstrated that when artesunate, a derivative of artemisinin, is used in combination with other medicines, the cure rate for Plasmodium falciparum (the most severe form of malaria) exceeds 80%, accompanied by a significant reduction in recurrence rates and gametocyte infection rates. By 2013, out of the 87 countries where Plasmodium falciparum malaria was prevalent, 79 had adopted artemisinin-based combination therapies (ACTs) as the first-line treatment for this deadly form of malaria.

Artemisinin has paved the way for the development of a new generation of anti-malaria medicines. It originates from TCM, and its discovery has saved millions of lives worldwide, particularly in developing countries. It is believed that through the sustained efforts of researchers and health care workers, global malaria control and ultimately its eradication will be attainable goals.

8　China's Health Resource Planning

Formulating health resource planning is a pivotal instrument for materializing the Healthy China Initiative and significantly contributes to the construction of China's medical and health service system. China's health resource planning encompasses a diverse array of categories, spanning from talent cultivation, infrastructure, pharmaceutical resource allocation, to capital within the health domain. This chapter will first provide an overview of China's health resource planning. It encompasses the delineation of health resources, their categorization, allocation methodologies, as well as the fundamentals of health resource planning such as its concept, types, and formulation principles. Subsequently, the chapter delves into the indicators employed in China's health resource planning, utilizing these metrics as a foundation to elaborate on the planning formulation process. This intricate procedure encompasses defining strategic objectives, and formulating health resource development strategies and budget. Finally, a case study of China's health talent team construction planning is presented to help readers understand the specific forms of China's health resource planning.

8.1　Overview of China's Health Resource Planning

8.1.1　Concepts Related to Health Resource Planning

Health resources encompass the aggregate of various elements utilized or consumed in the provision of health services, comprising human resources, funds, infrastructures, equipment, medications, information, knowledge, and technological resources. Illustrative measures of a nation's or region's health vitality include the quantity of health institutions, hospital beds, health personnel, allocated health funds, and the ratio of health funds to Gross Domestic Product (GDP). Health resources are important indicators to measure the health status of a country or region and the material and technical foundations upon which health programs rest.

These resources can be further categorized into health human resources, health material resources, health financial resources, and health information and technology. Health human resources are individuals capable of delivering health services, encompassing both active practitioners and those undergoing training for future engagement. Health material resources include physical assets such as facilities, equipment, and medicines dedicated to health delivery. Health financial resources pertain to monetary inputs for health provision, stemming from governmental, societal, and personal sources, and are commonly referred to as "health expenditure." Health information and technology revolve around data, patents, norms, procedures, and other knowledge-based assets relevant to health.

In China, the allocation of health resources is executed through three principal modalities: first, planned allocation, wherein the government takes the responsibility of deciding resource distribution; second, market allocation, driven by market dynamics like pricing and competition, determining resource allocation patterns; third, a hybrid model combining planning and market mechanisms, enabling collaborative governance of resource allocation by both the government and market forces.

Health resource planning embodies a systematic approach aimed at defining the developmental objectives, scale, and pace of health resources, grounded in considerations such as the natural ecology, socioeconomic progression, population health challenges, and health demands. It endeavors to devise comprehensive plans for the rational allocation of these resources, with the overarching goal of augmenting the quality and availability of health services and optimizing the effectiveness and efficiency of resource usage. Enhancing resource allocation efficiency through meticulous planning constitutes a globally recognized practice and a cornerstone strategy for the Chinese government in ensuring equitable and efficient health resource allocation to address public health necessities. In devising such plans, the government meticulously considers three key dynamics: first, macro-micro relations, reflecting the interplay between national oversight of society-wide health resources and institutional-level health resource management; second, stock-increment balance, examining the interdependence between existing and forthcoming health resources; third, equity-efficiency nexus, striking a balance between the dual values of equity and efficiency in health resource allocation decisions.

8.1.2 Types of Health Resource Planning in China

China's health resource planning can be classified according to planning levels, planning subjects and planning periods (Figure 8-1).

In terms of planning levels, China' health resource planning is divided into national and regional tiers. National planning sets the tone by outlining developmental objectives, guiding principles, and strategic frameworks for the nation's health undertakings, thereby serving as a guiding framework. Conversely, regional planning is more nuanced, tailoring health development directions, models, and objectives according to the specific socioeconomic context and health profile of each area. It involves the rational distribution of medical and health institutions across various tiers, functions, and sizes, culminating in a cohesive blueprint for regional health progress. In China, the state often initiates regional

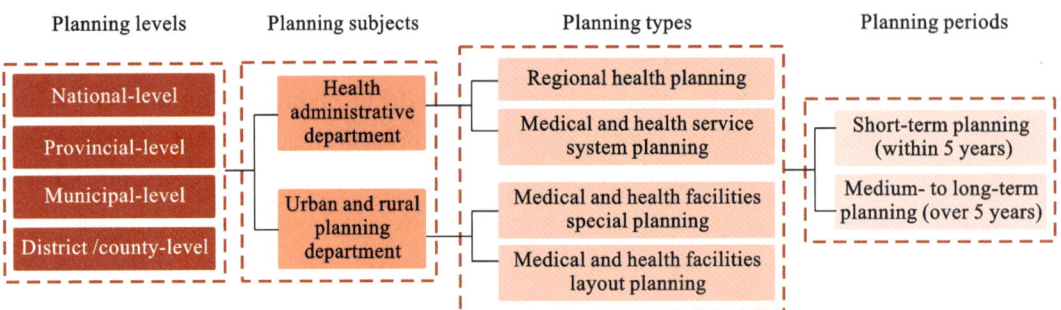

Figure 8-1　Types of health resource planning in China

planning directives, establishing resource allocation guidelines for defined periods. Subsequently, provincial health administrative departments establish baseline standards, followed by prefectural and county-level health administrative departments defining localized goals, allocation benchmarks, key tasks, and implementation guarantees. Execution of the regional health planning underpins the macroeconomic regulation of the health undertakings by governments at all tiers and facilitates comprehensive industry management in health.

Regarding planning subjects, the demarcation in China's health resource planning splits into two branches. The first, spearheaded and led by health administrations across all levels, encapsulates regional health planning and medical and health service system planning. It revolves around intra-system resource allocation, service provision, and developmental management. The second, handled by urban and rural planning departments, focuses on the land allocation and spatial arrangement for medical and health facilities through specialized plans and layout strategies such as medical and health facilities special planning and medical and health facilities layout planning. This chapter primarily delves into the former category—planning spearheaded and led by health administrative departments across all levels for execution.

When viewed through the lens of planning periods, China's health resource planning is bifurcated into short-term planning and medium- to long-term planning. Short-term planning, exemplified by that aligned with the national five-year economic and social development plans such as the "14th Five-Year Plan for National Health," the "14th Five-Year Plan for National Medical Security," the "14th Five-Year Plan for Health Standardization," set forth during the 14th Five-Year Plan period, encapsulates the period from 2021 to 2025. Conversely, medium- to long-term planning, epitomized by the "Outline of the Healthy China 2030 Plan" issued by the Central Committee of the Communist Party of China and the State Council on October 25, 2016, covers a longer time frame. As the inaugural national-scale, medium- to long-term health strategy since the founding of the People's Republic of China, it outlines ambitious goals spanning from enhancing population health, optimizing demographic structure and health literacy, restructuring a modern medical and health systems, fostering comprehensive health service models, propelling medical and health reforms, and bolstering the health industry's growth.

8.1.3 Principles for the Formulation of China's Health Resource Planning

To ascertain the precision and viability of health resource planning, governments worldwide adhere to a set of principles that not only conform to the health sector's developmental trajectories but also align with their unique political landscapes in formulating health resource planning. Universally embraced principles guiding the formulation of health resource planning encompass five main tenets: the first is the target-oriented principle, which delineates, actionable, quantifiable, achievable and assessable objectives; the second is the process-oriented principle, adhering to a scientific planning methodology entailing situational analysis, goal formulation and adjustment, strategy development and execution, and performance monitoring; the third is the coordination principle, emphasizing harmonious integration among diverse health institutions and personnel, fostering judicious and productive resource allocation; the fourth is the systemic principle, necessitating a holistic and dynamic examination of the health system's multifaceted internal and external factors and their reciprocal impacts, and finally establishing a complete health planning system; and the fifth is the sustainability principle, ensuring alignment with socioeconomic progress and public health needs, supporting the health sector's enduring expansion while safeguarding environmental and resource integrity.

China, anchored in its distinct national context and cumulative experience, has distilled its health resource planning approach into five tailored principles.

First, the coordination principle. It underscores that China's health resource planning should be coordinated with the national economic and social development. The government must calibrate health development aspirations, scale, and pace according to regional disparities, factor in socioeconomic influences on the development of health undertakings and population health, leverage conducive conditions and seize development prospects, dynamically adjust to socioeconomic transformations to tackle health challenges posed by industrialization, urbanization and demographic aging, and determine the number, scale and distribution of medical and health institutions scientifically and reasonably on a health needs-oriented basis. It also necessitates stakeholder collaboration, ensuring diverse viewpoints are incorporated to forge consensus. The solution of many health problems requires the joint efforts of the government and society. Therefore, it is necessary to strengthen the interaction, communication and coordination among all parties.

Second, the systemic principle, also known as the integrity principle. It underscores that health planners should view the health system or its components as an interconnected whole, recognizing that health system functionality is intertwined with broader societal systems. Similarly, each part of the health system is interconnected with others. The formulation of health resource planning, therefore, goes beyond simple allocation, aiming to enhance the health system's operational effectiveness holistically. To ensure that health resources are used more effectively, cooperation both within the health system and with external systems must be strengthened. This requires coordinated efforts between the government and market forces, with the government assuming a pivotal role in systemic design, planning, financing, service provision, and oversight to uphold public health's welfare orientation and cater to varied health service demands.

Third, the sustainability principle. As important planning to guide the operation of the health system, the concept of sustainable development should be emphasized in the process of formulating health resource planning. One of the objectives of health resource planning is to address health issues. Health resource planning must contemplate both immediate and future health necessities, addressing prevailing issues while averting emerging ones. Sometimes, the government formulates a certain plan to address a specific existing health issue. Due to the high level of attention from the government, the function of the plan is effectively implemented, and the health issue is resolved. However, once the issue is resolved, the implementation of the plan often ceases, leading to the recurrence of the same health issue after some time.

Fourth, the differentiated guidance principle. China has a large population and a vast territory, with significant regional economic disparities. There are substantial differences in the quantity and distribution of health resources, the level of health services, and the health status of the population across different regions. When formulating health resource planning, it is necessary to consider the specific conditions of different regions, systems, institutions, and organizations, as well as the health needs of the population, the level of economic and social development, and the current status of health resources. The quantity and distribution of health resources across different regions, types, and levels should be rationally coordinated, and allocation standards should be developed accordingly. This principle is reflected in setting goals, choosing strategies, and allocating resources, which includes clearly defining and implementing the functions and tasks of medical and health institutions at various levels and types, implementing the strategy of "centralized control with peripheral development" based on factors such as population size, distribution, age structure, transportation conditions, and diagnosis and treatment needs, as well as rationally allocating the number of medical and health institutions in each region, and promoting the balanced distribution and homogeneous development of medical resources in each region.

Fifth, the principle of balancing equity and efficiency. Equity and efficiency are fundamental to the government's agenda, with efficiency enabling the sustainability of health initiatives and equity reflecting the purpose of the health undertakings development. Thus, the formulation of health resource planning requires achieving a balance between equity and efficiency, optimizing resource usage while upholding universal access to health resources and health services, particularly for marginalized communities. Specifically, this involves securing universal access to basic medical and health services to promote fairness and justice, coupled with the optimized, cost-effective allocation and usage of health resources to harmonize equity and efficiency.

8.2 Formulation of China's Health Resource Planning

8.2.1 Health Resource Planning Targets

Health resource planning targets serve as metrics, quantitatively or qualitatively reflecting the efficacy of planning execution. They play a pivotal role in guiding regional health advancements, optimizing health resource allocation and activities, assessing health resource planning outcomes, bolstering health strategies and policies, propelling enhancements in health service quality, and safeguarding public health.

In China, health resource planning targets are bifurcated into two types: obligatory targets and anticipated targets. Obligatory targets denote compulsory targets to be attained by the planning cycle's conclusion, embodying the government's accountability, commitments, and directives to subordinate levels. Governments are duty-bound to harness public resources and administrative authority to guarantee the fulfillment of obligatory targets. Conversely, anticipated targets represent the government's desired achievements by the planning horizon, expressing its policy intent. Here, the government employs policy levers to orient, regulate, and mediate societal resources to attain or remain proximal to these benchmarks. The targets can further be categorized based on the type of health resources, encompassing health workforce allocation targets, targets of bed allocation in medical and health institutions, health expenditure allocation targets, and others.

Within health workforce allocation targets, quantitative and structural targets coexist. Notable targets consist of the number of health technicians per 1 000 population, reflecting the aggregate of locally active health professionals across various medical and health institutions, encompassing practitioners, assistant practitioners, registered nurses, lab technicians, and health supervisors, and excluding managerial staff; the number of practitioners and assistant practitioners per 1 000 population, pinpointing qualified physicians engaged in direct medical or preventive care, again excluding managerial staff per 1 000 population; the number of registered nurses per 1 000 population, indicating the count of certified nursing personnel per 1 000 population; the number of other health technical personnel (for specific types of specialized practitioners and public health practitioners, the numbers are generally calculated per 10 000 population, such as the number of mental health practitioners per 10 000 population and the number of pediatricians per 10 000 population); the composition and dispersion of the health workforce, mirroring the caliber and rationality of human workforce allocation, with health resource planning necessitating criteria for professional mix, educational attainment, and hierarchical titles.

　　Similarly, targets of bed allocation in medical and health institutions incorporate both quantitive and structural targets. Key targets encompass the number of beds in medical and health institutions per 1 000 population (allocation targets of total number of beds in medical and health institutions in one region) and the bed allocation structure and distribution. According to the current situation and existing problems of bed distribution in medical and health institutions in one region, supplementary targets may be introduced to meet the special needs, such as dedicated beds for rehabilitation, mental health, or pediatrics, either per 1 000 population or as a percentage of total beds. For instance, to invigorate social medical services, the "13th Five-Year Plan on Health and Wellness" targeted over 30% of hospital beds in social hospitals by 2020. To bolster primary health undertakings, the health resource planning may delineate bed capacities for medical and health institutions at various tiers (Table 8-1).

Table 8-1　The level of targets related to China's health resource planning in 2025

Main targets	Current situation in 2020	Goals for 2025	Target attribute
Number of beds in medical and health institutions per 1 000 population	6.46	7.40-7.50	Guided
Including: Municipal-level and above public hospitals	1.78	1.90-2.00	Guided
County-level public hospitals and primary medical and health institutions	2.96	3.50	Guided
Number of beds in public hospitals specialized in TCM per 1 000 population	0.68	0.85	Guided
Number of practitioners and assistant practitioners per 1 000 population	2.90	3.20	Anticipated
Number of practitioners and assistant practitioners of TCM per 1 000 population	0.48	0.62	Anticipated
Number of registered nurses per 1 000 population	3.34	3.80	Anticipated
Number of pharmacists per 1 000 population	0.35	0.54	Anticipated
Doctor to nurse ratio	1:1.15	1:1.20	Anticipated
Bed to health personnel ratio	1:1.48	1:1.62	Anticipated
Proportion of second-level and above general hospitals with geriatric medicine departments (%)	—	≥60.00	Anticipated

Continued

Main targets	Current situation in 2020	Goals for 2025	Target attribute
Suitable bed number for county-level general hospitals	—	600-1 000	Guided
Suitable bed number for municipal-level general hospitals	—	1 000-1 500	Guided
Suitable bed number for provincial-level and above general hospitals	—	1 500-3 000	Guided

Notes: 1. Hospital beds include beds in the same level of maternal and child health care hospitals and specialized disease prevention and treatment centers (institutes).

2. "Provincial-level hospitals" include those held by provinces, autonomous regions, and municipalities directly under the central government; "municipal-level and above hospitals" includes provincial-level and above hospitals and municipal-level hospitals, among which "municipal-level hospitals" include those held by prefecture-level cities, regions, prefectures, and leagues; "county-level hospitals" include those held by counties, county-level cities, municipal districts, and banners.

3. Suitable bed number refers to the bed number of a single practice point in a general hospital.

Source: National Health Commission

Health expenditure allocation targets are similarly composed of both quantitative and structural targets. Quantitative targets shed light on the magnitude and directional shifts in health spending, exemplified by the total health expenditure. Conversely, structural targets delve into the allocation and utilization patterns of health expenditure, along with the equity in health service provision, as illustrated by the proportion of government health expenditure within the total health expenditure (Table 8-2).

Table 8-2　Main targets for the development of national medical security in China during the 14th Five-Year Plan period

Category	Main targets	2020	2025	Target attribute
Insurance coverage	Basic medical insurance coverage rate (%)	>95	>95[1]	Obligatory
Fund security	Basic medical insurance (including maternity insurance) fund income (trillion yuan)	2.5	Income scale is more in line with the level of economic and social development	Anticipated
	Basic medical insurance (including maternity insurance) fund expenditure (trillion yuan)	2.1	Expenditure scale is more in line with the level of economic and social development, as well as the basic medical needs of the people	Anticipated

Continued

Category	Main targets	2020	2025	Target attribute
Guarantee level	Proportion of hospitalization expenses within the scope of basic medical insurance for urban employees (%)	85.2	Maintain stability	Anticipated
	Proportion of hospitalization expenses within the scope of basic medical insurance for rural and non-working urban residents (%)	70	Maintain stability	Anticipated
	Proportion of hospitalization medical expenses assistance for key beneficiaries meeting the regulations (%)	70	70	Anticipated
	Proportion of personal health expenditure to total health expenditure (%)	27.7	27	Obligatory
Fine management	Proportion of hospitalization expenses based on disease diagnosis related groups and diagnosis related groups to total hospitalization expenses (%)	—	70	Anticipated
	Proportion of the amount of drugs purchased by public medical institutions through provincial-level centralized procurement platforms to the total amount of drugs (excluding TCM decoction pieces) purchased (%)	Around 75	90	Anticipated
Fine management	Proportion of the amount of high-value medical consumables purchased by public medical institutions through provincial-level centralized procurement platforms to the total amount of high-value medical consumables purchased (%)	—	80	Anticipated
	Drugs procured through centralized volume-based purchasing (variety)	112	>500[2]	Anticipated
	High-value medical consumables procured through centralized volume-based purchasing (category)	1	>5[3]	Anticipated

Continued

Category	Main targets	2020	2025	Target attribute
High quality service	Direct settlement rate of hospitalization expenses across provinces [4] (%)	>50	>70	Anticipated
	Online availability rate of medical security government services (%)	—	80	Anticipated
	Availability rate of government service windows for medical security (%)	—	100	Obligatory

Notes: 1 refers to the basic medical insurance coverage rate maintained at over 95% annually during the 14th Five-Year Plan period.

2 refers to the centralized volume-based procurement of over 500 varieties of drugs at the national and provincial levels in various provinces (autonomous regions, municipalities directly under the central government) by 2025.

3 refers to the centralized volume-based procurement of high-value medical consumables at the national and provincial levels in various provinces (autonomous regions, municipalities directly under the central government) by 2025, with a quantity of 5 or more categories.

4 refers to the proportion of hospitalization expenses directly settled across provinces to the total number of inpatients seeking medical treatment across provinces and regions.

Source: General Office of the State Council of the People's Republic of China

Furthermore, the ambit of health resources extends to encompass elements such as facilities, equipment, information, and technological advancements. In China, governments at all levels customarily undertake the planning of substantial medical equipment, exemplified by stipulating the allocation of advanced apparatuses like electronic computed tomography scanners and magnetic resonance imaging machines on a per 10 000 population basis within a given region. In 2019, a pivotal initiative was launched by the National Health Commission and the National Administration of Traditional Chinese Medicine, unveiling the "National Standards and Norms for the Informatization Construction of Primary Medical and Health Institutions (Trial)." This comprehensive framework outlined a meticulous structure comprising 4 primary, 58 secondary, and 212 tertiary targets, including the target that primary medical and health institutions should provide internet-based medical and health services, and have eight functions such as appointment, payment, diagnosis and treatment suggestions, and doctor-patient communication.

8.2.2 Formulation Process of China's Health Resource Planning

In the formulation of the health resource planning by Chinese governments at various levels, a holistic approach is imperative, necessitating the thorough examination of both intrinsic and extraneous determinants. Health resource allocation targets must stem from an appraisal of the population's health service necessities, with a clear demarcation of the discrepancy between present conditions and anticipated objectives, guiding subsequent planning endeavors. The process initiates with a diagnostic phase of issues, succeeded by the drafting of a strategic blueprint. Upon approval, the establishment of steering and working committees follows, with defined roles, team training, and financial provisions set in place.

Phase Ⅰ: comprehensive health situation analysis. Initiating health resource planning necessitates an exhaustive examination of the health landscape, encompassing political, economic, social, and environmental dynamics. This analysis transcends the immediate health system, embracing the broader health industry evolution. It also goes beyond the immediate situation, including both past and future contexts. Data gathering could employ techniques like surveys, existing literature reviews, health record audits, and stakeholder symposia for a dynamic, multi-faceted analysis.

The Chinese health administrative departments' health situation analysis encompasses four dimensions: the present status analysis from natural, political, social, and economic perspectives, usually being carried out by common methods such as issue ranking, trend projection, standard analysis, and expert evaluation; retrospective analysis on population, disease, health service needs and demands, health resource utilization and so on; prospective analysis, that is, forward-looking forecasts on economic, demographic, and epidemiological trends; major obstacles analysis, namely, identification of barriers impeding health issue resolutions and industry progress to formulate targeted policies and measures.

The six commonly used analytical methodologies underpin this analysis process are as follows: descriptive analysis detailing the distribution and change pattern of health services or health events in a social population; factor analysis to identify issues and influencing factors in population health and health services via single-factor analysis and multiple-factor analysis; mathematical modeling analysis to elucidate functional relationships between health services and relevant influencing factors; systematic analysis treating health challenges as interconnected systems to analyze system elements, diagnose the issues, reveal the cause of the issues, and put forward the feasible solution to the issues; input-output analysis, including cost-benefit and cost-effectiveness analyses, to explain the relationship between health service input (health resources) and output (health service utilization); composite evaluation analysis to research on the correlations among population health status, health service needs, health resources, and health service utilization.

Phase Ⅱ: defining population health objectives. Objective-setting for health resource planning embodies the strategic intent of health administrative departments. The three-stage process adopted by health administrative departments when setting objectives includes outlining the thematic focus (the overall direction), pinpointing priority sectors and putting forward strategic initiatives and specific measures, and establishing core targets (qualitative and quantitative targets) that serve as a basis for post-evaluation according to the baseline level. Therefore, the objectives of health resource planning are hierarchical, forming a system composed of overarching objectives, specific objectives, and targets. The overarching objectives define the long-term orientation and development direction, reflecting the expected health outcomes for the population to be achieved during the planning period. Specific objectives include the characteristics, quality, quantity, time frames, and the population and regions involved. Targets are the concrete embodiment of the objectives and serve as the measures by which the achievement of the objectives are evaluated.

Phase Ⅲ: assessing health resource needs and setting planning objectives. This step entails understanding the type, volume, timing, and allocation of required resources. When formulating health resource planning, it is necessary to draw from principles like efficiency-driven investment and economically scaled planning, prioritizing existing resources before considering additional allocations, taking into account financial feasibility, respecting the opinions of financial personnel, and developing flexible planning. Then the health resource planning objectives should be determined based on the above assessment. Commonly used calculation methods include health service demand method, health need method, service objective method, and health resources to population ratio method. The 2020 document "National Health Commission Planning Management Measures (Trial)" specifies that the formulation of health and wellness plans should involve fundamental work such as conducting current situation surveys, gathering information, and conducting research studies. It emphasizes the importance of thoroughly investigating major issues, setting priority objectives, proposing significant projects and action measures, and conducting comprehensive evaluations. Preliminary foundational research is crucial for planning, while the development positioning of the planning is a prerequisite for its overall approach.

Phase Ⅳ: crafting resource development strategies and implementation steps. Four core strategies—self-reliance, social resource mobilization, financial channel broadening, and optimization of the allocation of existing health resources—are adopted. Implementation measures must detail content, rationale, scope, responsible entities, and timelines.

Phase V: supervision and assessment framework. This phase outlines four key steps: establishing planning implementation and evaluation bodies, defining roles and responsibilities, devising detailed execution plans, and creating assessment and monitoring mechanisms inclusive of defining the content, methodology, timelines, and responsible personnel for the implementation of the health resource planning.

Phase Ⅵ: budget presentation. The main considerations for preparing the budget for China's health resource planning are as follows: prioritizing key areas to ensure major objectives and health strategies are met; aligning the budget with local economic development levels, ensuring it does not exceed fiscal and individual payment capacities; conducting cost-benefit and cost-effectiveness analyses, directing more funds towards disease response activities and reserving funds for health resource distribution adjustments; for one-time investment budgets, conducting feasibility studies and considering maintenance costs and personnel salary increases; identifying funding sources, including self-owned funds; developing annual rolling budgets due to the long planning period.

Phase Ⅶ: feasibility assessment. After the draft plan for regional health resource planning is formed, it is necessary to organize relevant departments and experts from within and outside the region to review, discuss, and provide feedback on the draft plan. It is also important to communicate the core ideas of the draft plan to the public. A set of feasibility assessment targets should be established to provide experts participating in the evaluation with comparable information. The planning staff should avoid influencing or guiding the experts' opinions as much as possible. The draft plan should be revised, supplemented, and improved based on experts' feedback. If conditions permit, it is advisable to use computer simulations to test the feasibility of the draft plan before making further modifications to form the final draft plan for approval.

Phase Ⅷ: legislative approval. The planning concludes with adherence to legal protocols to have legal effect, which means the draft plan should be passed by the health resource planning leading group, validated by the people's government, and considered and adopted by the standing committees of the people's congresses. The process underscores the government's accountability, collaborative governance, health sector stewardship, societal engagement, and legal safeguards.

Case Study　The 14th Five-Year Plan for the Construction of China's Health Talent Team

Throughout the duration of the 13th Five-Year Plan, China witnessed a notable rise in both the aggregate and per capita numbers of its health personnel. By the conclusion of 2020, the country was home to 13.48 million health personnel, comprising 4.09 million practitioners and assistant practitioners and 4.71 million registered nurses. To bolster this momentum and reinforce the health talent pipeline, thereby furnishing robust human capital for the Healthy China Initiative, the National Health Commission unveiled the "14th Five-Year Plan for Health Talent Development" in August 2022. The overarching ambition for this plan is threefold: to propel enhancements in talent service capabilities alongside a more balanced talent structure, to refine talent management systems and mechanisms, and to foster a nurturing ecosystem conducive to talent growth. Main planning targets for health talent development during this strategic interval are encapsulated within Table 8-3.

Table 8-3　Main planning targets for health talent development in China during the 14th Five-Year Plan period

Main targets	Unit	2020	2025
Total number of personnel	10 000 people	1 347.5	1 600
Practitioners and assistant practitioners	people/1 000 population	2.90	3.20
Practitioners and assistant practitioners of TCM	people/1 000 population	0.48	0.62
Registered nurses	people/1 000 population	3.34	3.80
Pharmacists	people/1 000 population	0.35	0.54
General practitioners	people/10 000 population	2.90	3.93
Professional public health institution personnel	10 000 people	92.5	120

1. Talent Allocation

Strengthen the development of health technical professionals. Focusing on the allocation of practitioners and nurses, personnel numbers and composition are calibrated based on health service demands and practitioner workload standards. Expand practitioner ranks to reach 4. 5 million practitioners and assistant practitioners by 2025. Reinforce nursing staff to achieve 5. 5 million registered nurses by 2025. Elevate pharmacist allocation and training to reach 770 000 pharmacists in medical and health institutions. Bolster technical expertise in medical imaging, laboratory, pathology, etc. , and define allocation norms, roles, competencies, and professional standards.

Strengthen the development of public health workforce. By 2025, the number of personnel in professional public health institutions should reach 1. 2 million, with 250 000 in disease control and prevention institutions. Set up public health positions scientifically, adjust the structure of senior, intermediate, and junior positions in public health institutions, increase the proportion of intermediate and senior positions, and improve the compensation and benefits of personnel.

Strengthen the development of primary health workforce. Accelerate the training of general practitioners, aiming to reach 550 000 general practitioners by 2025, with 3. 93 general practitioners per 10 000 population. Strengthen the development of village clinic workforce, promote the transition of village doctors to practitioners and assistant practitioners, and by 2025, have approximately 45% of village doctors as practitioners or assistant practitioners.

Strengthen the development of TCM workforce. By 2025, the number of practitioners and assistant practitioners of TCM should reach 0. 62 per 1 000 population, with 150 000 TCM pharmacists nationwide. Establish a talent training model that aligns with the characteristics of TCM, promote TCM talent development through major projects, and implement the TCM Special Talent Training Program (Qihuang Program).

Strengthen the development of workforce to address population aging. Actively respond to population aging and changes in population policy, and meet the health service needs of key groups such as the elderly, pregnant women, and infants. Coordinate the allocation of various talent resources for prevention, medical care, nursing, rehabilitation, and palliative care. Strengthen the development of talent for elderly health services, childcare services, and maternal and child health services.

2. Talent Cultivation

Develop a clinical medicine talent training system with "5 + 3" as the main structure and "3+2" as the supplement. Improve the on-the-job training system and encourage village doctors to participate in formal education. Increase support for higher medical schools in central and western regions, and reduce disparities in training levels between regions, institutions, and disciplines.

Implement a high-level medical talent program to focus on cultivating a group of leading clinical medicine professionals who work on the front lines of medical care, possess excellent medical skills, and are capable of successfully diagnosing and treating difficult and critical conditions. Additionally, these professionals should have significant scientific value, notable social benefits, substantial social impact, and be recognized by peers. By 2025, the full-time equivalent of 180 000 medical research and development personnel in the health system should reach 180 000 annually. Utilize national high-level young talent programs, medical science and technology innovation platforms, and science and technology projects to foster high-level, innovative, and multi-disciplinary clinical talents and build outstanding young innovation teams. Continue to improve the selection of young and middle-aged experts with outstanding contributions, and categorize high-level talents effectively.

Adapt to changes in disease spectrum and medical service needs by focusing on enhancing the training and development of clinical specialists in critical care, oncology, cardiovascular and cerebrovascular diseases, and other key areas. Prioritize support for diseases with high provincial mortality rates and high referral rates by enhancing technical and talent support from national-level high-quality hospitals to provincial-level hospitals, addressing gaps in specialized disciplines, and improving diagnostic and treatment capabilities at the provincial level. Strengthen the talent development in county-level medical institutions, with a focus on building specialist teams in oncology, cardiovascular, and cerebrovascular fields.

3. Talent Utilization

Improve the personnel mechanism for public institutions, and implement open recruitment and competitive appointments. Deepen the reform of the income distribution system in public hospitals, implementing a performance-based approach where more effort leads to more rewards and higher performance results in better compensation. Innovate the management model for public medical and health institutions' staffing, reasonably determine the total number of personnel, and make dynamic adjustments. Explore various personnel mechanisms and government service purchase methods.

Enhance the three-stage medical talent training system, including college education, post-graduate education, and continuing education, with organic connections and standardized norms. Improve medical education quality based on industry demand to balance the supply and demand of medical talents.

Reasonably develop personnel staffing standards for public medical and health institutions and establish a dynamic evaluation and adjustment mechanism. Strengthen talent collaboration between hospitals, primary medical and health institutions, and professional public health institutions. Improve professional title evaluation standards, enhance title management and service methods, adhere to the principle of demand-based use, refine job settings, and clarify job responsibilities, qualification requirements, and competency standards. Expand the autonomy of medical and health institutions in job settings and personnel hiring, optimize the job structure, and increase the proportion of intermediate and senior professional and technical positions.

Establish a sound compensation system suited to the characteristics of the medical and health industry. Improve the income and expenditure structure of public hospitals, increasing the proportion of personnel expenses. Optimize the compensation structure for medical staff, raising the level of guaranteed wages. Allow public health institutions to exceed current salary control levels for public institutions. Implement performance-based salary policies for primary medical and health institutions to improve the income levels of primary health personnel.

9 Health Financing and Total Health Expenditure in China

The contradiction between limited health resources and people's increasing need for health services will always exist. Health financing is not merely about raising funds but also effectively allocating and utilizing them. Securing adequate funds and their effective allocation and utilization is crucial for the efficient operation of the health service system and maximizing its functional effectiveness. Based on its developmental history and current state, China has adopted a government-led, multi-source collaborative financing strategy. According to the *China Health Statistical Yearbook 2022*, in 2021, Chinese total health expenditure was 7 684.5 billion yuan, accounting for 6.72% of the GDP. Personal health expenditure accounted for 27.60%, which is below the global average with per capita health expenditure at 5 440.0 yuan.

This chapter covers three major areas: health financing in China, allocation and utilization of health funds in China, and total health expenditure.

9.1 Health Financing in China

As previously mentioned, health resources encompass the aggregate of various elements utilized or consumed in the provision of health services, including health human resources and health material resources. Health funds are the monetary expression of health resources, which flows into the health field in monetary form and then achieves its consumption and compensation through various forms of health services, thus flowing out of the health sector and producing the improvement of the health of the population. This process is known as the movement of health funds. In a sense, studying health financing involves examining the patterns of fund movements within the health sector.

9.1.1 Overview of Health Financing

9.1.1.1 The Concept of Health Financing

The World Health Organization defines health financing activities as the total activities of raising, allocating, and utilizing funds for health in a way that is adequate, fair, and efficient. This includes four aspects: how funds are raised for health services, how funds are allocated and how services are organized, how the efficiency of fund utilization is enhanced, and how to control the unreasonable increase of health expenditure. Health financing entails the activities of raising funds for health services and studying the collection, reasonable allocation, and effective utilization of funds within a certain period and social context. It involves fund-raising, risk-sharing, and service purchasing functions. Evaluation of health financing mainly focuses on assessing different financing methods.

9.1.1.2 Objectives of Health Financing

The World Health Organization and United Nations Children's Fund proposed the primary health care (PHC) strategy in the "Declaration of Alma-Ata" in 1978, urging countries to provide their residents with the most basic, universally accessible, socially equitable, and affordable for both the public and the government health care services. The objectives of health financing include both intermediate objectives and ultimate objectives. The intermediate objectives focus on equity, efficiency, risk sharing, and sustainability of health financing, while the ultimate objectives include improving health status, financial risk protection, and patient satisfaction.

9.1.2 Raising of Health Funds in China

9.1.2.1 Health Financing Sources in China

Internationally, sources of health financing are divided into two major categories: public health expenditure and private health expenditure. The former, also known as broad government health expenditure, can be further subdivided into government budget (tax revenue) and social health insurance expenditure, reflecting the role of government organizations and institutions as funding entities in health financing. Private health expenditure refers to funds raised by individuals or their employers through voluntary health insurance or community insurance (not government-sponsored or mandatory), including commercial health insurance expenditure and personal health expenditure; costs incurred by non-governmental health institutions are also included in private health expenditure.

In China, government health expenditure, social health expenditure, and personal health expenditure are the three main sources of total health expenditure. Government health expenditure includes expenses at all government levels for medical and health services (including medical services and public health services), medical insurance administrative affairs, and other government investments in the medical and health sector. Social health expenditure refers to contributions to health from all sectors of society excluding government spending, including social medical security payments (excluding government subsidies), commercial health insurance premiums, social donations, fees from privately-run medical institutions, and administrative and public service fee revenue. Personal health expenditure refers to cash payments made by residents when receiving various medical and health services. Figure 9-1 shows a comparison of health financing sources in China with international health financing sources, and Figure 9-2 illustrates changes in the structure of health financing in China from 2000 to 2021.

	Category		Specific content	Category	
International health financing sources	Public health expenditure (broad government health expenditure)	Government budget (tax revenue)	Government expenditure on medical services, public health services, health surveillance, etc.	Government health expenditure	Health financing sources in China
		Social health insurance expenditure	Government subsidies for social health insurance1		
			Social health insurance premiums paid by individuals (and their employers)	Social health expenditure	
	Private health expenditure	Commercial health insurance expenditure	Commercial health insurance premiums		
		Other non-governmental organization expenditure	Non- governmental organization health expenditures and social donations, etc.		
		Personal health expenditure	Residents' cash payments when receiving medical and health services	Personal health expenditure	

Figure 9-1 Comparison of health financing sources in China with international health financing sources

Note: 1 refers to basic medical insurance for urban employees and basic
medical insurance for rural and non-working urban residents.

Source: *Health Systems in Transition* by Meng Qingyue et al. ,2015

9.1.2.2 Chinese Statutory Health Financing System

Chinese statutory health financing system covers basic medical insurance, medical assistance and disease emergency assistance systems, public health systems, and major illness insurance for urban and rural residents. Among them, basic medical insurance and the medical assistance system together form the basic medical security system covering both urban and rural residents. Specifically, employees in urban areas are covered by basic medical insurance for urban employees, while non-working urban residents and rural residents are covered by basic medical insurance for rural and non-working urban residents. The medical assistance and disease emergency assistance systems act as a safety net for impoverished populations in urban and rural areas, subsidizing the cost of basic medical insurance and providing further aid for medical expenses not covered by basic medical insurance after reimbursement. The public health systems are primarily funded by the governments and offer basic public health services free of charge to all residents. The major illness insurance for urban

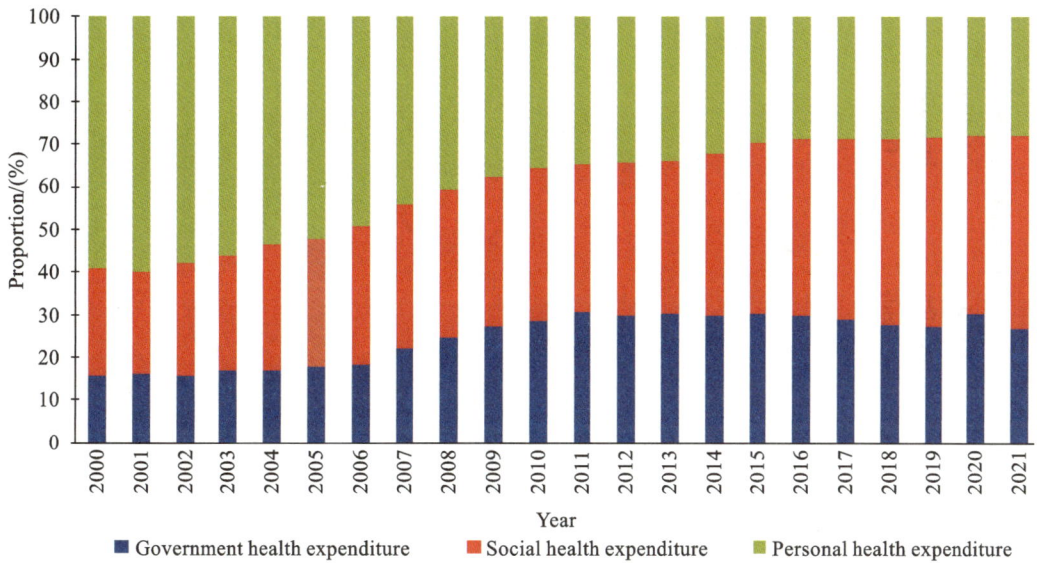

Figure 9-2   Changes in the structure of health financing in China from 2000 to 2021
Source:China Health Statistical Yearbook 2022

and rural residents is an institutional arrangement that provides further protection against high medical costs incurred by patients with serious illnesses. Table 9-1 provides an overview of Chinese statutory health financing system.

9.2   Allocation and Utilization of Health Funds in China

Once health funds have been mobilized,the next task is how they are utilized and for whom,which determines who has access to health services,what type of health services are accessed,and the quantity and quality of health services. Governments need to consider in which institutions to invest,and for which services within an institution they should invest. The question of how to fulfil the functions of health financing to promote effective service delivery in the health service system and the improvement of the overall health of the population is not only a question in the field of economics,but also,to a large extent,a political,social and ethical one.

9.2.1   Overview of Allocation and Utilization of Health Funds

The allocation of health funds involves scientifically and rationally optimizing the allocation of health funds through government macro-control and market regulation, ultimately directing them towards various sectors of the health service system. The structure of health fund allocation describes where health resources ultimately flow,including

Table 9-1　Overview of Chinese statutory health financing system

System		Coverage			Financing			Utilization of funds
		Scope (population)	Breadth (services)[1]	Depth (costs)[1]	Government health expenditure	Social insurance fees	Fiscal transfer payments	Medical insurance funds[1]
Basic medical insurance	Basic medical insurance for urban employees	Urban employees	Inpatient, outpatient, and retail drug costs at designated institutions	There are starting payment criteria, co-payment and maximum payment limits for eligible fees listed on the insurance medicines/medical service/diagnostic and treatment items catalog		Individuals and employers jointly bear at least 2% and 6% of employee wages, respectively		Individual accounts + social pooling funds
	Basic medical insurance for rural and non-working urban residents[2]	Non-working urban residents (including students) and rural residents	Mainly inpatient, whereas outpatient services are also covered in eligible areas		✓	Premiums paid by individuals and government subsidies	✓	Social pooling funds
Medical assistance and disease emergency assistance systems		Impoverished population			✓		✓	
Public health systems		All residents			✓		✓	
Major illness insurance for urban and rural residents						✓		Major illness insurance social pooling funds

Notes: 1 indicates differences exist between regions and medical insurance systems.

2 is managed and subsidized by central and local governments. Despite its voluntary nature, it is essentially considered a public or social insurance, hence included under social health expenditure.

Source: *Health Systems in Transition* by Meng Qingyue et al., 2015

which institutions, projects, or regions. The main users of health funds include hospitals, community health institutions, and public health institutions, which are both payees of health funds and providers of health services. Expenditures take various forms, such as diagnostic and treatment fees, inspection fees, medication fees, health education fees, preventive care fees, and construction fees of public health emergency response institutions.

9.2.2 Structure of Health Fund Allocation in China

9.2.2.1 Integration of Health Funds in China

(1) Fiscal Transfer Payments

In 1994, China established a tax-sharing fiscal management system and a corresponding transfer payment system. There are two basic types of transfer payments: general transfer payments and special transfer payments. The Central Committee of the Communist Party of China issues general transfer payments to ensure funding for welfare sectors like education and social security. Special transfer payments are allocated by the Central Committee of the Communist Party of China to achieve specific policy goals and development strategies, or to compensate local governments for delegated tasks, with local finances required to utilize the funds according to specified purposes.

(2) Medical Insurance Funds

China manages its two major basic medical insurance funds separately, settling accounts with medical institutions within designated pooling areas. These funds are centrally managed by medical insurance administrative institutions and are uniformly adjusted to cover expenses such as medication fees, surgery fees, nursing fees, and basic diagnostic fees for insured individuals. Medical insurance management departments in these pooling areas annually prepare budget forecasts for revenue and expenditure. Revenue budgets consider factors such as local economic development, wage levels, insurance coverage, and financing ratios. Expenditure budgets take into account the age structure of the insured, disease spectrum, growth in medical costs, benefit coverage, security levels, and fund balances.

The basic medical insurance for urban employees implements the management of designated medical institutions and retail pharmacies. Individual accounts can be used to cover the individual's share of general outpatient expenses and hospitalization costs, and drugs purchased at designated retail pharmacies. They may also be used to cover eligible medical expenses for family members who have been linked through the family pooling system. The social pooling funds pay for inpatient medical expenses, outpatient treatment for serious illnesses that comply with regulations, and gradually included general outpatient expenses. Medical expenses below the deductible are paid from individual accounts or out-of-pocket; costs above the deductible and below the maximum payment limit are primarily paid by social pooling funds, with the individual bearing a certain percentage. The specific deductible, maximum payment limit, and the individual's share of expenses between these thresholds of social pooling funds are determined by the pooling area. In China, there are different provisions for different levels of medical institutions in the setting of the deductible. Typically, first-level hospitals have the lowest deductibles, followed by second-level hospitals, with third-level hospitals having the highest. A similar trend exists for co-payment ratios, with first-level hospitals having the lowest co-payment rates (highest reimbursement rates), thus encouraging patients to seek treatment at appropriate levels and utilize health resources efficiently.

The national basic medical insurance drug catalog, diagnosis and treatment item catalog, and medical service facility catalog, along with respective management methods, define the scope and standards for basic medical services. The national basic medical insurance drug catalog is divided into Class A and Class B. Class A drugs, which are uniformly standardized across China, are included in the basic medical insurance fund's payment scope and are reimbursed according to the payment standards of the basic medical insurance. Class B drugs, where the insurance fund covers part of the cost, require the patient to pay a certain proportion of the expenses before being included in the insurance fund's payment scope and reimbursed according to the payment standards of the basic medical insurance. The "National Basic Medical Insurance, Work Injury Insurance, and Maternity Insurance Drug List (2022)" includes a total of 2 967 drugs, consisting of 1 586 Western medicines and 1 381 Chinese patent medicines.

(3) Medical Assistance Fund

Medical assistance is financed through government appropriations and social donations, catering to the different medical needs of the assisted individuals. Medical assistance includes subsidizing the individual contribution to basic medical insurance for rural and non-working urban residents and further subsidizing unaffordable out-of-pocket expenses for individuals and their families that remain after payments from basic medical insurance, major illness insurance, and other supplementary insurance. Members of urban and rural low-income households, households enjoying "five guarantees" and other registered impoverished residents automatically qualify for medical assistance. Using relevant documentation, they only need to pay the out-of-pocket part at designated medical institutions, with the rest covered by medical assistance fund and settled immediately with the institutions. Unregistered eligible beneficiaries must initially pay the full medical costs and later apply for reimbursement from civil affairs departments.

(4) Disease Emergency Assistance Fund

Since 2013, provincial-level and municipal-level governments in China have been establishing disease emergency assistance fund at their respective levels, encouraging contributions from all sectors of society. The fund aids patients within China suffering from acute, severe illnesses or injuries who need emergency care but cannot pay and whose identities may be unknown. For eligible emergency treatment expenses, medical institutions can apply for subsidies from the disease emergency assistance fund, which implements direct payment. Fund management institutions review and summarize payment applications from medical institutions before submitting them to the corresponding financial departments for disbursement from social security funds directly to the medical institutions.

9.2.2.2 Services Purchased with Health Funds in China

(1) Basic Medical Services

According to the regulations of basic medical insurance, patients can only receive reimbursements from the medical insurance fund when they seek treatment at designated medical institutions or pharmacies. Patients use their social security cards to directly claim reimbursements from the fund. At non-designated institutions or pharmacies, insured individuals can receive medical services at their own expense.

Basic medical insurance involves setting deductibles, co-payment ratios, and maximum payment limits to share medical costs with patients. For service providers, medical insurance institutions implement prior approvals, concurrent reviews, and post-use audits to reduce unnecessary services provided by medical institutions. Some regions have experimented with payment methods such as service unit, capitation, and total budget control to grant medical institutions greater financial autonomy. Medical insurance administrative institutions manage designated medical institutions and retail pharmacies through the establishment and implementation of designated service agreements. These agreements regulate the management of designated medical institutions and retail pharmacies and clarify the rights and obligations of these institutions and pharmacies and the medical insurance administrative agencies.

(2) Public Health Services

Government and community-driven medical and health institutions that meet certain standards and requirements and have the requisite service capabilities can apply to provide public health services. To ensure that residents in the same area have access to essentially equal public health services, local governments and relevant departments determine the public health services for their jurisdiction as the content of government service purchase based on local economic and social development, fiscal payment capacity, and residents' basic public health needs. Individual public health services, such as immunization plans, may be funded by calculating the per capita cost of service recipients to determine fixed subsidies per unit. Group public health services, such as health education, may have their comprehensive costs calculated to set comprehensive project subsidies or package all public health service projects into a single comprehensive project subsidy.

The flow of health funds in China is illustrated in Figure 9-3.

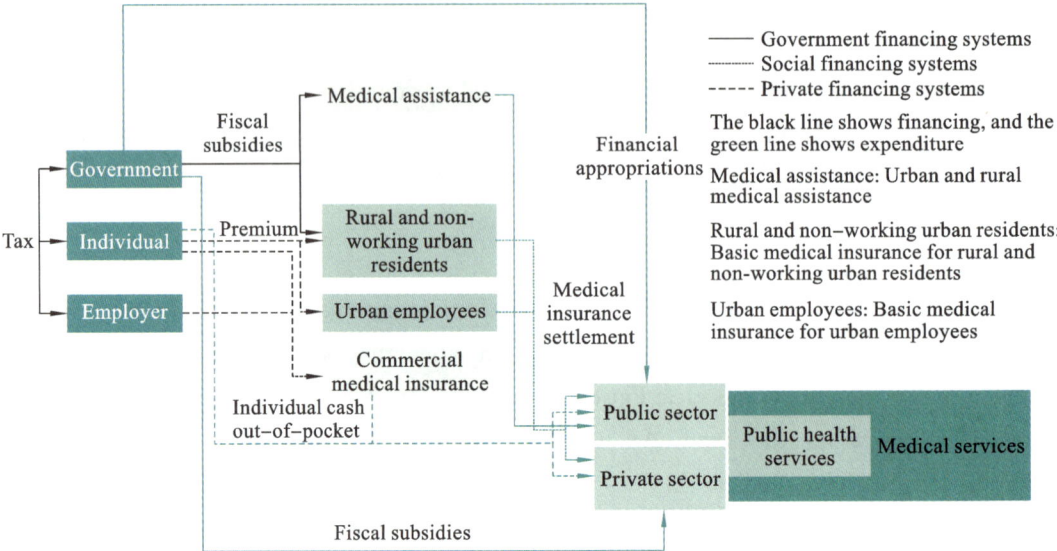

Figure 9-3　The flow of health funds in China

9.2.3　Main Users of Health Funds in China

9.2.3.1　Medical Institutions

In China, the financing of public health services is primarily through fiscal appropriations from local health departments, which are distributed based on capitation. Some paid service items are directly charged to the users (such as flu vaccines, which are not included in the national basic public health services). For some primary health care services and emergency services, public medical institutions may receive partial budget allocations from local health departments and charge patients based on service items. If the patient is insured, local medical insurance funds settle accounts with the institutions using mixed payment methods. In terms of medical cost settlement, the service recipient (patient) pays according to service items, and this payment method is also applied to basic medical insurance fund payments, as shown in Table 9-2.

Table 9-2　Payment mechanisms for providers

Provider	Payer				
	Local government	Local social medical insurance fund[1]	Private/Commercial medical insurance	Cost sharing	Direct payment
Primary public medical institutions	Subsidy	Mixed payment[2] (globe budget, capitation, fixed quota, fee-for-service, etc.)	Fee-for-service	Fee-for-service	Fee-for-service

Continued

Provider	Payer				
	Local government	Local social medical insurance fund[1]	Private/Commercial medical insurance	Cost sharing	Direct payment
Second-level and third-level public medical institutions	Subsidy	Mixed payment[2] (globe budget, fee-for-service, etc.)	Fee-for-service	Fee-for-service	Fee-for-service
Private medical institutions	None	Mixed payment[2]/None	Fee-for-service	Fee-for-service	Fee-for-service
Retail pharmacies	None	Fee-for-service	None	Fee-for-service	Fee-for-service
Public health service institutions or medical institutions providing preventive services	Subsidy	None/Fee-for-service	None/Fee-for-service	None/Fee-for-service	Fee-for-service for paid services

Notes: 1 typically includes capitation for outpatient services, service unit for inpatient services, with both globe budget and fee-for-service applicable to both outpatient and inpatient services.

2 refers to the use of mixed payment methods for different service types under a medical insurance system (e. g. , capitation for outpatient services, globe budget for inpatient services).

Source: *Health System in Transition* by Meng Qingyue et al. , 2015

In 2011, the Ministry of Human Resources and Social Security released the "Opinions of the Ministry of Human Resources and Social Security on Further Advancing the Reform of Medical Insurance Payment Methods," which outlined the current objectives of the payment method reform as follows: to enhance total budget control through the management of fund budgets and to explore the payment method of globe budget. Building on this foundation, the reform seeks to explore capitation in conjunction with the implementation of outpatient pooling, and DRGs in conjunction with the security offered for major diseases in both inpatient and outpatient settings. The plan involves establishing and improving the negotiation and consultation mechanisms between medical insurance administrative institutions and medical institutions, along with risk-sharing mechanisms, to gradually develop a payment system that aligns with the evolution of the basic medical insurance system, emphasizing both incentives and constraints.

9.2.3.2　Medical Staff

In China, medical staff, as employees of hospitals, have their salaries and benefits closely tied to the medical institutions they work for, with human resource costs primarily compensated through service revenues. Beyond the basic salary, workload has historically been a major criterion for assessing medical staff's bonus income. Theoretically, performance metrics, patient satisfaction, and the completion rate of medical insurance indicators have been progressively included in evaluations, significantly impacting the bonus income of medical staff. With the advancement of health system reforms, the "Opinions of the Central Committee of the Communist Party of China and the State Council on Deepening the Reforms of the Medical and Health System" proposed implementing a comprehensive performance appraisal and job performance wage system focusing primarily on service quality and workload to effectively motivate medical staff.

Starting from October 1, 2009, public health institutions and primary medical and health institutions in China began implementing performance wage reforms, with the full implementation of the performance wage system by 2010. Central and local governments provide fiscal subsidies for the reform of the performance wage system. Performance wages are divided into two parts: basic performance wages and bonus performance wages. Basic performance wages, constituting about 60% to 70% of the total performance wages, reflect factors such as regional economic development, price levels, and job responsibilities, and are generally issued monthly. Bonus performance wages primarily reflect workload and actual contributions and are disbursed based on assessment results, allowing for flexible distribution methods and approaches. Depending on the circumstances, performance wages may include position allowances and comprehensive goal assessment rewards. Over the long term, the setting of performance wages helps to curb excessive prescribing and other irrational medical behaviors, enhancing efficiency, service quality, and patient satisfaction. However, the negative effects of performance wages cannot be overlooked, as it could erode trust between colleagues and weaken team cohesion.

9.3　Total Health Expenditure

9.3.1　Overview of Total Health Expenditure

Total health expenditure is a comprehensive monetary measure used to reflect the total amount of financial resources raised by the whole society for health services within a specific period (typically one year) in a country or region. It includes recurrent health expenditures and fixed capital formation costs. Recurrent health expenditures represent the monetary value of all medical and health products and services ultimately consumed by residents within the accounting period. Fixed capital formation costs refer to the value of assets acquired by health service providers (net of the disposal value of similar assets) within the accounting period, which are repeatedly used or have a useful life of more than one year in the provision of health services.

Total health expenditure is a societal concept, encapsulating all health care spending by the whole society, including internal expenditures within the health sector as well as those by other units and individuals. It also includes gratuitous aid and donations to the health sector from various community groups and international organizations. Total health expenditure serves as an informational tool capable of effectively analyzing and evaluating the equity and efficiency of a nation's or health system's performance, providing crucial information and objective evidence for government health policy decisions.

9.3.2 Health Expenditure Accounting

The System of Health Accounts (SHA) aligns with the principles and systems of national economic accounting, targeting the entire health system to establish health expenditure accounting indicators and an accounting framework, specifically to study the financial operations within the health system. SHA allows for the calculation of a country or region's health expenditures and guides the accounting of sub-accounts in health, such as disease expenditures, expenditures by different age groups, public health expenditures, and pharmaceutical expenditures.

SHA divides the dimensions of health expenditure accounting into core and extended dimensions based on the funding, production, and consumption phases of medical and health services. Core dimensions include service functions, service providers, and financing schemes, addressing three fundamental questions: what types of medical and health products and services are consumed, which health service providers deliver these products and services, and which financing schemes compensate for these products and services. The funding phase of the extended dimensions further clarifies where the funds for the funding schemes originate and how they are raised. The production phase addresses the resource costs and capital investments consumed by health service providers in producing medical and health products and services, while the consumption phase answers who consumes the medical and health products and services, including the distribution of health expenditures by disease, age, gender, region, and economic status. Health expenditure accounting methods include source-based method, institution-based method, function-based method, expenditure-based method, and matrix balancing accounting method, with adjustments made by countries based on their existing systems and health policy analysis needs. The SHA2011 accounting framework is shown in Figure 9-4.

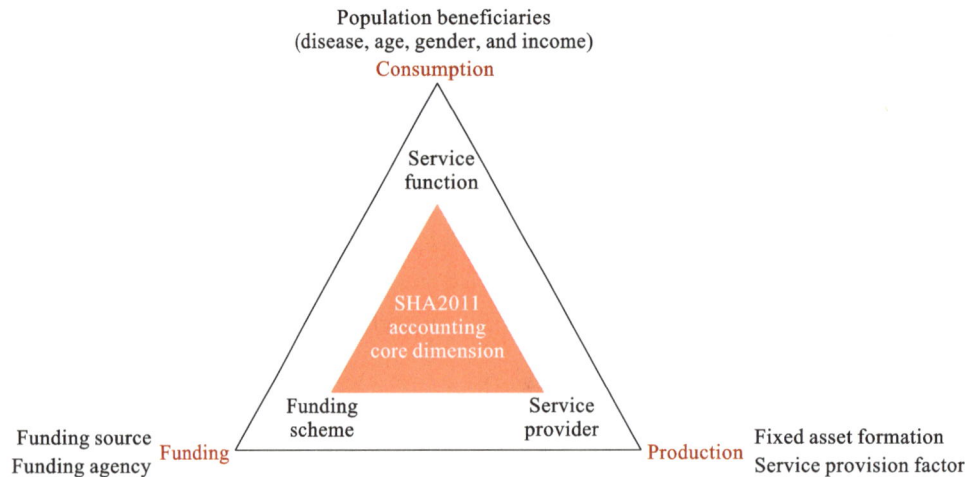

Figure 9-4 The SHA2011 accounting framework

9.3.3 Total Health Expenditure in China

In 2021, the total funding for health expenditure in China reached 7 684.5 billion yuan, accounting for 6.72% of the GDP. The per capita health expenditure was 5 440.0 yuan. According to the classification of financing, in 2021, the government health expenditure was 2 067.6 billion yuan, accounting for 26.91% of the total health expenditure; social health expenditure was 3 496.33 billion yuan, accounting for 45.50% of the total health expenditure; personal health expenditure reached 2 120.57 billion yuan, making up 27.60% of the total health expenditure.

From 1980 to 2021, the average annual growth rate of Chinese total health expenditure was 16.57%; the proportion of total health expenditure relative to GDP increased from 3.15% to 6.72%, with an average annual growth rate of 1.87%.

Over the same period, the share of government health expenditure in total health expenditure decreased from 36.24% to 26.91%; social health expenditure's share increased from 42.57% to 45.50%; personal health expenditure's share rose from 21.19% to 27.60%.

The basic information of Chinese total health expenditure from 1980 to 2021 is shown in Table 9-3.

Table 9-3　Chinese total health expenditure from 1980 to 2021

Year	Total health expenditure (100 million yuan)				Composition of total health expenditure (%)			Urban and rural health expenditure (100 million yuan)		Per capita health expenditure (yuan)			Total health expenditure as a percentage of GDP (%)
	Total	Government health expenditure	Social health expenditure	Personal health expenditure	Government health expenditure	Social health expenditure	Personal health expenditure	Urban	Rural	Total	Urban	Rural	
1980	143.23	51.91	60.97	30.35	36.24	42.57	21.19			14.5			3.15
1985	279.00	107.65	91.96	79.39	38.58	32.96	28.46			26.4			3.09
1990	747.39	187.28	293.10	267.01	25.06	39.22	35.73	396.00	351.39	65.4	158.8	38.8	3.96
1995	2 155.13	387.34	767.81	999.98	17.97	35.63	46.40	1 239.50	915.63	177.9	401.3	112.9	3.51
2000	4 586.63	709.52	1 171.94	2 705.17	15.47	25.55	58.98	2 624.24	1 962.39	361.9	813.7	214.7	4.57
2005	8 659.91	1 552.53	2 586.41	4 520.98	17.93	29.87	52.21	6 305.57	2 354.34	662.3	1 126.4	315.8	4.62
2006	9 843.34	1 778.86	3 210.92	4 853.56	18.07	32.62	49.31	7 174.73	2 668.61	748.8	1 248.3	361.9	4.49
2007	11 573.97	2 581.58	3 893.72	5 098.66	22.31	33.64	44.05	8 968.70	2 605.27	876.0	1 516.3	358.1	4.29
2008	14 535.40	3 593.94	5 065.60	5 875.86	24.73	34.85	40.42	11 251.90	3 283.50	1 094.5	1 861.8	455.2	4.55
2009	17 541.92	4 816.26	6 154.49	6 571.16	27.46	35.08	37.46	13 535.61	4 006.31	1 314.3	2 176.6	562.0	5.03
2010	19 980.39	5 732.49	7 196.61	7 051.29	28.69	36.02	35.29	15 508.62	4 471.77	1 490.1	2 315.5	666.3	4.85
2011	24 345.91	7 464.18	8 416.45	8 465.28	30.66	34.57	34.80	18 571.87	5 774.04	1 804.5	2 697.5	879.4	4.99

Continued

Year	Total health expenditure (100 million yuan)				Composition of total health expenditure (%)			Urban and rural health expenditure (100 million yuan)		Per capita health expenditure (yuan)			Total health expenditure as a percentage of GDP (%)
	Total	Government health expenditure	Social health expenditure	Personal health expenditure	Government health expenditure	Social health expenditure	Personal health expenditure	Urban	Rural	Total	Urban	Rural	
2012	28 119.00	8 431.98	10 030.70	9 656.32	29.99	35.67	34.34	21 280.46	6 838.54	2 068.8	2 999.3	1 064.8	5.22
2013	31 668.95	9 545.81	11 393.79	10 729.34	30.10	36.00	33.90	23 644.95	8 024.00	2 316.2	3 234.1	1 274.4	5.34
2014	35 312.40	10 579.23	13 437.75	11 295.41	29.96	38.05	31.99	26 575.60	8 736.80	2 565.5	3 558.3	1 412.2	5.49
2015	40 974.64	12 475.28	16 50671	11 992.65	30.45	40.29	29.27	31 297.85	9 676.79	2 962.2	4 058.5	1 603.6	5.95
2016	46 344.88	13 910.31	19 096.68	13 337.90	30.01	41.21	28.78	35 458.01	10 886.87	3 328.6	4 471.5	1 846.1	6.21
2017	52 598.28	15 205.87	22 258.81	15 133.60	28.91	42.32	28.77			3 756.7			6.32
2018	59 121.91	16 399.13	25 810.78	16 911.99	27.74	43.66	28.61			4 206.7			6.43
2019	65 841.39	18 016.95	29 150.57	18 673.87	27.36	44.27	28.36			4 669.3			6.67
2020	72 175.00	21 941.90	30 273.67	19 959.43	30.40	41.94	27.65			5 111.1			7.12
2021	76 844.99	20 676.06	34 963.26	21 205.67	26.91	45.50	27.60			5 440.0			6.72

Notes: 1. This table shows accounting figures, and figures of 2001 are the preliminary accounting figures.

2. The figures are calculated on the prices of the indicated years.

3. Since 2001, the total health expenditure does not include funds for higher medical education, and since 2006, it includes funds for urban and rural medical assistance.

Source: *China Health Statistical Yearbook 2022*

10 Legal System and Supervision of Medicine and Health in China

Medical and health services are closely related to the health of billions of people and the well-being of countless households, making themselves a significant issue of people's livelihood. Deepening the medical and health system reform, accelerating the development of medical and health services, strengthening the construction of the legal system and supervision of medicine and health, adapting to the growing medicine and health demand of the people, and continuously improving the health quality of the people are inevitable requirements for implementing the Scientific Outlook on Development and promoting comprehensive, balanced, and sustainable economic and social development. They are also crucial measures to safeguard social fairness and justice, and enhance people's quality of life, and an important task in building a moderately prosperous society in all respects and a harmonious socialist society.

10. 1   Overview of China's Legal System for Medicine and Health

10. 1. 1   Concept and Characteristics of China's Legal System for Medicine and Health

The legal system for medicine and health in China refers to the total of legal norms that regulate various social relationships arising from citizens' health affairs. As an important component of China's legal system, it has the general properties of laws, such as normativity, state compulsion, state will, universality, and justifiability, as well as its own unique characteristics.

10. 1. 1. 1   Legislative Characteristics of China's Legal System for Medicine and Health

As China's health legal system gradually improves, the country's legal system for medicine and health has gradually become an essential component of the socialist legal system. First, China's legal system for medicine and health is constantly being refined and perfected around the core content of citizens' health rights and interests, demonstrating strong professionalism, scientific rigor, and technical expertise. Second, problem-oriented system improvement has become a new characteristic of China's legal system for medicine and health. As the systems at the level of health laws and administrative regulations tend to stabilize, the implementation of China's legal system for medicine and health and the issues arising from its implementation, as well as the revisions and even legislation driven by the feedback of implementation effects, have become the main topics in the construction of China's legal system for medicine and health. Additionally, significant progress has been made in the legal construction of TCM in China, elevating it to the level of a national development strategy and moving towards modernization.

10.1.1.2 Enforcement Characteristics of China's Legal System for Medicine and Health

First, the implementation of China's legal system for medicine and health are distinctly policy-oriented. Various specific measures are issued in the form of policies, and overall planning and special actions are implemented through policy methods. Second, the implementation of this system is grounded in the standard system. As an essential component of China's legal system for medicine and health, medical and health standards provide guidance for the implementation of this system. Third, the legal construction of China's drug regulatory system has been steadily advancing, and the overall objectives of it are gradually being implemented. Fourth, anti-monopoly efforts in China's pharmaceutical sector continue to escalate. The National Development and Reform Commission has gradually increased its law enforcement efforts against horizontal monopoly issues in the medicine and health sector. Fifth, China is actively building a working mechanism to connect drug administrative law enforcement with criminal justice, aiming to combat drug-related crimes and violations.

10.1.1.3 Judicial Characteristics of China's Legal System for Medicine and Health

First, judicial interpretations enhance the guidance of relevant laws. Second, judicial authorities severely combat drug-related crimes and offenses, establish institutionalized and normalized accountability mechanisms, and accelerate the construction of medical dispute early warning and response mechanisms. Third, judicial authorities attach great importance to the guiding role of typical case judgments. Guiding cases, typical cases, and others are published for reference in related cases, thus providing judicial guidance for the law enforcement and supervision of the legal system for medicine and health.

10.1.2 Basic Principles of China's Legal System for Medicine and Health

The basic principles of China's legal system for medicine and health are the overarching rules that guide and regulate the development of medicine and health law, including legislation, law enforcement, and judicial activities. Even when the law does not regulate certain health affairs, it should also play a role in guiding, regulating, and restricting such affairs. The basic principles of China's legal system for medicine and health include the following three aspects.

10.1.2.1 Safeguarding Citizens' Health

The purpose of medical and health laws and regulations across different departments and levels is to safeguard citizens' health. The right to health is one of the fundamental human rights, recognized and protected by the Constitution of China. The constitutional right to health can be specified through legislation on basic medical health and health promotion into citizens' rights to access public health service resources and basic medical service guarantees. Its manifestations include the right to basic medical services, the right to medical security, the right to medical assistance, and the right to emergency medical treatment.

10.1.2.2 Government Leadership

China's Constitution clearly states the government's basic obligation to provide medical and health services. The Law of the People's Republic of China on Basic Medical and Health Care and the Promotion of Health released in 2019 clarifies the overall government's leadership responsibility, mainly manifested in the government's investment in the establishment of public hospitals at all levels, the development of medical education, the establishment of social medical insurance system, the free provision of basic public health services and the provision of medical assistance to needy people. However, government leadership does not mean that the government shoulders everything. China adheres to the principle of combining government leadership and market-oriented mechanisms.

10.1.2.3 Putting Disease Prevention First

In accordance with the law of disease development and to improve the efficiency of the utilization of medical and health resources, China adheres to the principle of putting disease prevention first and combining prevention with treatment in the field of health. Its connotation includes national health investment tilted towards health care, emphasizing pre-risk control and prevention, establishing a sensitive mechanism for disease risk prediction, control and prevention, and so on.

10.1.3 Origin and Development of China's Legal System for Medicine and Health

It is widely believed that the earliest recorded evidence of ancient Chinese medicine and health law can be traced back to the Yin and Shang dynasties. In books such as *Han Fei Zi*, *The Book of Change*, *Spring and Autumn Annals*, *Rites of Zhou*, and *Zuo's Commentary*, there are ancient records of the importance placed on healthy descendants. *Rites of Zhou* extensively records medical management systems, including the organizations managing medicine, medical record-keeping, and physician assessment systems. Since the Tang and Song dynasties, health legislation has become more detailed. The *Tang Code* contains many provisions related to medicine and health, with criminal legal provisions for medical malpractice, fraud, dispensing errors, and harm caused by medicine, as well as regulations in the areas of food hygiene and health management. During the Song Dynasty, a specialized pharmaceutical agency was established to manage pharmaceutical affairs within and outside the palace, and a national pharmacy bureau was opened. In the period of the Republic of China, health legislation became specialized and specific, with regulations such as the "Regulations on the Prevention of Infectious Diseases" and the Medical Practitioners Law. After the founding of the People's Republic of China, the development of China's legal system for medicine and health went through four phases.

The first phase: from the founding of the People's Republic of China to the promulgation of the first Constitution in 1954. China attached great importance to the construction of health undertakings and the health legal system. Many health regulations were established to promote the development of medical and health services and safeguard the physical health of citizens. Apart from the "Common Program of the Chinese People's Political Consultative Conference," which served as a temporary constitution, a series of laws and regulations were issued, including the "Regulations on Health Organizations of the Central People's Government," the "Interim Measures for Inoculation," the "Provisional Regulations on the Management of Narcotic Drugs," and the "Interim Measures for Traffic Quarantine," marking the beginning of the development of China's legal system for medicine and health.

The second phase: from the promulgation of the first Constitution of China in 1954 to the eve of the reform and opening-up in 1978. Under the guidance of the Constitution, China successively promulgated a large number of laws and regulations related to medicine and health, such as the "Interim Measures for the Health and Epidemic Prevention Stations and Organizational Structure Regulations for Health and Epidemic Prevention Stations at All Levels" issued by the Ministry of Health in 1954, the "Management Measures for Infectious Diseases" issued by the Ministry of Health in 1955, the "Safety and Health Regulations for Factories" issued by the State Council in 1956, the "Frontier Health and Quarantine Regulations of the People's Republic of China" issued by the Standing Committee of the National People's Congress in 1957, the "Some Provisions on Strengthening Drug Administration" jointly issued by the Ministry of Health and other ministries in 1963, and the "Provisional Regulations on the Management of Poisonous Drugs and Restriction of Highly Toxic Drugs" jointly issued by the Ministry of Health and other ministries in 1964.

The third phase: from the beginning of the reform and opening-up in 1978 to 2013. The Constitution of the People's Republic of China in 1982 explicitly stipulated "developing medical and health services" and "protecting the health of the people," providing a constitutional basis for the legal system of medicine and health. Since then, the Standing Committee of the National People's Congress had successively enacted laws such as the Drug Administration Law of the People's Republic of China, the Frontier Health and Quarantine Law of the People's Republic of China, and the Food Hygiene Law of the People's Republic of China. At the same time, there were a lot of health administrative regulations approved and issued by the State Council, such as the "Measures for the Control of Narcotic Drugs," the "Measures for the Control of Psychotropic Drugs," and the "Regulations on the Handling of Medical Accidents." During this period, the health administrative departments formulated and issued thousands of health regulations and normative documents. Local health legislation was also relatively common.

The fourth phase: from 2014 to the present. The legislation in this phase is a deepened development of the third phase and a proactive adjustment made under the guiding ideology of comprehensively promoting the construction of a healthy and law-based China. The focus of legislation is to strengthen the legal construction in health, while ensuring traditional medical and health services, and enhance the legal construction and supervision in the field of medical devices. In 2019, the Standing Committee of the National People's Congress enacted the Law of the People's Republic of China on Basic Medical and Health Care and the Promotion of Health, ending the situation in which the development of medical and health care and the guarantee of basic medical and health care services for citizens had no legal basis, giving the health sector of China its own "basic law."

10.2　Main Components of China's Legal System for Medicine and Health

Due to China's vast territory and varying levels of development across different regions, coupled with the extensive and complex nature of health activities, the adjustment of health legal relations relies not only on laws but also on administrative regulations, departmental rules, local laws and other normative documents. Even at specific implementation levels, a large number of normative documents are needed as supplements. These documents vary in rank and have different effects. The legal system for medicine and health in China is centered on the right to health and can be divided into three parts based on different objects: public health legal system, medical legal system, and medical security legal system. These laws, regulations, and normative documents basically cover all aspects involved in the development of China's health undertakings, including public health, disease prevention and treatment, medical administration, pharmaceutical administration, and other fields.

10.2.1　Public Health Legal System

10.2.1.1　Legal System for Prevention and Treatment of Infectious Diseases

The law on the prevention and treatment of infectious diseases is formulated and promulgated by the state, and its implementation is guaranteed by the state's coercive power. It regulates the various social relations arising from the efforts of the state, government, social organizations and citizens in the prevention, control, and elimination of the occurrence and prevalence of infectious diseases, as well as the protection of human health and public health activities. In February 1989, China promulgated the Law of the People's Republic of China on Prevention and Treatment of Infectious Diseases. This law was revised in August 2004, providing clear and specific provisions on the policies and principles for the prevention and treatment of infectious diseases, prevention of infectious diseases, epidemic reporting, notification and announcement, epidemic control, medical treatment, supervision and management, safeguard measures, and legal responsibilities. It serves as an important legal basis and fundamental guideline for standardizing and institutionalizing the control and prevention of infectious diseases.

10.2.1.2   Legal System for Public Health Emergency Response

The public health emergencies refer to the unexpected and sudden public health events that cause or may cause significant harm to the health of the general public. These events include major infectious disease outbreaks, outbreaks of diseases of unknown origin, severe food poisoning and occupational poisoning, and other public health incidents that severely affect the physical and mental health of the public. In May 2003, the State Council issued the "Regulations on Preparedness for and Response to Public Health emergencies." It summarizes the lessons learned from the prevention and treatment of SARS and establishes institutional arrangements for the scope and specific content of public health emergency management. It further institutionalizes the rapid response mechanism for dealing with public health emergencies from a legal perspective and strengthens corresponding responsibilities. In August 2007, the 29th Session of the Standing Committee of the 10th National People's Congress passed the Emergency Response Law of the People's Republic of China, which provides clear provisions on prevention, emergency preparedness, monitoring and early warning, emergency response and rescue, post-incident recovery and reconstruction, and other activities related to the response to emergencies. This law, together with the "Regulation on Preparedness for and Response to Public Health emergencies" and relevant departmental regulations, constitutes a relatively comprehensive legislative system for dealing with public health emergencies in China.

10.2.1.3   Legal system for Mental health

In China, the definition of mental health has both narrow and broad senses. Narrowly speaking, mental health specifically refers to the prevention, diagnosis, treatment, and rehabilitation of mental disorders. Broadly speaking, in addition to the above-mentioned activities, it also includes the promotion of mental health and corresponding safeguard measures. In October 2012, the 29th Session of the Standing Committee of the 11th National People's Congress passed the Mental Health Law of the People's Republic of China. This law is a legal instrument that regulates the treatment of patients with mental disorders, safeguards their legitimate rights and interests, and promotes their recovery. It is a compilation of legal norms that govern the various social relations arising from the efforts of the state, government, social organizations, and citizens in maintaining and enhancing mental health, preventing and treating mental disorders, promoting the recovery of patients with mental disorders, and safeguarding human health. It was officially implemented in May 2013.

10. 2. 2   Medical Legal System

10. 2. 2. 1   Legal System for Medical Institution Management

Currently, in terms of medical institution management in China, there are two main legislative models: specialized legislation and comprehensive legislation. Specialized legislation primarily involves formulating administrative regulations, rules, and other normative documents, such as the "Regulations on the Administration of Medical Institutions" and the "Implementation Details of the Regulations on the Administration of Medical Institutions," which clearly stipulate matters related to the nature, purpose, planning and approval, registration, practice, and supervision of medical institutions. These two documents are the core legal documents governing the management of medical institutions. The regulations on medical institution management are not only supported by specialized legislative documents, but also scattered throughout other comprehensive legislative documents, such as the Drug Administration Law of the People's Republic of China and the Law of the People's Republic of China on the Prevention and Treatment of Occupational Diseases, which contain relevant legal provisions concerning the management of medical institutions.

10. 2. 2. 2   Legal System for Medical Practice Management

Medical practice refers to the services provided by medical professionals utilizing their specialized medical knowledge and skills to patients, including diagnosis, treatment, nursing, prevention, rehabilitation, and other services aimed at safeguarding physical health and life safety. In terms of the management of medical practice, Chinese legal documents cover a wide range, from laws to administrative regulations, to local laws and regulations, and even include relevant diagnosis and treatment norms and guidelines as supplements, basically forming a complete management system. There are specific management regulations governing everything from professional practice management to facility management, as well as pharmaceuticals, medical devices, emergency rescue, and specific diagnosis and treatment practices.

10. 2. 2. 3   Legal System for the Management of Health Professionals

The law of medical practitioners is a compilation of legal norms that govern the various social relations arising from the physician qualification examination, practice registration, and medical practice activities. The Law of the People's Republic of China on Medical Practitioners was passed by the 3rd Session of the Standing Committee of the 9th National People's Congress in June 1998 and came into effect in May 1999. It applies to professional medical staff who work in medical, preventive, and health care institutions, have legally obtained the qualification of medical practitioners or assistant medical practitioners, have obtained a physician practice license through registration, and engage in corresponding medical, preventive, and health care services. This includes medical practitioners in family planning technical service institutions and foreign medical practitioners who temporarily practice medicine in China.

A nurse refers to a health professional who has obtained a nurse practice license through registration, engages in nursing activities in accordance with regulations, and fulfills the responsibilities of protecting life, alleviating pain, and promoting health. Currently, China's legislation on nursing work is still not perfect, the implementation of some legitimate rights and interests of nurses is insufficient, and the quality of nursing in some primary medical and health institutions is not good. Although the ratio of doctors to nurses has been optimized, some medical and health institutions prioritize medical treatment while neglecting nursing, and there is still a phenomenon of reducing the number of nurses, which poses many potential hazards to medical safety and makes it imperative to improve the legislation for nurse management. The relevant departments of the State Council, people's governments at all levels, and their relevant departments should take measures to improve nurses' working conditions, guarantee their compensation, strengthen the construction of the nursing team, and promote the healthy development of the nursing industry. The relevant departments of the State Council and local people's governments at or above the county level should take measures to encourage nurses to work in urban and rural primary medical and health institutions.

Rural doctors refer to health personnel who have not yet obtained the qualification of medical practitioners or assistant medical practitioners but have obtained the rural doctor practice license issued by the local health administrative agencies. They are registered to engage in preventive, health care, and general medical services in rural medical and health institutions. In August 2003, the State Council promulgated the "Regulations on the Practice of Rural Doctors," marking the entry, education, training, and management of rural doctors onto a legal track. This file stipulates that the country implements a rural doctor practice registration system, and the health administrative departments of the people's government at the county level is responsible for the registration of rural doctors.

A licensed pharmacist refers to a pharmaceutical technician who has passed the national unified examination, obtained the certified pharmacist license, and has been registered and certified. Licensed pharmacists engage in professional activities in drug production, distribution, use and other units. Currently, China implements a registration system for licensed pharmacists, only and other those who are registered can practice. Those who are not registered are not allowed to practice as licensed pharmacists. The NMPA is the administrative body responsible for the qualification registration of licensed pharmacists nationwide, while the drug regulatory agencies of various provinces (autonomous regions, municipalities directly under the central government) are the registration agencies for licensed pharmacists within their respective jurisdictions. To apply for registration, one must obtain the certified pharmacist license, abide by laws and regulations, adhere to the professional ethics of pharmacists, be physically healthy and able to persevere in working as a licensed pharmacist, and obtain the approval of the unit where they work.

10. 2. 2. 4 Legal System for Pharmaceutical Affairs Management in Medical Institutions

The relevant laws and regulations on pharmaceutical affairs management in China are centered on the Drug Administration Law of the People's Republic of China and the "Regulations for the Implementation of the Drug Administration Law of the People's Republic of China." They supervise and manage drugs throughout the drugs' entire lifecycle, including research and development, production, distribution, and use, to ensure drug quality and medication safety. The Drug Administration Law of the People's Republic of China is formulated to strengthen drug management, guarantee drug quality, safeguard the public's medication safety and legitimate rights and interests, and protect and promote public health. All units or individuals engaged in drug research and development, production, distribution, use, and supervision and management activities within the territory of China must abide by this law.

10. 2. 3 Medical Security Legal System

10. 2. 3. 1 Basic Medical Insurance System for Urban Employees

The basic medical insurance system for urban employees refers to a social medical insurance system implemented through national legislation, targeting all employers and their employees as well as flexible employment personnel. Its funding is primarily raised through contributions from both employers and in-service employees, as well as individual contributions from flexible employment personnel, to ensure the basic medical needs of insured individuals. The basic medical insurance system for urban employees is a significant component of China's basic medical insurance system. In December 1998, after summarizing the pilot experience from various localities, the State Council issued "The Decision of the State Council on Setting up Basic Medical Insurance System for Urban Employees," which proposed to initiate the establishment of the basic medical insurance system for urban employees nationwide from early 1999. This marked the gradual replacement of the government-funded and labor protection medical systems, which had been implemented in urban areas in China for nearly half a century, with the new medical insurance system for employees. In October 2010, the Social Insurance Law of the People's Republic of China, passed by the 17th Session of the Standing Committee of the 11th National People's Congress of China, listed "basic medical insurance for employees" as one of the specific types of basic medical insurance.

10. 2. 3. 2 Basic Medical Insurance System for Rural and Non-Working Urban Residents

The basic medical insurance system for rural and non-working urban residents refers to a social insurance legal system under which the state provides basic medical care to rural and non-working urban residents in need of treatment due to illness or non-work-related injuries. Based on the principles of comprehensive coverage, basic protection, multiple levels, and sustainability, China has established a basic medical insurance fund for rural and non-working urban residents through diversified financing methods such as government subsidies and individual contributions, aiming to achieve social mutual assistance and safeguard the medical insurance rights and interests of rural and non-working urban residents. The basic medical insurance system for rural and non-working urban residents in China originated from the basic medical insurance system for non-working urban residents and the new rural cooperative medical care system. In 2016, the State Council integrated the two systems and established a unified basic medical insurance system for rural and non-working urban residents.

For a long time, China's medical and health sector has involved numerous departments, and poor coordination between them has been a significant bottleneck hindering the deepening of medical reform. In 2018, the State Council conducted institutional reform and established the National Health Commission, upholding the concept of comprehensive hygiene and comprehensive health, initiating a new round of super-department reform. This concept aligns with the advocacy of a legal perspective in China's health sector, as it can clarify responsible entities, reduce internal frictions and resistances in medical reform, smoothen coordination, and assist the government in playing a stronger leadership role in actively promoting reform. China attaches great importance to the connection between health legalization and deepening reform, actively promotes the revision and improvement of laws and regulations, and implements the Law of the People's Republic of China on Basic Medical and Health Care and the Promotion of Health to safeguard the development of the medical and health industry.

10.3　Medicine and Health Supervision and Management in China

10.3.1　Overview of Medicine and Health Supervision in China

10.3.1.1　Concept, Function, and Role of Medicine and Health Supervision

Medicine and health supervision is an important guarantee for safeguarding the life and health rights of all citizens. It refers to the administrative law enforcement activities conducted by relevant government administrative departments in accordance with health laws and regulations, including the supervision and inspection of individuals, legal persons, and organizations engaged in health-related administrative permit matters and their implementation of health laws and regulations, as well as the handling of their behaviors.

The function of medicine and health supervision refers to the effectiveness that medicine and health supervision possesses or should exert, including regulatory, restrictive, preventive, and promotional functions. The regulatory function refers to the role of medicine and health supervision in standardizing people's behaviors, indicating what behaviors are legal or must be enforced by law through recognition of law-abiding individuals and punishment of violators. The restrictive function refers to the limitation of relevant rights and constraints on specific behaviors imposed by the supervisory actions of medicine and health supervision entities on the counterparts. The preventive function is the embodiment of the health policy of putting disease prevention first, which is a system that enforces and standardizes social health affairs or behaviors to prevent potential problems. Medicine and health supervision is not a passive and reactive activity, but an active and proactive involvement or integration into the entire operation process of the supervised entities, aiming to identify and eliminate potential health hazards in advance. The promotional function refers to the fact that medicine and health supervision can significantly promote the continuous improvement of various aspects, links, and fields of the social system, especially those related to health activities, effectively protecting people's health and continuously improving the level of productivity.

The role of medicine and health supervision is multifaceted. First, it promotes the modernization of the national governance system and governance capabilities. The medical and health system is a crucial component of modern national system, and the management in the field of medicine and health reflects a country's administrative governance capabilities and level. As the foundation and guarantee for the overall operation of the medicine and health management system, the medicine and health supervision system can effectively ensure the scientific development of the health undertakings on a legal track. It is one of the important means to standardize and maintain the medical and health system, and promote the development of the national governance system and socialist modernization. Second, it safeguards people's health rights and upholds the strategic position of national health. People's health is a significant indicator of national prosperity and strength. Optimizing health services, creating a healthy ecosystem, and providing comprehensive and lifelong health protection for the people serve as a solid foundation for enhancing people's well-being and achieving national rejuvenation. Medicine and health supervision is an important carrier and implementation means for national administrative departments to oversee and manage the development of the health undertakings and safeguard the health of the people. Third, it maintains the environment of the medical and health industry. Since the reform and opening-up, significant changes have occurred in the internal and external environments of China's medicine, health, and health care service supply markets. Market mechanisms inevitably have inherent drawbacks such as blindness, spontaneity, and profit-seeking tendencies. The purpose of medicine and health supervision and management is to correct market failures caused by improper market incentives. Regulating the behavior of various entities in the medical and health industry not only relies on self-moral constraints, industry rules, and social supervision, but also requires a combination of market regulation and government supervision to intervene in the economic operation and resource allocation of the medical and health service market, maintain public order, and ensure the quality of health services.

10.3.1.2   Principles of Medicine and Health Supervision

In China, the supervision of medicine and health follows the principle that "laws must be established, laws must be followed, law enforcement must be strict, and violations of the laws must be punished" in addition to the following principles.

(1) The Principle of Legality

The principle of legality is a fundamental requirement for law enforcement in modern countries and governments governed by law. It primarily includes the following aspects: the establishment of medicine and health supervision entities must be lawful, the possession of medicine and health supervision powers must be lawful, the exercise of medicine and health supervision powers must be lawful, and those who unlawfully exercise their supervision powers shall bear legal responsibilities.

(2) The Principle of Rationality

The principle of rationality refers to the necessity of ensuring that the establishment of medicine and health supervision entities, the possession of supervision powers, the exercise of supervision powers, the accountability of illegal acts, and the implementation of administrative relief are all just, objective, and appropriate. Specifically, it comprises two main aspects. First, the principle of fairness and justice requires equal treatment of all parties concerned without discrimination. Second, the principle of proportionality stipulates that medicine and health supervision entities should take into account both the achievement of supervisory objectives and the protection of the legal rights and interests of the supervised parties when carrying out their supervisory duties.

(3) The Principle of Due Legal Process

The principle of due legal process refers to the necessity for medicine and health supervision entities to follow proper legal procedures when conducting supervisory actions that affect the rights and interests of the supervised parties. This includes informing the supervised parties beforehand, explaining the basis and rationale for the actions, listening to their statements and defenses, and providing appropriate relief channels for the supervised parties afterwards.

(4) The Principle of Reliance Protection

The fundamental meaning of the principle of reliance protection is that medicine and health supervision entities should uphold their credibility in their actions or commitments, and should not change them arbitrarily or act inconsistently.

10.3.1.3   The Medicine and Health Supervision Entities

The medicine and health supervision entities serve as the organizational foundation for the state to exercise its functions of health supervision and management, and to achieve the objectives of health legislation. They are organizations that enjoy the power of national health supervision, can conduct health supervision activities in their own name, and independently bear legal responsibilities for the consequences of their actions. According to Chinese medicine and health laws and regulations, the medicine and health supervision entities in China consist of two main categories: health supervision administrative agencies and organizations authorized by laws and regulations.

Health supervision administrative agencies refer to state organs that are established in accordance with national laws to exercise the functions of national health supervision and management, including the health administrative departments of people's governments at all levels, drug regulatory agencies, and other health supervision agencies. Health administrative departments generally refer to the departments within governments at all levels that are responsible for medical and health administrative work, primarily overseeing policy formulation and environmental protection in the field of medical and health care. Specific law enforcement and operational work is carried out by subordinate institutions such as health supervision bureaus (offices) responsible for administrative law enforcement, centers for disease control and prevention responsible for the control and prevention of infectious diseases and chronic diseases, maternal and child health care hospitals responsible for maternal and child health, as well as hospitals at all levels and township health centers. Currently, drug supervision and management in China is primarily handled by the NMPA. Its responsibilities mainly include:

First, to supervise the safety of drugs (including TCMs and ethnic medicines, the same below), medical devices and cosmetics; to draw up regulatory policy plans, organize the drafting of laws and regulations, formulate departmental regulations, and supervise the implementation thereof; to research and formulate regulatory and service-related policies that encourage new technologies and new products for drugs, medical devices and cosmetics.

Second, to undertake standard management for drugs, medical devices and cosmetics; to organize the formulation and publication of the Chinese Pharmacopoeia and other drug and medical device standards, organize the drafting of cosmetic standards, organize the formulation of the classification management system, and supervise the implementation thereof; to participate in formulating the National Essential Medicine List, and assist in the implementation of the national essential medicine system.

Third, to regulate the registration of drugs, medical devices and cosmetics; to develop the registration system, conduct strict review and approval for marketing, improve measures to facilitate the review and approval process, and organize the implementation thereof.

Fourth, to undertake the quality management for drugs, medical devices and cosmetics; to formulate quality management standards for research and development and supervise the implementation thereof; to formulate production quality management standards and supervise the implementation thereof in line with NMPA's responsibilities; to formulate quality management standards for distribution and usage and guide the implementation thereof.

Fifth, to undertake post-market risk management for drugs, medical devices and cosmetics; to organize the monitoring, evaluation, and handling of drug adverse reactions, medical device adverse events, and cosmetic adverse reactions; to undertake emergency response management for drugs, medical devices and cosmetics in accordance with law.

Sixth, to undertake management of qualifications for licensed pharmacists; to formulate regulations of qualifications for licensed pharmacists, and guide and supervise the registration of licensed pharmacists.

Seventh, to organize and guide the supervision and inspection of drugs, medical devices and cosmetics; to develop the inspection system, investigate and punish illegal activities during the registration process for drugs, medical devices and cosmetics in accordance with law, and organize and guide the investigation and punishment of illegal activities during the manufacturing process in line with NMPA's responsibilities.

Eighth, to engage in international exchange and cooperation in the regulation of drugs, medical devices and cosmetics, and participate in developing relevant international regulatory rules and standards.

Ninth, to guide the work of drug regulatory departments of all provinces, autonomous regions, and municipalities directly under the central government.

Tenth, to complete other tasks assigned by the Central Committee of the Communist Party of China and the State Council.

The organizations authorized by laws and regulations to carry out medicine and health supervision and management refer to organizations other than administrative organs that are authorized by laws and regulations to exercise specific administrative functions in their own name, including social organizations, social groups, enterprises, and public institutions.

10.3.2 Main Content of Medicine and Health Supervision and Management in China

10.3.2.1 Supervision and Management of Medical Institutions

Supervision of medical institutions generally encompasses oversight of their establishment and practice, referring to the administrative law enforcement activities where the health supervision entities conduct inspections on whether the establishment approval, licensing of practice grades, and practice activities of medical institutions are lawful in accordance with relevant laws and regulations, and handle any illegal or improper acts during the establishment and practice of medical institutions. To ensure the quality and safety of medical care and protect the health of citizens, China has continuously strengthened the management of medical institutions and regulated the order of the medical service market. Since 1994, China has promulgated and implemented various laws and regulations related to the supervision of medical institutions, such as the "Regulations on the Administration of Medical Institutions," the "Implementation Details of the Regulations on the Administration of Medical Institutions," the "Measures for the Administration of Medical Cosmetology Services," and the "Measures for the Administration of Prescriptions," and has now formed a relatively complete legal and regulatory system for the supervision of medical institutions.

The establishment and approval process of medical institutions consists of three parts: planning for the establishment of medical institutions, approval for the establishment of medical institutions, and medical institution practice registration and related management such as cancellation, change registration and verification. First, the planning for the establishment of medical institutions is primarily the responsibility of the health administrative departments of local people's governments at or above the county level. The planning is based on the current situation of population, medical resources, medical needs, and distribution of medical institutions within the administrative area. Second, the approval for the establishment of medical institutions is premised on compliance with the planning layout and medical institution establishment plan within the administrative area. Any unit or individual wishing to establish a medical institution must obtain the approval of the health administrative department at or above the county level in the locality. After obtaining the Approval Certificate for the Establishment of a Medical Institution, they can proceed with other procedures at relevant departments. Finally, the practice registration of medical institutions mainly examines whether the medical institutions applying for practice possess the statutory qualifications for operations.

The supervision of medical institutions' practice generally refers to the oversight conducted by health administrative departments to ensure the legality of medical institutions' practice activities. It comprises three main aspects: supervision of practice licenses, supervision of practice activities, and supervision of practice norms, duties, and obligations. First, supervision of practice licenses includes both the supervision of practice access and the use of stamps and names. The former requires medical institutions to obtain the Practicing License of Medical Institution before conducting any medical activities, while the latter involves ensuring that the stamps, bank accounts, plaques, and names used in medical documents are identical to the approved and registered name of the medical institutions. Second, supervision of practice activities includes oversight of the scope of diagnosis and treatment, practicing medical personnel, and medical diagnostic and treatment activities. Lastly, supervision of practice norms, duties, and obligations requires medical institutions to adhere to relevant clinical diagnosis and treatment norms in their practice and fulfill related obligations such as providing preventive health care and medical support for sudden health events.

10.3.2.2 Supervision and Management of Health Professionals

Supervision of health professionals refers to the administrative law enforcement activities conducted by medicine and health supervision entities in accordance with health management laws and regulations to oversee and inspect health professionals, and to pursue the responsibilities of those who violate the law. Health professionals refer to those engaged in health technical work, specifically, professionals who have acquired medical and health knowledge through higher or secondary medical and health education or training, passed the review of health administrative departments, and are engaged in medical treatment, prevention, pharmacy, nursing, or other health technical work.

The supervision of health professionals primarily focuses on professional qualifications, qualifications for specialized technical services, and diagnostic and treatment practices of the health professionals.

First, the supervision of health professionals' professional qualifications primarily involves overseeing and managing their acquisition of corresponding qualifications. These qualifications refer to the knowledge, skills, abilities, and status qualifications that personnel providing specific health technical services to the public should possess. Health professionals often need to go through a series of rigorous review procedures to obtain these qualifications. Generally, the acquisition process begins with examinations or assessments, such as the medical practitioner qualification examination, the nurse licensing examination, and the licensed pharmacist qualification examination, and ends with registration in the health administrative department.

Second, the supervision of health professionals' qualifications for specialized technical services refers to the qualifications they further obtain under legal circumstances to perform specific specialized health technical services after registration or assessment, due to the numerous health service projects in a certain field and the different risk and complexity of each project.

Third, the supervision of health professionals' diagnostic and treatment practices directly affects the level of diagnostic and treatment practices and patients' health. Therefore, various countries and governments implement strict regulatory measures to standardize their practices. The primary means of regulation is the implementation of qualification licensing, which involves strict management of industry access, even down to the access of specific diagnostic and treatment practices. After health professionals obtain general industry access qualifications, the focus of health supervision lies in their specific behaviors, including their scope of practice and other areas.

10.3.2.3 Drug Supervision and Management

Drug supervision and management refers to the oversight and inspection activities conducted by drug regulatory agencies in accordance with their statutory authorities, covering various aspects of drug research and development, production, sales, use, pricing, and advertising. In China, the NMPA is in charge of drug supervision and management. The legal basis for drug supervision and management includes the Drug Administration Law of the People's Republic of China, the "Good Laboratory Practice for Non-Clinical Laboratory Studies," the "Good Clinical Practice," and the "Good Manufacturing Practice (Revised in 2010)," among others.

The main content of drug supervision and management includes drug management, licensed pharmacist management, and drug supervision and inspection, all conducted in accordance with relevant laws and regulations. These laws and regulations are normative documents formulated and issued in accordance with the law, covering issues such as national drug standards. Drug management primarily involves the supervision and management of drug market access, the production, circulation, and use of drugs, and drug quality, the investigation and handling of illegal drugs, and the supervision and management of market exit, etc. Licensed pharmacist management mainly involves the supervision and management of the professional access, professional conduct, and professional exit of pharmaceutical technicians practicing in key pharmaceutical technology professions. Drug supervision and inspection refers to the oversight and inspection conducted by drug regulatory authorities on drug research and development, production, distribution, and use activities in accordance with laws and regulations.

10.3.2.4   Supervision of Infectious Disease Prevention and Treatment

Supervision of infectious disease prevention and treatment refers to the administrative law enforcement activities carried out by the government's health administrative departments in accordance with health laws and regulations, including granting permits to individuals, legal persons, and organizations engaged in matters related to infectious diseases, overseeing and inspecting the implementation of laws and regulations for infectious disease prevention and treatment, and taking actions against any violations. The purpose of this supervision is to effectively prevent, control, and eliminate the occurrence and prevalence of infectious diseases, safeguard people's health, and uphold the unity and dignity of the national health legal system.

According to the Law of the People's Republic of China on Prevention and Treatment of Infectious Diseases, the health administrative department of the State Council is responsible for the prevention, treatment, and supervision of infectious diseases nationwide, and the health administrative departments of local people's governments at or above the county level are responsible for the prevention, treatment, and supervision of infectious diseases within their respective administrative regions. The supervision of infectious disease prevention and treatment generally includes prevention supervision, control supervision, and other aspects.

Case Study   The Promulgation of the Law of the People's Republic of China on Basic Medical and Health Care and the Promotion of Health

The Law of the People's Republic of China on Basic Medical and Health Care and the Promotion of Health was passed by the 15th Session of the Standing Committee of the

13th National People's Congress on December 28, 2019. The law includes the basic elements necessary for national health legislation, while also embodying new concepts such as "comprehensive hygiene," "comprehensive health," and "integrating health into all policies." The law came into effect on June 1, 2020.

The establishment of the Law of the People's Republic of China on Basic Medical and Health Care and the Promotion of Health is accompanied by the continuous deepening of the health system reform of China. With the gradual establishment of the basic medical and health system with Chinese characteristics, many fundamental and principled issues in the development of China's health undertakings urgently need to be regulated by a basic and comprehensive law. At the same time, the task of promptly elevating proven effective practices and specific systems to the level of law had emerged.

In terms of legislative objectives, the law primarily focuses on the following: first, implementing the provisions in the Constitution of the People's Republic of China on the state's development of medical and health undertakings and the protection of people's health; second, guiding the overall reform and development of China's medical and health services; third, promoting and ensuring the effective implementation of the construction of a healthy China. Under the guidance of the legislative approach that upholds government leadership, ensures basic services, strengthens grassroots-level services, and establishes mechanisms, the law makes macro legal norms and institutional designs in areas such as actively ensuring government investment, mobilizing participation from the entire society, comprehensively safeguarding people's health throughout their lives, significantly improving people's health levels, and significantly improving health equity. It fully plays the important role of law in leading, promoting medicine and health system reforms, and ensuring the construction of a healthy China.

This law is China's first fundamental and comprehensive law in the field of medical and health sector, reflecting the concept shift from "treating illnesses as the center" to "putting people's health at the center," providing legal guarantees for the reform and development of the medical and health undertakings. To date, the health rule of law has developed well as a comprehensive legal field involving multiple traditional legal departments, and the legal system of medicine and health composed of constitutional provisions, laws and regulations, regulatory documents, and standard guidelines has basically taken shape.

11 China's Medical and Health Information System

In the information era, the information construction in the medical and health industry has become a crucial national development strategy. As the core of medical and health informatization, the construction of information systems has a profound impact on improving the quality and efficiency of medical services, optimizing the allocation and utilization of medical resources, promoting the management and supervision of the medical and health, and enhancing the intelligent governance capabilities of public health. With the continuous progress and application of information technology, the construction of medical and health informatization in China has made great progress, but it is still necessary to continuously strengthen the construction and application of information systems, and improve the integration and innovative capabilities of information technology with the medical and health industry to promote sustainable and healthy development of medical and health undertakings. This chapter will discuss the importance of the medical and health information system, the development status of medical and health informatization in China, and the medical and health information management system in China, so as to provide insights into the current status, issues, and future directions of medical and health informatization in China.

11.1 The Importance of the Medical and Health Information System

11.1.1 Macro Level

With the establishment of a socialist market economy, the construction of medical and health information infrastructure is crucial for the development of the medical and health undertakings. Building a practical and shared medical and health information system can help authorities and researchers to access reliable information promptly, provide efficient medical and health management services and comprehensively improve medical and health quality, capacity, and management levels. Recently, many urban areas in China have advanced the construction of the medical and health information system. The "14th Five-

Year Plan for National Health Informatization" highlights that during the 13th Five-Year Plan period, significant efforts were made to integrate the strategies of Healthy China and Digital China, fully implement the 13th Five-Year Plan for national health informatization development, and accelerate the normative application of healthcare big data and innovative development of "Internet + Healthcare." This integration played a vital role in supporting the high-quality development of health undertakings. On a macro level, the importance of the construction of medical and health information system to the development of the medical and health undertakings is reflected in several aspects.

First, enhancing the spread of healthcare services and the rational allocation of resources. In the drive for medical reform and informatization, healthcare services in China are poised for deeper transformation. Although public hospitals remain the mainstay of medical and health service system in China, the key to promoting the upgrading of medical and health services is to address regional disparities in medical resources, and form a new pattern of medical treatment of "minor diseases at the grassroots level, major diseases to the hospital, and rehabilitation back to the community" by implementing measures such as hierarchical diagnosis and treatment and telemedicine. Among them, the hierarchical diagnosis and treatment information system, which leverages big data, cloud computing, mobile internet, and the Internet of Things is one of the very important construction content. This system can interconnect with the information system of various medical and health institutions, providing unified referral information services, optimizing workflows in medical institutions, encouraging residents to develop better medical-seeking habits, and enhancing the orderliness, accessibility, fairness, and cost-effectiveness of medical services, thereby optimizing regional health resource allocation.

Second, strengthening medical and health management and supervision. According to the requirements of the "Code of Practice for the Recording of the Entire Process of Administrative Law Enforcement in Healthcare" issued by the National Health Commission, establishing a sound health supervision system, accelerating the promotion of the "Internet + Transparent Supervision" model in health supervision, striving to build a comprehensive management service platform of smart health supervision, optimizing the law enforcement process, improving the efficiency of law enforcement, and truly achieving a leap from traditional to modern law enforcement modes, are crucial for safeguarding public health. By supervising and evaluating the behavior of medical institutions and health professionals, medical services can be standardized and normalized, so as to increase patient satisfaction. Achieving data-driven collaboration in public health management and data-supported intelligent decision-making applications can effectively support refined management of health supervision and enhance comprehensive supervision and enforcement capabilities. With the growing demand for internet-based medical services, the focus on China's smart health supervision is shifting towards comprehensive supervision. The use of big data for detailed analysis, the discovery of violations and timely investigation, and the efforts to achieve the transformation of supervision channels from offline to online, play an important role in the realization of the whole process of supervision.

Third, enhancing the capability of intelligent public health governance. The application of cutting-edge technologies such as block chain and artificial intelligence significantly boosts the resilience of public health information systems and shapes the future direction of health governance. Public health, fundamentally a process of social governance centered around "groups," requires distributed group participation to achieve the resilience of information systems. Intelligent public health governance represents an innovative form of public health management, relying on the informatization process of institutional structures and system reform and leveraging professional and independent knowledge for scientific and efficient public health governance. This approach is crucial for timely responses to major diseases and public health emergencies. In the future, public health information systems will become integral to smart cities, coordinated through smart city command centers, enabling intelligent city-wide management and offering efficient services across economic and social domains, including public health.

Fourth, facilitating the advancement and transformation of the medical and health industry. As the government continues to promote the reform of the medical and health system and the digital transformation of the medical and health industry, the medical information industry is undergoing significant upgrades and shifts. It is transitioning from focusing solely on medical service informatization to rapid development in health insurance informatization and pharmaceutical informatization, progressing towards integrated and collaborative informatization across the entire life-health industry chain. During this transformation, platforms based on cloud computing and big data, adopting middle platform thinking for digital transformation, are being rapidly deployed to support the construction and operation of core systems in medical treatment, medical insurance, and pharmaceuticals. These platforms also support the development and operation of various innovative medical applications. The digital transformation platform is expanding its services from independent medical or medical insurance departments to the entire industry chain, presenting both opportunities and challenges for upgrading and transforming the medical and health industry.

11.1.2　Micro Level

In May 2020, the General Office of the National Health Commission issued the "Notice of the General Office of the National Health Commission on Further Improving the Appointment Diagnosis and Treatment System and Strengthening the Construction of Smart Hospitals," calling for speeding up the establishment and improvement of the appointment diagnosis and treatment system, innovating and building the smart hospital systems, and vigorously promoting the development of internet-based diagnosis and treatment as well as internet hospitals, which prompted many hospitals to focus on their information system construction and accelerate the pace of informatization. Hospital informatization construction has become an essential means for hospitals to implement refined management, reduce operational costs, and reform medical treatment processes. During the 13th Five-Year Plan period, many hospitals aligned their informatization efforts with the national medical informatization development plan, Using third-party platforms to integrate medical data, strengthen information management levels, and promote the informatization and paperless operation in various functional departments. On a micro level, the importance of medical and health information system construction for hospital management is evident in the following aspects:

First, optimizing medical-seeking processes and reducing waiting times. By implementing self-service registration and payment systems and outpatient queuing systems, hospitals can optimize outpatient medical-seeking processes, addressing the "Three Long, One Short" (long queues for registration, consultation, and payment, and short consultation times) problem. The introduction of intelligent medical devices like automatic diagnostic equipment and smart medicine cabinets allows patients to self-check and retrieve medications, thus reducing the workload on medical staff and enhancing efficiency. Online consultations and appointment registration via internet hospitals can further facilitate convenient medical-seeking access for patients, avoiding the traditional congestion and crowding in outpatient settings, and significantly improving medical-seeking efficiency and patient experience.

Second, establishing and implementing electronic medical record(EMR) to improve the quality of medical records. Establishing EMR is central to integrating data from various hospital function systems, such as hospital information system, laboratory information system, and picture archiving and communication system. EMR is at the core of hospital informatization construction. As EMR evolves, hospital informatization construction is shifting focus from billing processes to clinical workflows. EMR plays a crucial role in structuring clinical data, helping to integrate and analyze data comprehensively, showcasing patients' diagnosis and treatment processes, and providing essential data support for the management and control of personnel (personnel management and performance evaluation), finance (budget management and cost accounting), and materials (medication and supply management). Establishing and implementing EMR not only improves the quality of medical records but also aids doctors in accurate diagnosis and treatment, facilitating automated and intelligent hospital management, including unified management of medical records quality and personnel.

Third, promoting clinical informatization construction to enhance diagnostic and treatment quality and efficiency. Clinical informatization construction focuses more on patients than hospital informatization construction. At its core is the establishment of clinical information system centered around EMR, covering nursing, imaging, laboratory testing, and more. The primary goal of it is to assist doctors in providing rapid and accurate diagnosis and treatment, improving work efficiency while ensuring the quality and traceability of medical records. Currently, third-level hospitals in China lead in clinical informatization construction, particularly in clinical laboratory information management and medical imaging information management, with the highest penetration rates. In the future, clinical information systems will integrate new technologies such as big data and artificial intelligence, advancing from speeding up and improving informatization management to data integration and intelligent analysis, addressing core issues of medical resource shortages.

Given the growing emphasis on the development of medical and health undertakings in China, advancing health insurance informatization has been included in the "Outline of the 14th Five-Year Plan (2021-2025) for National Economic and Social Development and the Long-Range Objectives Through the Year 2035." This provides a broader and more robust foundation for strengthening information system construction and application, enhancing the integration and innovation capabilities of information technology with the medical and health industry, and achieving high-quality development in medical and health undertakings, thereby improving public health and well-being.

11.2 Development Status of Medical and Health Informatization in China

11.2.1 Policy Planning and Development Requirements for Medical and Health Informatization in China

11.2.1.1 Policy Planning

At the national level, China has continuously promoted the development of the information industry and progressively strengthened informatization construction in the medical and health sector. From the 10th Five-Year Plan to the 14th Five-Year Plan periods, China has clearly outlined the need to enhance information system construction in medical and health sector and issued policies to support and regulate the development of medical informatization. Key documents, such as the "Opinions of the Central Committee of the Communist Party of China and the State Council on Deepening the Reform of the Medical and Health System" and the "Outline of the 12th Five-Year Plan for the National Economic and Social Development of the People's Republic of China," have actively promoted the development of medical and health informatization, telemedicine systems, and the informatization of public hospitals. In recent years, medical and health informatization layout in China has accelerated, reflecting the government's strong emphasis on medical and health informatization. Through ongoing policy improvements and increased investment, sustained progress in medical and health informatization has been achieved.

At the policy level, China has introduced a series of guiding documents to support the development of medical and health informatization, including the "14th Five-Year Plan for

National Informatization," as shown in Table 11-1. These documents demonstrate the government's focus and support for the development of medical and health informatization, providing policy guidance for the industry's development. Practically, China actively promotes the construction and application of medical and health informatization infrastructure, strengthens data standardization and sharing, and fosters deep integration of medical and health informatization with other industries and fields, such as artificial intelligence, big data, and cloud computing. Additionally, China is enhancing legal frameworks to ensure the security and effectiveness of medical and health information.

Table 11-1 Examples of policy planning for China's medical and health informatization

Release date	Issuing department	Document title	Interpretation of the key content	Policy attribute
September 2020	National Health Commission, National Development and Reform Commission, Ministry of Education, Ministry of Industry and Information Technology, Ministry of Public Security, Ministry of Human Resources and Social Security, Ministry of Transport, Ministry of Emergency Management, National Healthcare Security Administration	Guiding Opinions on Further Improving Pre-Hospital Emergency Medical Services	Enhancing the informatization level of pre-hospital emergency infrastructure and supporting facilities	Normative
November 2020	General Office of the Ministry of Industry and Information Technology, General Office of the National Health Commission	Notice of the General Office of the Ministry of Industry and Information Technology and the General Office of the National Health Commission on Organizing the Application for 5G+ Healthcare Application Pilot Projects	Pilot promotion: promoting the pilot of replicable and scalable 5G smart healthcare new products, new formats, and new models	Supportive

Continued

Release date	Issuing department	Document title	Interpretation of the key content	Policy attribute
September 2021	General Office of the State Council	14th Five-Year Plan for National Healthcare Security	Achieving breakthroughs in healthcare security informatization and standardization, promoting the coding standards for medical insurance business and the application of electronic medical insurance credentials	Supportive
September 2021	National Health Commission, National Administration of Traditional Chinese Medicine	Action Plan to Promote High-Quality Development of Public Hospitals (2021-2025)	Building three-pronged smart hospitals and promoting the standardization and normalization of hospital information construction	Supportive
December 2021	Central Cyberspace Affairs Commission	14th Five-Year Plan for National Informatization	Actively exploring the use of informatization to optimize medical service processes, constructing major medical infrastructure platforms, accelerating the construction of dedicated medical clouds, promoting data sharing and mutual recognition and business collaboration across various levels of medical and health institutions, and building an authoritative, unified, and shared national health information platform at all levels	Supportive

Overall, from the 10th Five-Year Plan to the 14th Five-Year Plan periods, the implementation of medical and health informatization policies in China has achieved significant success, laying a solid foundation for the modernization of medical services. Future efforts will be needed to focus on enhancing technological innovation and practical exploration to improve the coverage and quality of medical and health informatization.

11.2.1.2　Development Requirements

The development requirements for medical and health informatization in China can be summarized as follows:

First, the informatization construction of medical institutions. The informatization construction of medical institutions has to meet the needs of medical quality management, pharmaceutical management, medical record management, patient management, and physician scheduling, ensuring the stable and reliable operation of the information platform. Additionally, medical institutions must comply with information security management requirements, strengthening data backup and recovery management to ensure data integrity, confidentiality, and availability.

Second, the informatization construction of pharmaceutical manufacturing enterprises. The informatization construction of pharmaceutical manufacturing enterprises requires establishing a comprehensive, efficient, and digital information management system to support the research and development, production, sales, and quality management of pharmaceuticals. The information platform for pharmaceutical manufacturing enterprises must meet accuracy, real-time, and security requirements and interface with regulatory authorities at various levels to ensure lawful and compliant operations.

Third, the informatization construction of pharmaceutical distribution and retail enterprises. The informatization construction of pharmaceutical distribution and retail enterprises requires creating an end-to-end information management chain to meet the needs of supply chain, inventory management, and business processing. Additionally, establishing e-commerce portals and mobile applications to provide online purchasing and payment services can meet the diverse needs of consumers.

Fourth, the informatization construction of medical insurance. The informatization construction of medical insurance involves advancing the informatization of medical insurance management, data statistics, fund settlement, and medical insurance card management, establishing a national medical security system to achieve information management and unified supervision. This requires building a robust medical insurance information platform to protect patient privacy security and information security.

Fifth, the informatization construction of medical device enterprises. The informatization construction of medical device enterprises necessitates developing comprehensive information management platforms for digital management of product research and development, production, and sales processes. At the same time, it is necessary to meet the requirements of the "Compliance with Medical Device Safety Management" to ensure product quality.

Sixth, the informatization construction of medical institution evaluation standards. The informatization construction of medical institution evaluation standards must comply with national medical institution evaluation standards and related regulations on medical quality management and accident management, ensuring the usability, safety, and reliability of information systems, thereby improving medical service quality and patient satisfaction.

In summary, the development of medical and health informatization should focus on enhancing the level of information technology, continuously strengthening talent development and technological innovation, promoting the application of information technology in medical and health sector, establishing a sound information security system, guiding the medical and health sector to gradually form scientific and standardized information application models, and improving medical service levels and the medical environment. The government should formulate policies and regulations that align with national conditions, providing policy support and security for the development of medical and health informatization, promoting the application of medical and health informatization standards, providing technical support for the interaction and interoperability of the medical and health information system, and facilitating the integration and optimization of the medical and health information system.

11. 2. 2 Development of Medical and Health Informatization in China

The development of medical and health informatization in China dates back to the early 1980s. At that time, China began to engage with computer technology, with some hospitals attempting to use it to improve medical service quality and management levels. However, the integration of computer technology with medical services was not mature, and its application was limited. In the 1990s, as information technology continued to advance and spread, medical and health informatization entered a rapid development phase. This period saw a focus on hospital informatization construction, with hospitals at various levels implementing hospital information systems and clinical information systems, applying them to areas like EMR, medical quality control, medical resource management, and medical insurance management. Meanwhile, China also introduced a series of policies to support the development of medical and health informatization, fostering its widespread adoption and application. With the advent of new technologies like mobile internet, cloud computing, and artificial intelligence, medical and health informatization is moving towards more intelligent, digital, and universal directions. Nowadays, China has made significant strides in the construction of medical and health informatization, with continued innovation and development in hospital informatization, digital medical treatment, and telemedicine. Future advancements in information technology and its application scenarios will make medical and health information system a crucial support for medical services and research.

11. 2. 3 Current Status of Medical and Health Informatization in China

With the arrival of the information age, the construction of medical and health informatization in China has become a significant issue. Although China has established a relatively complete medical and health informatization infrastructure, the application of new medical reform models still faces severe challenges. The primary issues in regional medical and health informatization construction in China include information silos, lack of standardized workflows, insufficient funding, and a shortage of skilled personnel. In terms of building residents' electronic health records, China has made substantial progress, with nearly half of the provinces achieving an archiving rate of over 90% for residents' electronic health records, indicating potential for further advancement. In clinical informatization, China actively promotes the use of EMR and advances the application of informatization in medical imaging, laboratory testing, and teleconsultation. Despite common issues of mismatched output and input, the scaling up of medical and health institutions and increasing demands for national policies have led to gradual increases in staffing and funding for EMR systems, which are crucial for enhancing medical quality and efficiency.

11.3 Medical and Health Information Management System in China

11.3.1 Structure of Medical and Health Information Management System in China

In 2010, the Ministry of Health proposed the "3521 Project" overall framework for health informatization during the 12th Five-Year Plan period. In 2013, this project evolved into the "4631-2 Project," which serves as the top-level design for the development of medical and health informatization in China. The "4631-2 Project" aims to integrate health resources and establish a comprehensive, multidimensional national medical and health information management system to enhance the quality and efficiency of health services. The "4631-2 Project" includes four levels of population health information platforms, six business applications, three basic databases, one converged network covering all types of medical institutions (including TCM institutions), and two standard systems. Figure 11-1 illustrates the overall framework of the "4631-2 Project" in China.

11.3.1.1 Regional Population Health Information Platforms

Regional medical informatization construction involves integrating information systems across various medical institutions within a specific region through the use of information technology and platforms, achieving information interconnectivity and collaborative operations. This is an important part of China's medical and health informatization construction, and one of the important measures to advance the medical and health system reform and improve medical service quality and efficiency.

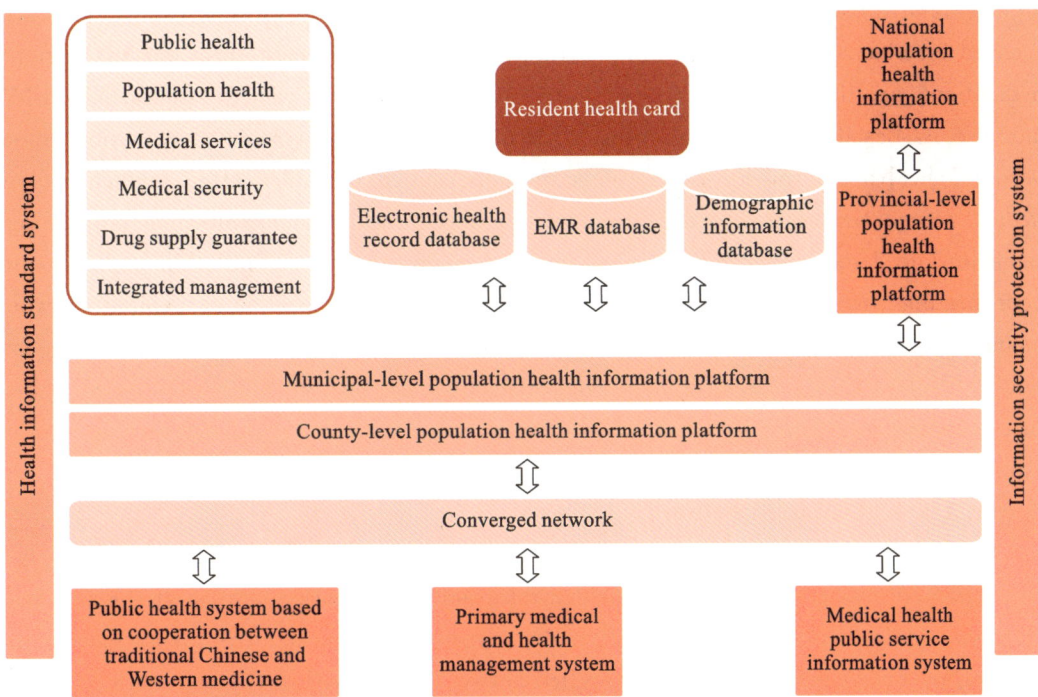

Figure 11-1 Overall framework of the "4631-2 Project" in China

To promote regional medical informatization construction, China has introduced significant initiatives for building regional population health information platforms. According to the "Guiding Opinions on Accelerating the Construction of Population Health Informatization," there should be comprehensive development of interlinked and interconnected four levels of population health information platforms, among which the regional population health information platforms are the most important and basic platforms to realize China's health modernization. The construction of regional population health information platforms will help improve the quality and efficiency of medical services, promote the popularization and application of medical information, and realize the goal of national health and medical and health modernization.

11.3.1.2 Business Applications

The "4631-2 Project" encompasses six business applications: public health, population health, medical services, medical security, drug supply guarantee, and integrated management. These applications fall within the scope of the implementation plan for medical and health informatization construction in China. Coordinating the construction and deepening of six key business application systems covering various areas of health and achieving interoperability among these systems can enhance the level of medical services, promote the improvement of the medical security system, standardize drug management, strengthen population health management, and improve medical management levels.

11.3.1.3 Basic Databases

The three basic databases include the electronic health record database, the EMR database, and the demographic information database. The electronic health record database is based on electronic health records, with data primarily sourced from various regional medical and health institutions' operational systems, including EMR system. The EMR database is based on EMR, storing structured lifelong electronic information about patients' health and medical conditions in numerous data tables after segmenting the medical record template according to business norms, so as to enable data storage and retrieval. The demographic information database is designed for population management, incorporating fields for household registration, residence, and management location (management location refers to specific management services for population monitoring and family development). These fields categorize information on household registration, residence, and management location, respectively, for statistical purposes, providing data on registered, permanent, and managed populations.

11.3.1.4　Converged Network

Following regional health planning requirements and localized management principles, the construction of a regional public health information network platform at the city level integrates various health administrative departments, disease control departments, and medical and health institutions into a unified network connected to the national public data network, forming a regional health information network.

11.3.1.5　Standard Systems

The standard systems within the "4631-2 Project" overall framework includes the health information standard system and the information security protection system. The health information standard system is a crucial part of the top-level design for health informatization. Health information standard system in China currently encompasses six categories: basic, data, application, technology, management, and security and privacy standards, as shown in Figure 11-2. The information security protection system ensures the security of medical data during generation, transmission, and integration processes. It was

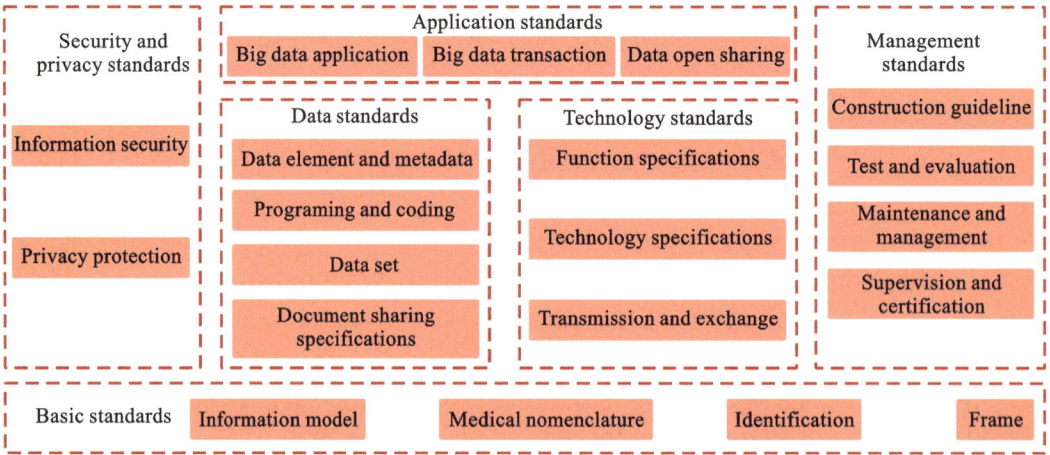

Figure 11-2　Framework of health information standard system in China

established in response to emerging issues such as the lack of medical information security standards, unreasonable network structures in medical institutions, information leakage led by network collaboration, and breaches of patient privacy.

11.3.2 Operation Mechanisms of Medical and Health Information Management System in China

Based on the "4631-2 Project," the "14th Five-Year Plan for National Informatization" in 2021 proposed to actively explore the use of informatization to optimize medical service processes, accelerate the construction of dedicated medical clouds, promote data sharing and business collaboration across information systems of various medical and health institutions, and build authoritative, unified, and interconnected national health information platforms. Accordingly, the operation mechanisms of medical and health information management system can be categorized as follows.

11.3.2.1 Health Data Governance

Health data governance is a core and most complex aspect of health information management, involving the construction of health information standard system, data collection and integration, data security and privacy protection, etc.

The construction of health information standard system is the foundation of health data governance. China has initially established a health information standard system, including basic, data, application, technology, management, and security and privacy standards. Basic standards provide guidance and overarching direction; data standards ensure unambiguous semantics; application standards guide data provision and application; technology standards set requirements for business application systems' technical levels and information network security and privacy protection technology levels; management standards are used to guide business application systems to reasonably apply relevant standards and to evaluate, supervise and manage the application of standards; and security and privacy standards regulate data security and privacy issues in health-related applications and services. Data collection and integration are critical components of health data governance. The health information management system collects and integrates relevant data through various information systems, such as EMR system and residents' health record system. China has established standardized residents' health records, including personal basic information, health check-up records, key population health management records, and other medical and health service records. Data security and privacy protection are also essential aspects of health data governance. The health information management system must establish robust data security and privacy protection mechanisms to safeguard the privacy and data security of patients and health service providers. China places a high priority on cybersecurity and, in terms of information security, is able to guide information sharing and network security development through relevant legal documents. Classifying the security levels of regional health information platforms and implementing platform rectifications are helpful to protect individual privacy and data security.

11.3.2.2 Construction of Health Information Platforms

The health information management system requires an open data-sharing and communication platform to enable data interconnectivity and sharing among various health institutions and service providers. This facilitates efficient and high-quality health services and provides comprehensive and accurate data support for decision-makers. The population health information platform is central to the "4631-2 Project," with municipal-level population health information platforms playing a crucial role in bridging and coordinating data sharing and interconnectivity between higher and lower levels. The construction of regional health information platforms must adhere to the "four unifications" principle: unified standards, unified deployment, unified special network, and unified platform. Unified standards require adherence to national information standard norms, strengthening the application and implementation of standards to achieve horizontal data integration and sharing among higher and lower units. Unified deployment involves centralized management of the regional health information platform project by the city health information center. Unified special network demands the unified operation of special networks across city, county, township, and village levels to facilitate interconnectivity and data sharing. Unified platform necessitates the development of interfaces for existing information systems in subordinate medical and health institutions, enabling regional health information interoperability and sharing.

11.3.2.3 Construction of Health Informatization Talent Team

To effectively promote the construction of health informatization talent team, the Office of the Ministry of Health successively issued the "Implementation Opinions on the Development of National Health Statistics and Informatization Talents" and the "Opinions on Strengthening the Construction of Health Statistics and Informatization Talent Teams" in 2011 and 2012. These documents set clear standards for staffing health informatization personnel in health administrative departments, hospitals above the second level, and public health institutions. In August 2022, the National Health Commission issued the "14th Five-Year Plan for Health Talent Development," aiming to improve talent management systems and mechanisms and create a conducive environment for talent development. Stakeholders in health information management include demand-side entities (health administrative departments, and medical and health institutions), supply-side entities (information technology companies), and maintenance entities, each with specific needs for health informatization talents. Therefore, China first adopts a demand-oriented mechanism for the cultivation and utilization of health informatization talents, with clear cultivation objectives and top-level planning for talent development. Additionally, a unified curriculum system is built to broaden the horizons of health informatization talents. Finally, a multi-level and multi-angle comprehensive practice training system is established to meet the need for cultivating versatile and application-oriented talents.

11.3.2.4 Promoting the Adoption of Health Informatization Application

Promoting the adoption of the application of health informatization is vital for improving health service quality and efficiency. Efforts should focus on building hardware facilities in primary medical and health institutions, enhancing their informatization levels to achieve comprehensive coverage of basic health services. In 2017, China issued the "Guiding Opinions of the General Office of the State Council on Promoting the Construction and Development of Medical Consortiums," advocating for the establishment of county-level medical communities and the concentrated construction of provincial-level, municipal-level, and county-level basic health data centers to achieve health information interconnectivity. These measures support the availability and reliability of information systems, providing robust support for the promotion of health informatization. Beyond hardware facilities, the imbalance in the talent workforce is a significant barrier to the widespread application of health informatization. Therefore, China has implemented various measures, such as formulating guidance on reforming training and promotion mechanisms for health information management talents and encouraging the transition of health informatization talents. These measures help enhance the capabilities of health informatization talents, advancing the construction and adoption of health informatization.

In China, health informatization application has become widespread, with the "Healthy Hubei" public service platform being a successful example. This platform aims to create a unified online health public service platform across Hubei province, integrating resources from hospitals at all levels into a single platform, offering functions such as appointment registration, outpatient payment, report inquiries, online consultations, and health monitoring. Users can conveniently access one-stop medical treatment and health services through a single platform. After several years of upgrades, the platform, building on the original "One-Stop Consultation," relies on the Hubei Provincial Health Medical Big Data Center to integrate advantageous medical and health resources across the province, create a people-centered smart health service system, provide comprehensive health services for convenience and public benefit and refined management throughout the life cycle, and promote "one-net" and "one-stop" medical treatment and health services to create a unified, province-wide health public service platform with a single entry point. As of December 2022, it has already brought together hundreds of medical institutions above the second level and thousands of registered doctors in Hubei province, with nearly 5 million registered users and over 20 million services provided (including more than 13 million pandemic-related services). Additionally, more than 5 million electronic health cards have been issued through the platform.

参考文献
References

1 中国卫生体系概况
Overview of China's Health System

［1］ 国家统计局.中国统计年鉴（2022）［M］.北京：中国统计出版社，2022.

［2］ 国家卫生健康委员会.中国卫生健康统计年鉴（2020）［M］.北京：中国协和医科大学出版社，2020.

［3］ 国务院办公厅.国务院办公厅关于印发"十四五"全民医疗保障规划的通知：国办发〔2021〕36 号［A/OL］.（2021-09-29）［2024-05-18］.https://www.gov.cn/zhengce/content/2021-09/29/content_5639967.htm.

［4］ 中华人民共和国国家卫生健康委员会.2021 年我国卫生健康事业发展统计公报［R/OL］.（2022-07-12）［2024-05-18］.https://www.gov.cn/xinwen/2022-07/12/content_5700670.htm.

3 中国医疗服务体系
China's Medical Service System

［1］ 国家统计局.中国统计年鉴（2022）［M］.北京：中国统计出版社，2022.

［2］ 国家卫生健康委员会.中国卫生健康统计年鉴（2020）［M］.北京：中国协和医科大学出版社，2020.

［3］ 国务院办公厅.国务院办公厅关于推进医疗联合体建设和发展的指导意见：国办发〔2017〕32 号［A/OL］.（2017-04-26）［2024-05-18］.https://www.gov.cn/zhengce/content/2017-04/26/content_5189071.htm.

［4］ 国务院办公厅.国务院办公厅关于印发"十四五"中医药发展规划的通知：国办发〔2022〕5 号［A/OL］.（2022-03-29）［2024-05-18］.https://www.gov.cn/zhengce/content/2022-03/29/content_5682255.htm.

［5］ 国务院办公厅.国务院办公厅关于印发"十四五"国民健康规划的通知：国办发〔2022〕11 号［A/OL］.（2022-05-20）［2024-05-18］.https://www.gov.cn/zhengce/content/2022-05/20/content_5691424.htm.

［6］ 李忠峰."十三五"财政卫生健康支出年增 7.5%［N/OL］.中国财经报（数字报刊），2020-10-29［2024-05-18］.https://114.118.9.73/epaper/index.html? guid=1732742846168956931.

［7］ 中华人民共和国国家卫生健康委员会. 2021 年我国卫生健康事业发展统计公报［R/OL］.（2022-07-12）［2024-05-18］. https://www. gov. cn/xinwen/2022-07/12/content_5700670. htm.

5 中国医疗保障体系
China's Medical Security System

［1］ 陈新中,俞云燕. 补充医疗保险体系建设及其路径选择［J］. 卫生经济研究,2010(1)：34-36.

［2］ 程晓明. 医疗保险学［M］. 2 版. 上海：复旦大学出版社,2010.

［3］ 刁孝华,谭湘渝. 我国医疗保障体系的构建时序与制度整合［J］. 财经科学,2010 (3)：77-84.

［4］ 顾海,吴迪."十四五"时期基本医疗保障制度高质量发展的基本内涵与战略构想［J］. 管理世界,2021 (9)：158-167.

［5］ 顾昕. 中国医疗保障体系的碎片化及其治理之道［J］. 学海,2017(1)：126-133.

［6］ 贾洪波,阳义南. 中国补充医疗保险发展：成效、问题与出路［J］. 中国软科学,2013 (1)：81-92.

［7］ 贾维周. 我国城市医疗救助制度的现况与对策研究［J］. 人口与经济,2008(1)：61-66.

［8］ 雷咸胜,崔凤. 城乡居民基本医疗保险制度整合与完善［J］. 西北农林科技大学学报(社会科学版),2016,16 (5)：1-7.

［9］ 李新伟,吴华章. 医疗救助制度的历史发展与现状［J］. 中国卫生经济,2009,28(12)：32-35.

［10］ 李珍. 社会保障理论［M］. 2 版. 北京：中国劳动社会保障出版社,2007.

［11］ 梁鸿,曲大维,赵德余. 中国城市贫困医疗救助的理念与制度设计［J］. 中国卫生资源,2007,10(6)：290-292.

［12］ 刘苓玲. 各国社会医疗救助制度及其对建立我国城市贫困人口社会医疗救助的启示［J］. 人口与经济,2006(1)：65-70.

［13］ 刘远立,程晓明,孟庆跃,等. 贫弱人群医疗救助基本服务包的设计［J］. 中国卫生经济,2003,22(6)：14-15.

［14］ 卢祖洵. 社会医疗保险学［M］. 北京：人民卫生出版社,2003.

［15］ 吕志勇,王霞. 商业健康保险与社会医疗保险系统耦合协调发展研究［J］. 保险研究,2013(9)：31-42.

［16］ 孟庆跃,杨洪伟,陈文,等. 转型中的中国卫生体系［M］. 日内瓦：世界卫生组织,2015.

［17］ 彭浩然,岳经纶. 中国基本医疗保险制度整合：理论争论、实践进展与未来前景［J］. 学术月刊,2020,52 (11)：55-65.

［18］ 仇雨临,王昭茜. 城乡居民基本医疗保险制度整合发展评析［J］. 中国医疗保险,2018(2)：16-20.

［19］ 仇雨临,翟绍果,郝佳. 城乡医疗保障的统筹发展研究：理论、实证与对策［J］. 中国软

科学，2011(4)：75-87.

[20]　孙祁祥,朱俊生,郑伟,等.中国医疗保障制度改革:全民医保的三支柱框架[J].经济科学，2007 (5)：8-17.

[21]　王保真.医疗保障[M].北京:人民卫生出版社,2005.

[22]　王超群.城乡居民基本医疗保险制度整合:基于 28 个省的政策比较[J].东岳论丛,2018, 39 (11)：83-92.

[23]　王虎峰.医疗保障[M].北京:中国人民大学出版社,2011.

[24]　王俊华.城乡基本医疗保险制度衔接模式比较研究[J].苏州大学学报(哲学社会科学版)，2009 (6)：21-24.

[25]　夏迎秋,景鑫亮,段沁江.我国城乡居民基本医疗保险制度衔接的现状、问题与建议[J].中国卫生政策研究,2010, 3 (1)：43-48.

[26]　姚岚,熊先军.医疗保障学[M].北京:人民卫生出版社,2013.

[27]　张廷新.论当前我国医疗保险制度改革[J].理论月刊,2001(3):63-64.

[28]　赵曼.中国医疗保险制度改革回顾与展望[J].湖北社会科学，2009 (7)：60-63.

[29]　朱坤,张小娟,朱大伟.整合城乡居民基本医疗保险制度筹资政策分析——基于公平性视角[J].中国卫生政策研究,2018, 11 (3)：46-50.

6　中国药品供应保障体系
China's Drug Supply Guarantee System

[1]　杨世民.药事管理学[M].6 版.北京:人民卫生出版社，2016.

[2]　张新平,刘兰茹.药品管理学[M].2 版.北京:人民卫生出版社,2023.

[3]　张志清.医院药事管理[M].北京:人民卫生出版社,2018.

7　中医药服务与管理
TCM Services and Management

[1]　国家卫生健康委员会.中国卫生健康统计年鉴(2021)[M].北京:中国协和医科大学出版社,2021.

[2]　贾二萍,熊巨洋,黎相麟,等.我国中医药健康服务现状及提升路径研究[J].中国医院,2020,24(3):25-27.

[3]　熊巨洋.完善中医药事业发展策略与机制研究[M].北京:科学出版社,2020.

[4]　泽桥医生.抗疟疾良药——青蒿素[EB/OL].(2022-03-08)[2024-05-18]. https://baijiahao.baidu.com/s? id=17267169973 18769683.

[5]　张元清,李婕,王亮.我国中医药服务发展现状、问题及对策建议[J].卫生软科学,2024,38(3):53-57.

8　中国卫生资源规划
China's Health Resource Planning

[1] 李晓梅,殷建忠.卫生规划制订与实践[M].北京:科学出版社,2017.

[2] 宋文舸.区域卫生规划编制的工作程序[J].中国卫生经济,1998,17(1):26-27.

[3] 王书平,黄二丹,甘戈."十四五"医疗卫生服务体系规划思路与发展定位思考及讨论[J].中国卫生经济,2021,40(5):8-11.

[4] 严晓玲,毛阿燕,胡广宇,等.我国卫生计生规划发展历程、存在问题与展望[J].卫生软科学,2017,31(12):40-43.

[5] 郑英,代涛,李力.部分国家医疗卫生服务体系规划的经验与启示[J].中国卫生政策研究,2015,8(5):8-12.

9　中国卫生筹资与卫生总费用
Health Financing and Total Health Expenditure in China

[1] 陈文.卫生经济学[M].4版.北京:人民卫生出版社,2017.

[2] World Health Organization. Guide to producing national health accounts:with special applications for low-income and middle-income countries[M].Geneva:World Health Organization,2003.

[3] World Health Organization. Health systems financing:the path to universal coverage[M].Geneva:World Health Organization,2010.

[4] World Health Organization,The World Bank. Global monitoring report on financial protection in health 2021[R/OL]. (2021-12-12) [2024-05-18]. https://iris. who. int/bitstream/handle/10665/350240/9789240040953-eng. pdf? sequence=1.

10　中国医药卫生法律制度与监督管理
Legal System and Supervision of Medicine and Health in China

[1] 陈云良.卫生法学[M].北京:高等教育出版社,2019.

[2] 樊立华.卫生监督学[M].2版.北京:人民卫生出版社,2013.

[3] 乐虹,赵敏.中国卫生法发展研究[M].武汉:华中科技大学出版社,2020.

[4] 袁杰,丁巍,赵宁.中华人民共和国基本医疗卫生与健康促进法释义[M].北京:中国民主法制出版社,2020.

[5] 张静,赵敏.卫生法学[M].北京:清华大学出版社,2014.

11　中国医药卫生信息体系
China's Medical and Health Information System

[1] 国务院办公厅.国务院办公厅关于推进医疗联合体建设和发展的指导意见:国办发

〔2017〕32 号［A/OL］.（2017-04-23）［2024-05-07］. https://www. gov. cn/gongbao/content/2017/content_5191699. htm.

[2]　胡红濮，秦盼盼，雷行云，等. 我国全民健康信息化发展历程及展望[J]. 医学信息学杂志，2019，40(7)：2-6.

[3]　湖北省卫生健康委员会. "健康湖北"微信公众号、支付宝双平台服务市民[EB/OL].（2022-12-10）［2024-05-07］. https://wjw. hubei. gov. cn/bmdt/dtyw/202212/t20221210_4450300. shtml.

[4]　马敬东，南京辉. 数字化转型背景下我国复合型卫生健康信息人才培养路径[J]. 医学信息学杂志，2022，43(3)：9-14.

[5]　王青兰，王喆，曲强. 新型国家公共卫生信息系统建设：提高系统韧性的思考[J]. 改革，2020(4)：17-27.

[6]　王帅，苏维. 我国区域医疗信息化发展现状、存在问题及对策研究[J]. 现代预防医学，2010，37(22)：4241-4243.

[7]　中华人民共和国国家卫生和计划生育委员会，国家中医药管理局. 卫生计生委 中医药局关于加快推进人口健康信息化建设的指导意见：国卫规划发〔2013〕32 号［A/OL］.（2014-02-20）［2024-05-07］. https://www. gov. cn/gongbao/content/2014/content_2600086. htm.

[8]　中华人民共和国国家卫生健康委员会. 国家卫生健康委关于印发卫生健康行政执法全过程记录工作规范的通知：国卫监督发〔2018〕54 号［A/OL］.（2019-01-09）［2024-05-07］. http://www. nhc. gov. cn/zhjcj/s5863/201901/e4f459fc8ce94021b0683679d78f0e0e. shtml.

[9]　中华人民共和国国家卫生健康委员会，国家中医药管理局，国家疾病预防控制局. 关于印发"十四五"全民健康信息化规划的通知：国卫规划发〔2022〕30 号［A/OL］.（2022-11-09）［2024-05-07］. http://www. nhc. gov. cn/cms-search/xxgk/getManuscriptXxgk. htm? id=49eb570ca79a42f688f9efac42e3c0f1.

[10]　中华人民共和国国家卫生健康委员会办公厅. 国家卫生健康委办公厅关于进一步完善预约诊疗制度加强智慧医院建设的通知：国卫办医函〔2020〕405 号［A/OL］.（2020-05-21）［2024-05-07］. http://www. nhc. gov. cn/yzygj/s3594q/202005/b2adae99376d4af0834fd8d43c5ddb4f. shtml.

[11]　中央网络安全和信息化委员会. 中央网络安全和信息化委员会印发《"十四五"国家信息化规划》[EB/OL].（2021-12-28）［2024-05-07］. https://www. gov. cn/xinwen/2021-12/28/content_5664872. htm.

[12]　周光华，徐向东，胡建平. 从卫生信息化到全民健康信息化的发展历程、特点及展望[J]. 中国卫生信息管理杂志，2019，16(4)：384-388,394.